In 1923 Friederich Lewy published a monograph containing neurological, psychiatric and neuropathological data on 43 patients with parkinsonism, of whom 21 were demented. Subsequent studies around the world have raised the profile of this form of dementia, suggesting that it may be more common than previously suspected – perhaps the second most common cause of degenerative dementia after Alzheimer's disease.

This book, which represents the first authoritative statement about dementia with Lewy bodies (DLB), arises from a workshop held in Newcastle, England, in October 1995, which brought together leading investigators with clinical and research experience of this condition. It includes review articles, case studies and recent research findings from the main centers studying DLB. The aims of the workshop, and of this volume, were to establish clinical diagnostic criteria and pathological protocols for DLB, and to explore evidence indicating that DLB patients may be more responsive to symptomatic therapy.

Covering the classification, cognitive manifestations, clinical diagnosis, epidemiology, genetics, neuropathology, neurochemistry and treatment of DLB, this is a landmark publication in clinical neuroscience. It presents new operational criteria for research on DLB, and will interest all those concerned with the problem of dementia in the elderly.

DEMENTIA WITH LEWY BODIES

DEMENTIA WITH LEWY BODIES

Clinical, pathological, and treatment issues

Edited by

R. H. PERRY
Department of Neuropathology, Newcastle General Hospital, Newcastle upon Tyne, UK

I. G. McKEITH
Institute for the Health of the Elderly, University of Newcastle upon Tyne, Newcastle upon Tyne, UK

E. K. PERRY
MRC Neurochemical Pathology Unit, Newcastle General Hospital, Newcastle upon Tyne, UK

Foreword by Jeffrey L. Cummings

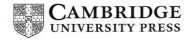

CAMBRIDGE
UNIVERSITY PRESS

PUBLISHED BY THE PRESS SYNDICATE OF THE UNIVERSITY OF CAMBRIDGE
The Pitt Building, Trumpington Street, Cambridge CB2 1RP, United Kingdom

CAMBRIDGE UNIVERSITY PRESS
The Edinburgh Building, Cambridge CB2 2RU, United Kingdom
40 West 20th Street, New York, NY 10011-4211, USA
10 Stamford Road, Oakleigh, Melbourne 3166, Australia

First published 1996

Printed in the United States of America

Typeset in Adobe Garamond

Library of Congress Cataloging-in-Publication Data

Dementia with Lewy bodies : clinical, pathological, and treatment
 issues / [edited by] Robert Perry, Ian McKeith, Elaine Perry.
  p.   cm.
 Includes index.
 "International Workshop on Dementia with Lewy Bodies held in
Newcastle in October 1995"–Acknowledgements.
 ISBN 0-521-56188-4 (hardback)
 1. Lewy body dementia–Congresses. I. Perry, Robert
II. McKeith, Ian. III. Perry, Elaine . IV. International
Workshop on Dementia with Lewy bodies (1995) : Newcastle upon Tyne,
England)
 [DNLM: 1. Lewy, Friederich Heinrich, 1885-1950. 2. Dementia,
Senile—pathology—congresses. 3. Parkinson Disease—pathology—
congresses. 4. Lewy Bodies—pathology—congresses. WT 155 D376
1996]
RC521.D457 1996
616.8'3–dc20
DNLM/DLC
for Library of Congress   96-16710
                                                                    CIP

*A catalog record for this book is available from
the British Library*

ISBN   0 521 56188 4 hardback

Dedicated to the memory of our colleagues,
Dorothy Irving and Tsunao Saitoh

Contents

Contributors

C. Ballard[*]
MRC Neurochemical Pathology Unit, Newcastle General Hospital, Newcastle upon Tyne, UK
C. Bancher
Ludwig Boltzmann Institute of Clinical Neurobiology, Lainz Hospital, Vienna, Austria
C. Bergeron[*]
Centre for Research in Neurodegenerative Disease, University of Toronto, Ontario, Canada
J. Bohl
Abteilung für Neuropathologie der Johannes Gutenberg-Universitat, Mainz, Germany
E. Braak
J. W. Goethe Universitat, Frankfurt/Main, Germany
H. Braak
J. W. Goethe Universitat, Frankfurt/Main, Germany
D. J. Brooks
MRC Cyclotron Unit, Hammersmith Hospital, London, UK
A. Brown
Department of Neuropathology, Newcastle General Hospital, Newcastle upon Tyne, UK
A. Burns[*]
Department of Psychiatry, Withington Hospital, Manchester, UK
E. J. Byrne[*]
Department of Psychiatry, Withington Hospital, Manchester, UK

[*] Workshop participant

D. B. Calne
*Neurodegenerative Disorders Centre, University of British Columbia,
Vancouver, British Columbia, Canada*
J. Carter[*]
Section of Old Age Psychiatry, Institute of Psychiatry, London, UK
D. F. Cohn
Department of Neurology, Ichilov Hospital, Tel Aviv, Israel
D. Collerton[*]
*Clinical Psychology Department, Bensham General Hospital, Gateshead,
UK*
M. Cornford
*Department of Pathology, UCLA Harbor Medical Center, Torrance, CA,
USA*
H. A. Crystal
Albert Einstein College of Medicine, Bronx, NY, USA
C. Davies
Bensham General Hospital, Gateshead, UK
P. Davies
Albert Einstein College of Medicine, Bronx, NY, USA
R. de la Fuente-Fernández
*Neurodegenerative Disorders Centre, University of British Columbia,
Vancouver, British Columbia, Canada*
R. A. I. de Vos[*]
*Streeklaboratoria Voor Pathologie en Medische Microbiologie, Enschede,
The Netherlands*
D. W. Dickson[*]
Albert Einstein College of Medicine, Bronx, NY, USA
L. M. Drach[*]
*Neurologisches Institut der Johann Wolfgang Goethe Universitat,
Frankfurt/Main, Germany*
S. A. Eagger[*]
Mental Health Unit, St. Charles Hospital, London, UK
A. Fairbairn[*]
Brighton Clinic, Newcastle General Hospital, Newcastle upon Tyne, UK
D. Galasko[*]
*Department of Neurosciences, UCSD School of Medicine, San Diego, CA,
USA*
K. Gedling
Section of Old Age Psychiatry, Radcliffe Infirmary, Oxford, UK

D. Hanger
Institute of Psychiatry, London, UK
L. A. Hansen[*]
Department of Neurosciences, UCSD School of Medicine, San Diego, CA, USA
J. Hardy
Albert Einstein College of Medicine, Bronx, NY, USA
C. R. Harrington[*]
Cambridge Brain Bank Laboratory, MRC Centre, Cambridge, UK
R. Harrison
Institute for the Health of the Elderly, Newcastle General Hospital, Newcastle upon Tyne, UK
R. J. Harvey
Dementia Research Group, National Hospital for Neurology and Neurosurgery, London, UK
T. Hope
Section of Old Age Psychiatry, Radcliffe Infirmary, Oxford, UK
Y. Ihara
Department of Neuropathology, Institute of Brain Research, University of Tokyo, Japan
P. G. Ince[*]
MRC Neurochemical Pathology Unit, Newcastle General Hospital, Newcastle upon Tyne, UK
D. Irving[†]
Department of Neuropathology, Newcastle General Hospital, Newcastle upon Tyne, UK
E. Iseki
Department of Psychiatry, Yokohama City University School of Medicine, Yokohama, Japan
E. N. H. Jansen[*]
Department of Neurology, Hospital Medisch Spectrum Twente, Enschede, The Netherlands
E. B. Jaros[*]
Department of Neuropathology, Newcastle General Hospital, Newcastle upon Tyne, UK
K. A. Jellinger[*]
Ludwig Boltzmann Institute of Clinical Neurobiology, Lainz Hospital, Vienna, Austria

[†] Deceased

P. Jenner
Biomedical Sciences Division, King's College London, London, UK
R. Katzman
Department of Neurosciences and the Alzheimer Disease Research Center, University of California at San Diego, La Jolla, CA, USA
J. Keene
Section of Old Age Psychiatry, Radcliffe Infirmary, Oxford, UK
P. J. Kelly
Department of Medical Statistics, University of Newcastle, Newcastle upon Tyne, UK
A. Korczyn*
Sackler School of Medicine, Tel Aviv University, Ramet Aviv, Israel
K. Kosaka*
Department of Psychiatry, Yokohama City University, Yokohama, Japan
S. Kuzuhara*
Department of Neurology, Mie School of Medicine, Tsu, Mie-Ken, Japan
M. Landon
Department of Biochemistry, University of Nottingham Medical School, Nottingham, UK
F. Lebert*
Centre Hospitalier Régional et Universitaire de Lille, Lille Cedex, France
G. Lennox*
Department of Neurology, University of Nottingham Medical School, Nottingham, UK
P. Liberini*
Division of Pharmacology, Universita degli studi di Brescia, Brescia, Italy
S. Lovestone*
Section of Old Age Psychiatry, Institute of Psychiatry, London, UK
J. Lowe*
Department of Histopathology, University of Nottingham Medical School, Nottingham, UK
K. Lowery
MRC Neurochemical Pathology Unit, Newcastle General Hospital, Newcastle upon Type, UK
K. Marder
Sergievsky Center, Columbia University, New York, USA
C. D. Marsden
Institute of Neurology, National Hospital for Neurology and Neurosurgery, London, UK

E. F. Marshall[*]
Department of Psychiatry, University of Newcastle, Newcastle upon Tyne, UK
R. J. Mayer
Department of Biochemistry, University of Nottingham Medical School, Nottingham, UK
R. Mayeux[*]
Sergievsky Center, Columbia University, New York, NY, USA
I. G. McKeith[*]
Institute for the Health of the Elderly, Newcastle General Hospital, Newcastle upon Tyne, UK
W. M. McMeekin
Department of Neuropathology, Newcastle General Hospital, Newcastle upon Tyne, UK
R. McShane[*]
Section of Old Age Psychiatry, Radcliffe Infirmary, Oxford, UK
I. Mena
Department of Radiology, UCLA Harbor Medical Center, Torrance, CA, USA
M. Memo
Brescia University School of Medicine, Brescia, Italy
B. Miller[*]
Department of Neurology, UCLA Harbor Medical Center, Torrance, CA, USA
T. Mizutani
Department of Neuropathology, Tokyo Metropolitan Institute of Gerontology, Tokyo, Japan
C. M. Morris
MRC Neurochemical Pathology Unit, Newcastle General Hospital, Newcastle upon Tyne, UK
A. D. Owen[*]
Pharmacology Group, King's College London, London, UK
F. Pasquier
Centre Hospitalier Régional et Universitaire de Lille, Lille Cedex, France
E. K. Perry[*]
MRC Neurochemical Pathology Unit, Newcastle General Hospital, Newcastle upon Tyne, UK
R. H. Perry[*]
Department of Neuropathology, Newcastle General Hospital, Newcastle upon Tyne, UK

M. A. Piggott*
MRC Neurochemical Pathology Unit, Newcastle General Hospital, Newcastle upon Tyne, UK

M. S. Pollanen
Centre for Research in Neurodegenerative Diseases and Department of Pathology, University of Toronto, Toronto, Canada

N. Quinn*
Institute of Neurology, National Hospital for Neurology and Neurosurgery, London, UK

M. Roth
Cambridge Brain Bank Laboratory, MRC Centre, Cambridge, UK

H. J. Sagar*
Department of Clinical Neurology, Royal Hallamshire Hospital, Sheffield, UK

A. Sahgal*
MRC Neurochemical Pathology Unit, Newcastle General Hospital, Newcastle upon Tyne, UK

T. Saitoh*†
Department of Neurosciences and the Alzheimer's Disease Research Center, UCSD, San Diego, CA, USA

D. P. Salmon*
Department of Neurosciences and the Alzheimer's Disease Research Center, UCSD, San Diego, CA, USA

A. H. V. Schapira
Royal Free Hospital, London, UK

D. J. Scoones
Department of Neuropathology, Newcastle General Hospital, Newcastle upon Tyne, UK

L. Souliez
Centre Hospitalier Régional et Universitaire de Lille, Lille Cedex, France

P. F. Spano
Brescia University School of Medicine, Brescia, Italy

L. J. Thal
Neurology Service, VA Medical Center, University of California, San Diego, CA, USA

P. Thompson*
Department of Old Age Psychiatry, Bensham General Hospital, Gateshead, UK

† Deceased

N. Turjanski[*]
MRC Cyclotron Unit, Hammersmith Hospital, London, UK
L. E. Urrutia
Department of Neurology, UCLA Harbor Medical Center, Torrance, CA, USA
A. Valerio
Brescia University School of Medicine, Brescia, Italy
S. Wach
Neurologisches Institut der J. W. Goethe Universitat, Frankfurt/Main, Germany
G. K. Wilcock[*]
Department of Care of the Elderly, Frenchay Hospital, Bristol, UK
C. M. Wischik
Cambridge Brain Bank Laboratory, MRC Centre, Cambridge, UK
H. Yamanouchi
Department of Neuropathology, Tokyo Metropolitan Institute of Gerontology, Tokyo, Japan
D. Yilmazer
J. W. Goethe Universitat, Frankfurt/Main, Germany
M. Yoshimura
Tokyo Metropolitan Medical Examiner's Office, Tokyo, Japan

Foreword

Lewy body dementia (LBD) burst on the scientific scene as a major concern for clinicians and pathologists little more than a decade ago. The Lewy body had previously been considered a common, if enigmatic, marker of idiopathic Parkinson's disease, but it suddenly became a focus of interest as ubiquitin stains revealed that up to 30 per cent of patients diagnosed clinically and pathologically with Alzheimer's disease have Lewy bodies in substantial numbers of cortical neurons. Is this a newly recognized dementing illness or a variant of Alzheimer's disease; what does the Lewy body tell us about deranged intracellular metabolism; do cortical Lewy bodies cause a dementia syndrome and if so how abundant must they be to produce cognitive impairment; is LBD clinically recognizable; what is the relationship between LBD and Parkinson's disease; does LBD have a different treatment response profile than Alzheimer's disease? These are the questions that the current volume strives to answer or at least to put into perspective and set the stage for future investigations.

Dementia with Lewy Bodies is organized into three sections: clinical aspects, pathology, and treatment. Prefaced by a fascinating biography of Lewy – who first described in 1913 the eosinophilic inclusions that came to bear his name – the clinical section addresses the current state of knowledge regarding the clinical syndrome associated with cortical Lewy bodies. Lewy body dementia and Alzheimer's disease are not differentiated by widely used clinical and research diagnostic criteria, and studies currently reported as describing the phenomenology and treatment of Alzheimer's disease almost certainly include a mixture of patients with Alzheimer's disease and patients with LBD. Means of distinguishing these two disorders are needed to allow studies of their mechanisms and treatment to advance.

The principal clinical features of LBD are described in the first section of the book and include fluctuations in cognitive abilities, vivid visual hallucinations, delusions, parkinsonism, gait abnormalities and falls, and an unusual sensitivity to neuroleptic medications. These symptoms may precede the occurrence of overt dementia and are most useful diagnostically when they occur before the dementia is severe. Attention, visuospatial skills, and psychomotor speed are more impaired in LBD than in Alzheimer's disease suggesting greater involvement of frontal-subcortical circuits, and imaging studies (structural, cerebral blood flow, metabolism) have identified greater frontal lobe involvement in LBD than in Alzheimer's disease. Electroencephalographic changes consisting of a slow background with superimposed bursts of frontally predominant slow waves are common in LBD. When present, they may aid in differentiating LBD from Alzheimer's disease.

The relationship between LBD and Parkinson's disease is as confusing as the relationship between LBD and Alzheimer's disease. All LBD patients eventually exhibit dementia, and cognitive impairment is increasingly recognized in Parkinson's disease. Lewy bodies are found in the cortex of nearly all patients with Parkinson's disease when they are carefully sought. All Parkinson's disease patients and many LBD patients have an extrapyramidal syndrome. Visual hallucinations occur spontaneously in LBD and are a frequent (often drug-related) phenomenon in Parkinson's disease. Both disorders are likely to worsen if the psychotic features are treated with neuroleptics. Neuropsychological features may aid differentiation of the diseases. The subcortical dementia of Parkinson's disease has more executive dysfunction and less profound language involvement than Alzheimer's disease; the dementia of LBD has features of both dementia syndromes. Genetic studies may also prove useful in distinguishing among these different conditions: Alzheimer's disease and LBD are associated with an increased prevalence of the apolipoprotein e-4 allele; Parkinson's disease with dementia has no increased representation of this genotype.

The second part of this volume addresses the neuropathology of LBD and other Lewy body diseases. The number of disorders known to have intracellular Lewy bodies is rapidly expanding. Primary Lewy body disorders include Parkinson's disease, LBD, primary autonomic failure, and Lewy body dysphagia; a number of other cortical and subcortical brain diseases may show Lewy bodies neuropathologically (e.g. Hallervorden–Spatz disease, subacute sclerosing panencephalitis, etc.) perhaps representing an epiphenomenon.

Cortical Lewy bodies are distributed preferentially in the frontal, cingulate, insular and temporal cortices. This does not coincide with the distribution of Alzheimer-type pathology which is most abundant in the hippocampus and cortex of the temporoparietal lobes. The tendency of Lewy bodies to involve limbic cortex correlates with the higher frequency of neuropsychiatric symptoms in LBD compared to Alzheimer's disease and Parkinson's disease. Patients with cortical Lewy bodies also have Lewy bodies in the brainstem where they may, in association with neurone loss, correlate with the occurrence of parkinsonism and the observed neuroleptic sensitivity of LBD.

Rapid advances have been made in understanding the neuropathology of LBD. Lewy bodies have been characterized and found to be comprised of neurofilament protein, ubiquitin, tubulin, microtubule-associated protein (MAP), and amyloid precursor protein. Controversy exists regarding how the presence of Lewy bodies should be interpreted; compelling arguments can be made that they represent a cytoprotective response by the cell or, conversely, that they are by-products of cellular injury. The presence of Lewy bodies may be associated with an increased cortical plaque density but there tends to be less neurofibrillary pathology in LBD than in Alzheimer's disease. This observation has given rise to the controversy regarding whether LBD is best regarded as a variant of Alzheimer's disease or is a unique disease that has a few pathological features in common with Alzheimer's disease.

Neurochemical features of LBD include a marked deficiency of cortical acetylcholine along with dopaminergic and noradrenergic deficits. In some cases, there appears to be relative serotonergic overactivity. The neurotransmitter changes reflect pathological involvement of the source nuclei in the basal forebrain and brainstem. The cholinergic deficits exceed those commonly observed in Alzheimer's disease.

Clinical and pathologic observations have a direct impact on pharmacologic intervention in LBD, and treatment is the focus of the third portion of this book. The sensitivity of LBD patients to neuroleptics makes this an ideal setting for the use of the novel antipsychotics that produce less D_2 dopamine receptor blockade. Risperidone and clozapine have been used successfully in this population. The cholinergic deficit may contribute to the neuropsychiatric as well as the cognitive deficits of LBD and cholinergic agents may have beneficial effects in both domains. Serotonin antagonists such as ondansetron have proved useful in the management of dopaminergic psychosis in Parkinson's disease and may be useful in LBD where there is a relative over-activity of serotonin function. Agents that slow the progress of LBD also warrant investigation. Neurotrophins such as nerve growth factor have neuroprotective effects on cholinergic cells and may have a role in ameliorating the cholinergic deficit of LBD. Neuroprotective drugs effective for reducing injury to cortical neurons and anti-amyloid agents that limit the production of cortical plaques also require study in LBD as they become available.

New neuropharmacologic issues have been raised by observations in LBD. First, given the marked cholinergic deficit of LBD, one would predict that treatment of parkinsonism in this disorder with anticholinergic agents would have adverse cognitive consequences. This requires further study. Second, levodopa administration produces visual hallucinations in some but not all patients with Parkinson's disease and hallucinations are more common in patients with dementia. Are drug-induced hallucinations clinical markers of cortical Lewy bodies? Only autopsy studies of patients that were thoroughly studied clinically will answer this question. Third, the tendency for levodopa and dopaminergic receptor agonists to cause hallucinations and delusions may render these agents problematic in the management of parkinsonism in LBD where psychotic features often occur spontaneously. Alternate strategies need to be identified. Fourth, recognition of the severe cholinergic deficit of LBD suggests that this disorder may respond to cholinergic treatment. Patients meeting criteria for LBD should be separately studied in trials of cholinesterase inhibitors and cholinergic receptor agonists.

Lewy body dementia has much to teach. Thorough investigation will improve current dementia classification, provide insight into the neuropathologic basis of neuropsychiatric phenomena, and enhance understanding of the neurogenetics and neuropathology of dementia. This volume provides a comprehensive introduction to the issues and will allow investigators to begin unraveling the lessons of LBD.

Jeffrey L. Cummings, M.D.
Professor of Neurology and Psychiatry
UCLA School of Medicine
Los Angeles, California

Acknowledgements

The International Workshop on Dementia with Lewy Bodies held in Newcastle in October 1995 was generously supported by Parke Davis and Company, The French Foundation for Alzheimer Research, Janssen-Cilag Ltd, Sandoz Pharma Ltd, Bayer AG, F. Hoffmann-La Roche AG, The Wellcome Trust, Eli Lilly and Company, Astra Arcus AB, Medical Research Council, Lederle Laboratories, Merck Sharp & Dohme Ltd.

The Editors are especially indebted to Newcastle City Health and Royal Victoria Infirmary and Associated Hospitals National Health Service Trusts for their support, to the Institute for the Health of the Elderly at the University of Newcastle upon Tyne for the provision of valuable resources and to its Director Jim Edwardson for his encouragement and guidance in the planning of the Workshop.

Neither the meeting nor the publication of this book would have been possible without the highly professional and continually creative administrative skills of Tanya Freeman who with the assistance of Alison Wright and Maureen Middlemist provided immense organizational expertise and encouragement to the Editors.

The Editors would also like to express their appreciation for the support of Dr Richard Barling, Cambridge University Press.

R. H. Perry
I. G. McKeith
E. K. Perry

Biographical note on F. H. Lewy

D . F . C O H N

Friederich (Fritz) Heinrich Lewy was born in Berlin, Germany on January 28, 1885, about 60 years after the death of Sir James Parkinson who described the shaking palsy.

Lewy's contribution to the pathology of the shaking palsy was so significant, particularly but not exclusively in describing the eosinophilic intracellular inclusion bodies in the brain, that we today speak of Lewy bodies and not eosinophilic inclusion bodies, in the same way that we speak of Parkinson's disease and not the shaking palsy. The term "Lewy bodies" was first coined by Trétiakoff in his thesis at the University of Paris in 1919.

According to the information available Lewy had a very successful career, even though he had to leave his native country in 1933 because he was Jewish. His father was a prominent hospital internist in Berlin, and in his family we find Paul Ehrlich who discovered the Salvarsan once used in the treatment of Lues. Lewy was a brilliant scientist, an excellent clinician and neuropathologist, and an outstanding teacher. He spent his first clinical semester in Zurich, where he studied neuroanatomy with von Monakow, and graduated in 1910 from the University of Berlin. From 1910 to 1912 he trained with outstanding teachers: Nissl, Alzheimer, and Spielmeyer in neuropathology in Munich; in clinical neurology with no less than Oppenheim and Cassierer in Berlin; neurophysiologic research with Magnus in Utrecht; and psychiatry with Kraeplin in Berlin.

Two years after graduating and training with the most prominent European neurologists of his time he was nominated director of the laboratories of the Neuropsychiatric Clinic at the University of Breslau which was recognized as an international Brain Institute. The outbreak of World War I interrupted his rapidly progressing career and he became a major in charge of field hospitals in France, Russia and later Turkey in the German army, his 'Fatherland' – which was later to betray him.

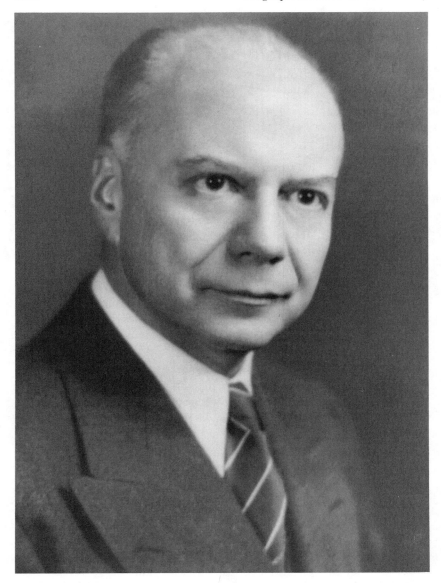

Friederich (Fritz) H. Lewy, 1885–1950. (From Historica Collections, College of
Physicians of Philadelphia, Philadelphia, PA.)

After the war he returned to Berlin and worked in the outpatient clinic of
Oppenheim and Cassierer until 1926 when he was appointed head of the
Department of Neurology at the Charite in Berlin. In 1923, at age 38, he

became Associate Professor of Neurology at the University of Berlin, and in 1926 he was nominated Director of the Institute of Neurology of Berlin, which he had to leave in 1933 when the Nazis came to power. He then spent one year in Britain and was afterwards invited by Frazier to the Medical School of the University of Pennsylvania in Philadelphia, USA.

In Philadelphia he was active as a Professor of Neurophysiology, Neuropathology and a consultant Neurosurgeon at the University of Pennsylvania until his death. During World War II he considered it his duty to join the armed services and became Chief of Neurology in the Army hospital at Framingham, Massachusetts. After the war he returned to the University of Pennsylvania.

Lewy's interest in neuropathology and especially movement disorders started very early in his career. In 1912, two years after graduation, we find the chapter about Paralysis agitans written by him in the *Handbuch der Neurologie* edited by Lewandowsky. In 1913 one year after this book was published the seventh convention of the German Society of Neurologists was held in Breslau (now Warsaw), Poland. On the first day, Oppenheim chaired the first session, and Lewy as the fifth speaker, described in detail, for the first time in public, the inclusion bodies which bear his name. His paper was published in the German journal *Deutsche Zeitschrift für Nervenheilkunde*.

He stated that at that time he had examined 60 brains of cases of Parkinson's disease. He described intra- and extracellular bodies free in the tissue and around arterial walls, which he thought to be breakdown products. These bodies were found in the dorsal motor nucleus of the vagus (the vegetative nucleus of the oblongata), in the nucleus basalis of Meynert, the nucleus lateralis thalami and the paraventricular nucleus. The bodies appeared to him as elongated or circular structures, which stained with eosin. Apart from these bodies he described further pathological findings, but was unable to correlate the site of these findings with the clinical picture of Parkinson's disease, although he assumed that the changes in the nucleus of the vagus were the cause of the vegetative symptoms. In 1923 he published a book about muscle tone and movement, *Die Lehre vom Tonus und der Bewegung*, in which he described the pathological findings of Parkinson's disease and tried to correlate them with clinical features of Parkinson's disease. In this book he described in detail the eosinophilic inclusion bodies and attempted to explain their development. He considered that axis cylinders became swollen and aggregated to produce compact basophilic cords. These swollen fibrils were then impregnated by eosinophilic cellular products and changed into elongated eosinophilic structures. In 1924 he contributed a chapter about the pathology of paralysis agitans in a German textbook of internal medicine, as at the time neurology was taught together with general medicine.

At the University of Pennsylvania in Philadelphia he continued his research work, investigating peripheral nerves and specifically the trigeminal nerve and trigeminal neuralgia. He was also consultant to the Commonwealth of Pennsylvania in occupational diseases of the peripheral nervous system. His research work included studies of the cerebellum, the hypothalamus, and action potentials in the central nervous system. He was subsequently appointed Associate Professor of Neuropathology in the Undergraduate and Graduate School of Medicine of the University of Pennsylvania. In clinical studies he viewed patients as individuals with a distinctive personality and expressed this view in his book *The Biology of the Personality*.

His wide knowledge, and academic and teaching abilities were internationally recognized. Early in his career in Germany he was secretary of the Neurologic Association. In the USA he was member of the following associations: the American Neurological Association, the American Association of Neuropathologists (of which he was Vice President in 1938), the American Physiological Society and the Association for Research in Nervous and Mental Diseases. In 1931 he was nominated Chairman of the Neurological Section of the International Hospital Association. He became chairman of the Board of Trustees of the American Academy of Neurology. The Argentine Society of Normal and Pathological Anatomy appointed him as a member and the Argentine Society of Neurology, Psychiatry and Neurosurgery made him an honorary member. He was also a Fellow of the American College of Physicians and the College of Physicians of Philadelphia, Fellow of the American Medical Association and Member of the Philadelphia Neurological and Physiological Societies.

Lewy was an excellent teacher[*] and greatly appreciated by his students as was stated in the yearbook of the University of Pennsylvania, *Scope*, in 1938: 'The neurosurgical conferences conducted on Tuesday afternoons by Dr. F. H. Lewy, provided some of the most interesting and instructive

---

[*] An old Jewish tale tells of a discussion among sages about the importance of the teacher in education. One of them named Chatam Sofer pointed to Moses of the Old Testament and his incomparable wisdom – acquired from the best teacher ever, God himself. Lewy had the best teachers of his time but they were, of course, mortal.

hours of our surgical trimester. Their popularity with classmates was attested by the fact that they were always exceptionally well attended, even by students not on service. Students in the future would profit considerably if more conferences of this type were conducted in other branches of surgery and medicine.'

In 1940 as a leading neurologist and scientist of his time, with a special interest in Parkinson's disease, he was well aware of, and competently described, the difficulties in research in general and researching this disease in particular:

'When I had investigated my first two dozen cases of Parkinson, I was convinced that I knew where the cause of tremor and rigidity was located, when I examined pathologically the seventh dozen of Parkinson brains I was completely confused because you seem to be able to prove just as well one theory as the contrary one'.

Born as Friéderich Heinrich Lewy in Berlin on January 28, 1885, he died as Fred Henry Lewy in Pennsburg Pennsylvania, aged 65, on October 5, 1950.

Abbreviations

Aβ	amyloid β-protein
ACh	acetylcholine
AD	Alzheimer's disease
AD-F	Alzheimer's patients with frontal behavioural features
AD-P	Alzheimer's disease syndrome with parieto-temporal hypoperfusion
AGE	advanced glycation endproducts
ALS	amyotrophic lateral sclerosis
ANCOVA	analysis of covariance
ANOVA	analysis of variance
APOE (ApoE)	apolipoprotein E
APP	amyloid precursor protein
ATD	Alzheimer-type dementia
ATP	Alzheimer-type pathology
BDI	Beck Depression Inventory
BDNF	brain derived neurotrophic factor
BDS	Blessed Dementia Scale
BPRS	Brief Psychiatric Rating Scale
BEAM	brain electrical activity mapping
CAMCOG	Cambridge Cognitive Examination
CAMDEX	Cambridge Examination for Mental Disorders in the Elderly
CBD	corticobasal degeneration
CD(R)	compound stimulus (reversal)
CDR	Clinical Dementia Rating
CERAD	Consortium to Establish a Registry for Alzheimer's Disease
ChAT	choline acetyltransferase

CLB (cLB)	cortical Lewy body(ies)
CLPA	conditional learning (pattern-location) paired associates
CNS	central nervous system
CSF	cerebrospinal fluid
CSF SLI	CSF somatostatin-like immunoreactivity
CT	computed tomography
CVLT	California Verbal Learning Tests
DA	dopamine
DAT	dementia of Alzheimer type
DCI	disabling cognitive impairment
DEP	depression
DI	Diagnostic Interview Schedule
DLB	dementia with Lewy bodies
DLBD	diffuse Lewy body disease
DLT	dementia of Lewy body type
DMTS	delayed matching to sample
DNOS	dementia not otherwise specified
DOPAC	dihydroxyphenylacetic acid
DRS	Dementia Rating Scale
DSM-IIIR, DSM-IV	Diagnostic and Statistical Manual of Mental Disorders (3rd edn revised; 4th edn)
EDR	extradimensional shift reversal
EDS	extradimensional shift
EEG	electroencephalogram
EMG	electromyogram
eMMS	extended Mini Mental State (examination)
EPS	extrapyramidal (motor) signs
FDA	Food and Drug Administration
FDG	^{18}F-fluorodeoxyglucose
FTD	fronto-temporal dementia
GABA	γ-aminobutyric acid
GSH	glutathione
5HIAA	5-hydroxyindoacetic acid
HMPAO	hexamethy-propyleneamine oxime
5HT	serotonin (5-hydroxytryptamine)
HVA	homovanillic acid
ICC	idiopathic clouding of consciousness
IDED	intra- and extra-dimensional (set-shifting)
IDPN	β,β'-iminodipropionitrile

IDR	intradimensional shift reversal
IDS	intradimensional shift
ILBD	incidental Lewy body disease
IP	idiopathic parkinsonism
IPD	idiopathic Parkinson's disease
ISH	in situ hybridization
α-KGDN	α-ketoglutarate dehydrogenase
KS	Korsakoff's syndrome
LB	Lewy body(ies)
LBD	Lewy body dementia (disease)
LBV	Lewy body variant
LN	Lewy neurites
MAP	microtubule-associated protein
MB	Mallory body
MCP	multicatalytic protease
MID	multi-infarct dementia
MMSE	Mini-Mental State Examination
MPP	1-methyl-4-phenylpyridinium
MPTP	1-methyl-4-phenyl-1,2,3,6-tetrahydropyridine
MRI	magnetic resonance imaging
MTS	Mental Test Score
MTS	matching to sample
NA	noradrenaline
NART	National Adult Reading Test
nbM	nucleus basalis of Meynert
NF	neurofilament
NFT	neurofibrillary tangles
NGF	nerve growth factor
NIA	National Institute of Aging
NIH.	National Institutes of Health
NINCDS–ADRDA	National Institutes of Neurological and Communicative Disorders – Alzheimer's Disease and Related Disorders Association
NINDS–AIREN	National Institute of Neurological Disorders and Stroke : Association Internationale pour la Recherche et l'Enseignement en Neurosciences
NMDA	N-methyl-D-aspartate
NT-3	neurotrophin-3
OPCA	olivopontocerebellar atrophy
PBE	Present Behavioural Examination

PBHI	Post Behavioural History Interview
PCP	phenocyclidine
PD	Parkinson's disease
PEPD	postencephalitic PD
PET	positron emission tomography
PHF	paired helical filaments
PPT	pedunculopontine tegmental (nucleus)
PR	pattern recognition
PSP	progressive supranuclear palsy
(Q)EEG	(quantitative) electroencephalograph
QNB	quinuclidinyl benzoate
rCBF	regional cerebral blood flow
RDC	Research Diagnostic Criteria
REM	rapid eye movement
RFLP	restriction fragment length polymorphism
SD(R)	simple discrimination (reversal)
SDAT	senile dementia of Alzheimer type
SDLT(SDLBT)	senile dementia of Lewy body type
SMTS	simultaneous matching to sample
SOD-1	superoxide dismutase-1
SP	senile plaques
SPECT	single photon emission computerized tomography
SPM	statistical parametric mapping
SS	spatial span
SWM	spatial working memory
THA	tetrahydroaminoacridine
UCLA ADC	University of California at Los Angeles Alzheimer Disease Center
UPDRS	Unified Parkinson's Disease Rating Scale
VaD	vascular dementia
VSMTS	visual search matching to sample
WAIS(R)	Wechsler Adult Intelligence Scale (revised)
WCST	Wisconsin Card Sorting Test
WISC(R)	Wechsler Intelligence Scale for Children (revised)
b.i.d.	bis in die (twice a day)
t.i.d.	ter in die (three times a day)
q.i.d.	quarter in die (four times a day)
p.o.	per oram (by mouth)

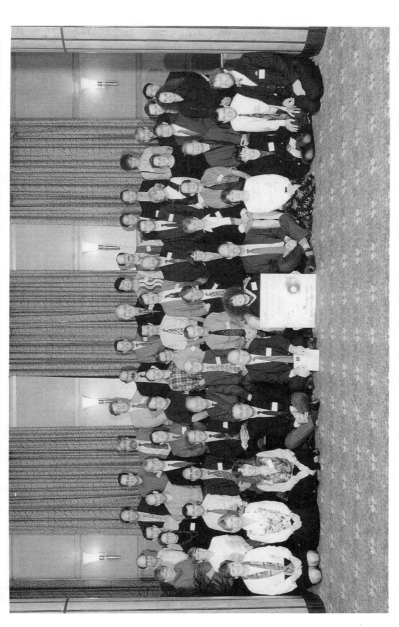

International Workshop on Dementia with Lewy Bodies 5–7 October 1995, Newcastle upon Tyne, UK. *Front row:* Freeman, Wright, Havercroft, Emre, Korczyn, Perry, Fleming, Piggott, Lebert, Ballard, Perry. *Seated:* Middlemist, Lowe, Liberini, Sagar, Jellinger, Wilcock, de Vos, Jansen, Campbell, Jaros, Harrington, Eagger. *Standing:* Marshall, Galasko, Bergeron, Dickson, McShane, Altstiel, Burns, Quinn, Collerton, Byrne, McKeith, Ince, Thompson, O'Brien, Lippa, Carter, Kuzuhara, Turjanski. *Back row:* Miller, Lovestone, Sahgal, Salmon, Sirinathsinghji, Fairbairn, Edwardson, Saitoh, Drach, Kosaka, Collins, Ward, Hansen, Cross, Lee.

Introduction

R . H . P E R R Y , I . G . M c K E I T H
and E . K . P E R R Y

The history of dementia associated with Lewy bodies (DLB) began not long after the history of Alzheimer's disease. Alois Alzheimer described neurofibrillary tangles in a case of presenile dementia in 1907 and Friederich Lewy first described cytoplasmic inclusions in neurons of the substantia innominata in cases of parkinsonism in 1912. In 1923, Friederich Lewy published a monograph containing neurological, psychiatric, and neuropathological data on 43 patients with parkinsonism amongst whom 21 were demented (see also Förstl & Levy, 1991). Dementia associated with Lewy bodies was later described by Hassler (Hassler, 1938) and over two decades later in 1962, Woodard (see also Woodard, 1985) reported a series of psychiatric cases in which Lewy bodies were identified at autopsy – he called these cases of "Lewy body disease". An isolated case was also reported in 1961 by Okazaki (Okazaki et al., 1961). Then in the early 1970s, the concept of 'incidental Lewy body disease' arose from the findings of Forno (1969) on long-stay psychiatric patients – cases that in retrospect most likely included cases of DLB. Dating from 1976, Japanese neuropathologists including Kosaka (see Kosaka, 1990) were responsible for describing the detailed clinical and pathological features of demented patients with cortical Lewy bodies which they termed 'Diffuse Lewy body disease' and divided into subgroups such as cortical type or brainstem type, based on the distribution of Lewy bodies and clinical presentation primarily with dementia or parkinsonism.

From the late 1980s onwards several groups raised the profile of this form of dementia by suggesting that it may be more common than previously suspected. In Newcastle, senile dementia of Lewy body type was reported as the second most common cause of dementia in the elderly after Alzheimer's disease (AD) (Perry et al., 1989 and 1990). A similar

1

prevalence was apparent in the Nottingham, UK series and the San Diego group reported Lewy bodies in around 20% of cases of Alzheimer's disease and defined this subgroup as the Lewy body variant of Alzheimer's disease (Hansen et al., 1990). Pathologically, ubiquitin antisera greatly aided the identification of cortical Lewy bodies and, in addition to Lewy bodies, distinct ubiquitinated neurites now termed Lewy neurites were identified in the hippocampus by Dickson (1991). Retrospective clinical assessment of confirmed DLB cases revealed distinct cognitive and other psychiatric features, in the different surveys (Byrne et al., 1989; Hansen et al., 1990; McKeith et al., 1992). Parallel with this emerging concept of a distinct kind of dementia associated with Lewy bodies has been the increasing awareness that in Parkinson's disease, the archetypal Lewy body disease, cognitive impairment in elderly cases is perhaps more the rule than the exception although categorical dementia is less common. Clinical manifestations of diseases associated with Lewy bodies are in fact diverse (see Chapter 26), although based on some of the most recent prevalence studies, dementia may be at least as common if not more so than parkinsonism.

Conceptually, individuals and research groups have increasingly struggled with the apparently competing notions that when dementia and Lewy bodies concur this represents Parkinson's disease, Alzheimer's disease, a combination of the two, or a related, but separate entity and a variety of different terminologies have arisen (see Chapter 16). Although it would be unrealistic to suppose that all who attended the workshop held in Newcastle in October 1995 departed totally satisfied by the new proposed nomenclature, the agreed term DLB at least has the merit of not favouring any of the previous forms of nomenclature! Most agreed that whatever it is called, it is best considered more a syndrome than a disease entity.

We organized the workshop not so much with a view to seeking any rigid consensus on particular issues, but primarily to bring together all those with clinical and research experience in dementia involved with cases in whom Lewy bodies have been identified at autopsy and to raise awareness of the condition through publication of this book. The idea for such a project arose from the realization based on our experience and those of other groups in the UK, USA and Japan that DLB may be the second most common form of degenerative dementia, after Alzheimer's disease. To verify this, the need for establishing clinical diagnostic criteria and readily applicable pathological protocols is obvious and until now there has been no organized opportunity for independent researchers to exchange viewpoints and explore areas of common agreement. A further incentive was preliminary clinical evidence and biological data indicating that DLB patients may be more responsive to symptomatic, for example, transmitter-orientated, therapy.

We were delighted at the positive response from all invitees on the need for such a meeting and their willingness to attend, some travelling across the world to Newcastle where there is a history of dementia research dating back to the 1960s. It was equally encouraging to receive such generous sponsorship from research organizations, notably the French Foundation, a full list of sponsors is provided, and the pharmaceutical industry notably Parke Davis (see Acknowledgements). This support enabled the group to interact for several days in the pleasant environment of a new hotel built around the city's Old Council Chambers situated by the river Tyne.

Following the first open day, with plenary lectures on clinical, epidemiological, genetic, pathological, neurochemical and pharmacological apects of DLB (including experts on Parkinson's disease) attended by over 170 participants, the remaining time was spent in closed workshop discussions. Workshop participants divided initially into three groups: clinical, pathological, and treatment; and the outcome of their discussions is summarized briefly at the end of each of these sections in this book. Then the task of exploring and attempting to reach consensus on clinical diagnosis criteria for DLB and pathological protocols occupied two main groups of participants for the rest of the time in lively and generally good-humoured discussions, some running well beyond the scheduled periods! By the end of the workshop these goals had been achieved to the satisfaction of the majority (and the results have been published in *Neurology* (McKeith et al., in press). Summaries of the clinical criteria and pathological guidelines are included in Appendices 1 and 2.

We hope the contents of this book will interest all those concerned with the problem of dementia in the elderly who are increasingly aware of the clinical, genetic, pathological and even therapeutic heterogeneity of Alzheimer's disease. We know that there will be some within the Parkinson's disease realm who will consider DLB as belonging to their precinct. The group was well aware that patients presenting with parkinsonian movement disorder and subsequently diagnosed as being demented would continue to be classified as Parkinson's disease (PD) with dementia by neurologists. To those who would still consider a primary diagnosis of dementia with Lewy bodies as PD we would suggest that since dementia is not an invariant feature of all cases of idiopathic Parkinson's – only of some primarily elderly cases – and that since the newly available genetic data in DLB indicate an APO E4 frequency as high as in AD, DLB may be in a separate category. Moreover as DLB *presents* in the elderly *with dementia* (with or without extrapyramidal disorder) the disease or syndrome needs to be brought to the attention of psychogeriatricians and geriatricians. Only further research at the different levels examined in this text and new approaches and insights generated by attracting attention from other areas of expertise will resolve these issues of nosology/classification. The operational criteria produced are primarily for research application and will be subject to revision, for example at subsequent workshops (the next is planned for late 1997 in San Diego, California). If this first volume plays any part in stimulating debate and promoting new investigative research it will have more than served its purpose. We will then, with continued exchange of experience, learn if DLB has really come of age with, like Alzheimer's disease itself, a very long incubation period between its original identification and widespread impact in the field.

References

Byrne, E.J., Lennox, G., Louin, J. & Godwin Austen, R.B. (1989). Diffuse Lewy body disease: clinical features in 15 cases. *J. Neurol. Neurosurg. Psychiatry.*, **52**, 709–17.

Dickson, D.W., Ruan, D., Crystal, H. et al. (1991). Hippocampal degeneration differentiates diffuse Lewy body disease (DLBD) from Alzheimer's disease: Light and electron microscopic immunocytochemistry of CA2-3 neurites specific to DLBD. *Neurology*, **41**, 1402–9.

Forno, L.S. (1969). Concentric hyalin intraneuronal inclusions of Lewy type in the brains of elderly persons (50 incidental cases): relationship to parkinsonism. *J. Am. Geriatr. Soc.*, **17**, 557–75.

Förstl, H. & Levy, R. (1991). FH Lewy on Lewy bodies, parkinsonism and dementia. *Int. J. Geriatr. Psychiatry*, **6**, 757–66.

Hansen, L., Salmon, D., Galasko, D., Masliah, E., Katzman, R. & De Teresa, R. (1990). The Lewy body variant of Alzheimer's disease: a clinical and pathologic entity. *Neurology*, **40**, 1–8.

Hassler, R. (1938). Zur pathologie der paralysis agitans und des post enzephalitischen parkinsonisms. *J. Psychologie Neurologie*, **48**, 387–476.

Kosaka, K. (1990). Diffuse Lewy body disease in Japan. *J. Neurol.*, **237**, 197–204.

Lewy, F.H. (1912). Paralysis agitans. I. Pathologische anatomie. In *Handbuch der Neurologie*, Vol. 3, ed. M. Lewandowsky, pp. 920–33. Berlin: Springer.

Lewy, F.H. (1923). Die Lehre vom tonus und der Bewegung. Zugleich systematische untersuchungen zur klinik, physiologie, pathologie and pathogenese der paralysis agitans. Berlin: Julius Springer.

McKeith, I.G., Perry, R.H., Fairbairn, A.F., Jabeen, S. & Perry, E.K. (1992). Operational criteria for senile dementia of Lewy body type (SDLT). *Psychol. Med.*, **22**, 911–22.

McKeith, I.G. et al. (1996). 'Consensus Guidelines for the Clinical and Pathological Diagnosis of Dementia with Lewy Bodies (DLB).' Report of the CDLB International Workshop. *Neurology* (in press).

Okazaki, H., Lipton, L.S. & Aronson, S.M. (1961). Diffuse intracytoplasmic ganglionic inclusions (Lewy type) associated with progressive dementia and quadriparesis in flexion. *J. Neurol. Neurosurg. Psychiatry*, **20**, 237–44.

Perry, R.H., Irving, D., Blessed, G., Perry, E.K. & Fairbairn, A.F. (1989). Clinically and pathologically distinct form of dementia in the elderly. *Lancet*, **i**: 166.

Perry, R.H., Irving, D., Blessed, G., Fairbairn, A.F. & Perry, E. (1990). Senile dementia of Lewy body type: a clinically and neuropathologically distinct form of Lewy body dementia in the elderly. *J. Neurol. Sci.*, **95**, 119–35.

Woodard, J.S. (1962). Concentric hyalin inclusion body formation in mental disease analysis of twenty-seven cases. *J. Neuropath. Exper. Neurol*, **2**: 442–9.

Woodard, J.S. (1985). *Correlative Observations in Dementia.* Orange, California: California Medical Publications.

Part one:

Clinical issues

1

The clinical diagnosis and misdiagnosis of Lewy body dementia

G . G . L E N N O X and J . S . L O W E

Summary

Dementia associated with Lewy bodies (here termed Lewy body dementia) is potentially recognizable in life. Clinical features such as fluctuations in cognitive performance, recurrent visual hallucinations and systematized delusions and spontaneous parkinsonism are all suggestive of the diagnosis and may occur before the dementia is established. Early gait disturbance, unexplained falls and sensitivity to neuroleptic treatment are also useful clinical pointers. The dementia itself is characterized by deficits in memory and language, together with a greater degree of impairment of attention, visuospatial skills and psychomotor processing than is seen in Alzheimer's disease. Two sets of clinical diagnostic criteria based upon some of these features have been proposed and validated by the Nottingham and Newcastle groups; both demonstrate good specificity but the Newcastle criteria appear to have superior sensitivity. A new set of consensus criteria, combining the most valuable features of both existing efforts, would represent an important advance in the clinical diagnosis of Lewy body dementia.

1.1 Introduction

There is an increasing consensus that the syndrome of dementia associated with Lewy bodies may be recognizable in life and distinguishable from other dementia syndromes such as Alzheimer's disease. This distinction would be valuable for research, especially for drug trials. But an accurate diagnosis of Lewy body dementia is even more important in routine clinical practice. Patients with Lewy body dementia may present with psychiatric rather than cognitive symptoms, including hallucinations, delusions or fluctuating confusional states; early recognition in these patients may allow a safer and more rational approach to investigation and treatment. In patients with established dementia, these same manifestations pose particular management pitfalls which are at least potentially avoidable. Finally, in comparison with Alzheimer's disease, Lewy body dementia may respond to a different range of therapies but at present almost certainly carries a worse prognosis.

It is primarily these differences, directly affecting clinical care, which have stimulated existing efforts to design clinical diagnostic criteria for Lewy body dementia. For clinicians, diagnostic criteria must be simple and robust and must not rely upon scarce or sophisticated investigational resources such as complex neuropsychometry or functional neuroimaging. In everyday practice, criteria should be sufficiently broad to alert clinicians to the possibility of Lewy body dementia even in atypical cases. For research workers, however, criteria must be above all accurate, even if this is achieved at the expense of excluding some patients who do in fact have the disease.

In this chapter we will discuss the ways in which Lewy body dementia can be diagnosed at the bedside (or, in this time of community care, at the hearthside), and the main problems of misdiagnosis revealed by validation studies of the existing diagnostic criteria (Byrne et al., 1991; McKeith et al., 1992) and by continuing clinicopathological studies in Nottingham.

1.2 Clinical diagnostic criteria in related disorders

At this point it is useful to consider attempts to devise diagnostic criteria for Parkinson's disease and Alzheimer's disease. Whereas Lewy body dementia results from predominantly cortical Lewy body disease, Parkinson's disease is the commonest manifestation of subcortical Lewy body disease (less common manifestations including progressive supranuclear palsy, dystonia, autonomic failure and isolated dysphagia) even though mild cortical involvement eventually occurs in most if not all cases (Hughes et al., 1992). Alzheimer's disease is relevant both as the major differential diagnosis in Lewy body dementia and because of the pathological similarities between the two disorders which have generated considerable nosological debate.

1.2.1 Diagnostic criteria for Parkinson's disease

Description of the characteristic motor signs of Parkinson's disease began in 1817 and was completed as soon as the technique of neurological examination was established in the first half of this century. Most medical students believe they can recognize the typical tremor, bradykinesia, rigidity, posture and gait disturbance which accompany brainstem Lewy body formation.

However, two recent studies have shown that only about 75% of patients given the diagnosis of Parkinson's disease by neurologists turn out to have brainstem Lewy bodies at post-mortem examination (Rajput et al., 1991; Hughes et al., 1992). Even the retrospective application of the stringent UK Parkinson's Disease Society Brain Bank criteria does not exclude patients with a wide range of other pathological processes affecting the substantia nigra and other basal ganglia, such as multiple system atrophy, progressive supranuclear palsy, arteriosclerotic disease and even a tangle-only process resembling Alzheimer's disease (Daniel & Lees, 1991).

The basic problem is that clinical features generally merely reflect the anatomical distribution of the pathology rather than its nature. Eliciting subtle clinical features with, for example, detailed neuropsychometry has the same limitation. This is probably also true of additional features such as response to treatment. Thus, Parkinson's disease characteristically responds to levodopa therapy, but so too do other diseases when they are confined to the substantia nigra and spare its targets in the basal ganglia, such as some cases of early multiple system atrophy or vascular disease.

It is only when the distribution of the pathology is relatively characteristic that we can begin to make an accurate diagnosis on clinical grounds. Where several pathological processes all have a tendency to affect the same group of structures, clinical diagnosis is always likely to be inaccurate unless supplemented by a specific biological marker such as a genetic polymorphism or mutation.

It is, however, interesting to note that in the absence of such markers, the single most useful clinical pointer to the diagnosis of Parkinson's disease is classical resting tremor; the anatomical basis of this manifestation is not fully understood. The same can be said for the striking fluctuations in mental performance seen in Lewy body dementia.

1.2.2 Diagnostic criteria for Alzheimer's disease

Matters are more complicated in Alzheimer's disease, because the established diagnostic criteria were devised before the general recognition of Lewy body dementia as a separate (if related) entity. Burns (1991) has reviewed the earlier studies that validated, for example, the widely accepted NINCDS–ADRDA criteria against various forms of pathological diagnosis of Alzheimer's disease, noting a consistent diagnostic accuracy of more than 80%. Tierney and colleagues (1988) found that differences in the pathological definition of Alzheimer's disease produced some variation in the sensitivity of the clinical criteria (between 81 and 88%) but had little effect on specificity; they did not consider cortical Lewy bodies. One of only two studies to report 100% accuracy for the NINCDS–ADRDA criteria (Morris et al., 1988) nonetheless identified brainstem Lewy bodies in 38% and cortical Lewy bodies in 8% without classifying them separately. One could therefore conclude from the earlier studies that the NINCDS–ADRDA criteria successfully diagnose patients with either Alzheimer's pathology or Lewy body pathology (or both) in more than 80% of cases.

Two recent validation studies have made a distinction between cases with Alzheimer's pathology alone and cases with Lewy body pathology (with or without plaques and tangles). Burns and colleagues (1990) performed a clinicopathological study of 50 patients who had fulfilled the NINCDS–ADRDA for either probable or possible Alzheimer's disease; 6 (12%) cases had cortical Lewy bodies either with (3 cases) or without (3 cases) plaques and tangles in sufficient density to support a second diagnosis of Alzheimer's disease. A larger study by Galasko and colleagues (1994) looked at 137 cases fulfilling the came criteria for probable or possible Alzheimer's disease; 38 (24%) had cortical Lewy bodies either with (29 cases) or without (4 cases) plaques and tangles in sufficient density to fulfil the NIA criteria (Khachaturian, 1985) for Alzheimer's disease. They found an even higher proportion of cases with cortical Lewy bodies in patients diagnosed by DSM-IIIR criteria as having a mixture of Alzheimer's disease and vascular dementia: 7 (37%) out of 19 cases.

One can therefore conclude that the NINCDS–ADRDA criteria do not reliably distinguish between Alzheimer's disease and Lewy body dementia. This is scarcely a criticism of these criteria, since they were not designed with this aim in mind. It does, however, suggest that diagnostic criteria that succeed in identifying cases of Lewy body dementia should be considered as exclusion criteria in the diagnosis of Alzheimer's disease.

1.3 The clinical diagnosis of Lewy body dementia

The clinical features of Lewy body dementia have been reviewed elsewhere (Chapter 4). The core feature of progressive dementia has been well described and is reviewed in detail elsewhere in this volume. Several of the early cohort studies (Byrne et al., 1989; Hansen et al., 1990; Perry et al., 1990) identified additional clinical features which are particularly suggestive of Lewy body dementia. These include unexplained fluctuations in cognitive performance (sometimes amounting to delirium), spontaneous parkinsonism or severe parkinsonian reactions to neuroleptics, psychotic features including visual hallucinations and recurrent falls. It is worth emphasizing that the diagnostic value of these clinical features largely depends upon their occurrence early in the course of the disease, either before the onset of dementia or when dementia remains mild.

In everyday clinical practice, a history of fluctuations in cognitive performance can usually be elicited from the patient's family. Characteristically these episodes of confusion will have been attributed to intercurrent infection or cerebrovascular disease; the patient may have recovered fully between these episodes. Milder fluctuations in patients with persisting cognitive impairment, described as good days and bad days, can be distinguished from diurnal changes in performance due to fatigue by their longer duration; they must also be distinguished from the functional deterioration that follows a change in surroundings (like a holiday or admission to hospital) in such patients. They can be detected using serial Mini-Mental State Examinations (MMSE) (Williams et al., 1993) but more extensive serial psychometry has not yet been reported.

The significance of parkinsonism must also be judged in relation to the stage of the patient's illness (Burkhardt et al., 1988; Crystal et al., 1990). Parkinsonism presenting before dementia is an important clinical guide, particularly if it conforms to criteria for Parkinson's disease and if the subsequent dementia has other features of Lewy body dementia. Conversely, parkinsonism occurring late in the disease course, when dementia is severe, has less diagnostic value; at this stage a wide range of cortical degenerations, including Alzheimer's disease, cause gait disturbance and rigidity. An additional difficulty with these two parkinsonian features is the subjective nature of their assessment. Even experienced eyes may find it hard to make a distinction between parkinsonian gait disturbance and the gait apraxia seen in almost any disease affecting the frontal lobes. Similarly, rigidity may be hard to distinguish from *gegenhalten*, the phenomenon of increasing active movement when the examiner is trying to assess passive movements, commonly perceived as an inability to relax. Nonetheless, rigidity is common in Lewy body dementia and probably more so than in Alzheimer's disease (Förstl et al., 1993).

Bradykinesia is a more specific and useful sign of parkinsonism, providing the examiner can be sure that the patient is able to understand and attend to the task. It is characterized not just by a slowing of simple repetitive movements, but also a tendency for the movements to fragment and to diminish in amplitude over a short period of time. Classical parkinsonian rest tremor is the most reliable sign of all, but the least common in patients presenting with dementia. This sinusoidal and rhythmic movement disorder must be carefully distinguished from the brief but often repetitive shocklike jerks of spontaneous multifocal myoclonus which occurs in a great many cerebral degenerations. Atypical postural and action tremors are also frequent but less specific.

Drug treatment is a serious confounding factor. As McKeith and colleagues have pointed out (McKeith et al., 1992), patients with Lewy body dementia may be unduly sensitive to neuroleptic medication. This may in itself provide a dangerous clue to the diagnosis (see Chapter 29). Milder parkinsonian reactions to neuroleptics are of very limited diagnostic value, although clinical experience suggests that the few patients who develop an extensive parkinsonian syndrome including a classical rest tremor generally do have brainstem Lewy bodies.

Falls are common in Lewy body dementia (Ballard et al., 1993). It is not clear whether this reflects parkinsonism, non-specific gait disturbance and instability, autonomic failure, impulsivity or wandering. These issues are discussed in Chapter 6.

Psychotic features are also common in Lewy body dementia and are occasionally an isolated manifestation of Lewy body pathology. They include complex visual hallucinations, typically taking the form of unthreatening people or animals, a range of systematized delusions and auditory hallucinations. These features are again discussed in detail in Chapter 6. In older patients presenting with Parkinson's disease before the onset of dementia, drug treatment is again a potential confounding influence. All antiparkinsonian drugs, especially anticholinergics, can precipitate visual hallucinations which generally resolve when the treatment is cut back. The hallucinations are nonetheless a warning sign and dementia frequently ensues after a few months or years.

1.4 Clinical diagnosis criteria for Lewy body dementia

Many groups have suggested that these clinical features are potentially sufficiently characteristic to allow the diagnosis of Lewy body dementia in life (e.g. Crystal et al., 1990). Both the Nottingham (Byrne et al., 1991) and the Newcastle (McKeith et al., 1992) groups have proposed operational clinical diagnostic criteria based upon them, which are summarized in Table 1.1.

Both sets of criteria follow the model of the NINCDS–ADRDA for Alzheimer's disease in seeking to exclude patients with stroke or other causes of dementia or parkinsonism by thorough clinical and laboratory investigation. The Newcastle criteria exclude patients with evidence of cerebral ischaemic damage on imaging; this is probably too stringent, given the increasing ability for both CT and MR imaging to detect trivial lacunar disease and the tendency of most neuroradiologists to report degenerative subcortical white matter disease as 'chronic ischaemia'.

The Nottingham criteria follow the NINCDS–ADRDA model further by defining two levels of diagnostic certainty: probable Lewy body dementia and possible Lewy body dementia, the former requiring three or more major parkinsonian features and the latter encompassing patients presenting with more unusual neuropsychiatric features and/or a lesser degree of parkinsonism. The Newcastle criteria lay less emphasis on parkinsonism, allowing the diagnosis of Lewy body dementia in patients without any parkinsonian features providing certain other features are present. With the benefits of hindsight, the Newcastle approach is probably more appropriate. Certainly it is now clear that Lewy body dementia is not the only cause of dementia and episodic confusion in patients with pre-existing Parkinson's disease (Hughes et al., 1993). It is, however, the commonest cause, and requiring parkinsonism to be mild in the Newcastle criteria has led some raters falsely to exclude Lewy body dementia in cases with moderate or severe parkinsonism (McKeith et al., 1994).

Both sets of criteria emphasize the presence of fluctuating cognition and episodic confusion; indeed this is required for a probable Nottingham diagnosis and for a Newcastle diagnosis. This causes problems, both because a minority of patients do not show this feature and because it is

Table 1.1. *Selected aspects of operational clinical diagnostic criteria for dementia associated with Lewy bodies*

Nottingham criteria (Byrne et al., 1991)
1. Probable LBD
   Either
      (i) gradual onset of DSM-IIIR dementia with prominent attentional deficits or early unexplained apparent acute confusional states
      (ii) classical Parkinson's disease with subsequent dementia as above
      (iii) simultaneous onset of both dementia (as described) and parkinsonism with three or more of tremor, rigidity, postural change, bradykinesia and gait abnormality
2. Possible LBD
   Either dementia (as described) with acute onset and rapid progression ± plateaux, frequently associated with psychiatric symptoms *or* dementia (as described) with subsequent parkinsonism with one or two of tremor, rigidity, postural change, bradykinesia and gait abnormality
Newcastle criteria (McKeith et al., 1992)
1. Fluctuating cognitive impairment affecting both memory and higher cortical functions (e.g. language, visuospatial ability, praxis or reasoning skills). The fluctuation is marked with the occurrence of both episodic confusion and lucid intervals and is evident either on repeated tests of cognitive function or by variable performance on daily living skills.
2. At least one of the following:
      (a) visual and/or auditory hallucinations which are usually accompanied by secondary paranoid delusions;
      (b) mild spontaneous extrapyramidal features or neuroleptic sensitivity syndrome (i.e. exaggerated adverse responses to standard doses of neuroleptics)
      (c) repeated unexplained falls and/or transient clouding or loss of consciousness.
3. Despite the fluctuating pattern the clinical features persist for weeks or months (unlike delirium) and progress often rapidly, to severe dementia

---

operationally difficult to define. McKeith et al. (1994) have shown that this can create particular problems for inexperienced raters.

The Newcastle criteria do, however, include a wider range of clinical manifestations, such as visual and/or auditory hallucinations and repeated unexplained falls, which might be predicted to improve their specificity.

The two sets of criteria do not necessarily identify the same patients within any given population (Shergill et al., 1994; Chapter 14). Two further studies have attempted to validate the criteria by applying them retrospectively to sets of case notes from patients with Alzheimer's disease, Lewy body dementia and multi-infarct dementia. Byrne (1995) describes a study of case notes of variable quality; both sets of criteria were applied. She reports moderate inter-rater reliability, low sensitivity for both criteria (Nottingham probable 0.17, Newcastle 0.15) and high specificity (Nottingham probable 0.95, Newcastle 0.93). Combining the Nottingham probable and possible groups increased sensitivity (0.38) but decreased specificity (0.76) (Byrne, personal communication). Overall there were low positive and reasonable negative predictive values. McKeith et al. (1994) applied the Newcastle criteria to 50 sets of case notes from their centre, finding that inter-rater reliability was very high amongst experienced old-age psychiatrists. Both this and the sensitivity fell with less-experienced clinicians. Despite including two such raters, the overall performance was very satisfactory, with a mean sensitivity of 0.74 and a mean specificity of 0.95.

It is possible that improved criteria could be devised by combining the most useful features of both existing sets of criteria, such as fluctuations, visual hallucinations, and a broad range of parkinsonian features occuring either spontaneously or in response to neuroleptic therapy. New criteria would, of course, require both retrospective and prospective validation.

1.5 Misdiagnosis of Lewy body dementia

The limitations of the existing criteria have already been discussed. Neither Nottingham or Newcastle criteria (or indeed a mixture of the two) are able to detect the minority of patients who present with an illness closely resembling typical Alzheimer's disease, nor the subgroup of unknown size that presents with an isolated psychosis.

Continuing clinicopathological studies in Nottingham have shown that diagnostic errors are now rare and take two main forms. First, inexperienced clinicians still tend to diagnose vascular dementia in patients with episodic confusion and parkinsonism, even though this picture is much more likely to be due to Lewy body dementia, especially if it is followed by progressive dementia. Secondly, neurologists tend to diagnose Lewy body dementia in most if not all cases of Parkinson's disease developing dementia with fluctuations and visual hallucinations; although in our series Lewy body dementia remains the most common pathological substrate of dementia in Parkinson's disease, occasional cases have either brainstem Lewy bodies and cortical Alzheimer's disease, or Alzheimer's lesions in both locations. Very occasional cases of clinically diagnosed Parkinson's disease complicated by dementia have a tau-related process with tangles and dystrophic neurites resembling Steele–Richardson–Olszewski disease.

1.6 The role of ancillary investigations

The San Diego group drew attention to neuropsychometric differences between groups of patients with pathologically confirmed Alzheimer's disease and Lewy body dementia (Hansen et al., 1990); they have extended these observations in this volume (Chapter 8). The Lewy body patients tend to show greater deficits of attention, psychomotor speed and visuospatial ability. Similar findings have been described in clinically-diagnosed patients by Sahgal and colleagues (1992) in a range of tests of visual attention and spatial working memory (Chapter 9). Taken together these findings suggest that Lewy body patients have greater frontal lobe dysfunction than patients with Alzheimer's disease. It is not yet clear whether these differences are sufficiently large and robust to form a useful adjunct to clinical diagnosis in individual cases.

There are similar problems with neuroimaging. Förstl et al. (1993) identified a greater degree of frontal lobe atrophy in patients with pathologically confirmed Lewy body dementia compared with similarly demented patients with Alzheimer's disease. Although this finding supports the neuropsychometric studies, current methods for evaluating regional patterns of atrophy are laborious and unreliable, making them difficult to employ in routine clinical diagnosis. Furthermore, relatively selective frontal lobe atrophy also occurs in other degenerative disorders causing dementia and parkinsonism, including Steele–Richardson–Olszewski disease and variants of Pick's disease.

There is as yet no consensus concerning the role of functional neuroimaging. One would predict from the neuropsychological studies that Lewy body patients would show greater degrees of frontal hypometabolism. This hypothesis has been supported by Miller and colleagues (Chapter 10) in a small study using single photon emission tomography, with partial pathological confirmation, but not by Turjanski and Brooks (Chapter 11) in a small positron emission tomography study of clinically diagnosed Lewy body dementia cases.

All of these ancillary investigations share a fundamental limitation. They identify the distribution of pathology with increasing precision, but provide little or no information about the underlying pathological process. Genetic studies may be more informative. We now think of the causes of Alzheimer's disease in terms of a set of specific pathogenic mutations (including APP, S182 and STM2 mutations) and a set of background genetic risk factors (including apolipoprotein E polymorphisms). The causes of Lewy body formation and the factors determining the distribution of this pathology throughout the nervous system are likely to have a similar complex genetic basis.

Several studies have suggested that the apolipoprotein E ϵ4 genotype is more frequent in patients with Lewy body dementia (particularly those with plaques and tangles) than in non-demented Parkinson's disease or normal controls (Benjamin et al., 1994; Galasko et al., 1994): presumably the ϵ4 allele is acting as a risk factor for cortical plaque and/or tangle formation in Lewy body disease. Mutant alleles of the cytochrome P450 gene CYP2D6B may act as a risk factor for brainstem Lewy body formation in a similar way (Rempfer et al., 1994). This gene does not, however, account for autosomal dominant families with Parkinson's disease and Lewy body dementia, and clearly further genes causing Lewy body formation await discovery. It is likely that there will also be an additional set of genetic risk factors which determine whether Lewy body pathology is expressed mainly in the brainstem to cause Parkinson's disease or in the cortex to cause Lewy body dementia. It remains to be seen whether this matrix of genetic influence will be sufficiently simple to help in clinical diagnosis.

References

Ballard, C.G., Mohan, R.N.C., Patel, A. & Bannister, C. (1993). Idiopathic clouding of consciousness: do the patients have cortical Lewy body disease? *Int. J. Geriatr. Psychiatry*, **8**, 571–6.

Benjamin, R., Leake, A., Edwardson, J.A. et al. (1994). Apolipoprotein E genes in Lewy body and Parkinson's disease. *Lancet*, **343**, 1565.

Burkhardt, C.R., Filley, C.M., Kleinschmidt-DeMasters, B.K. et al. (1988). Diffuse Lewy body disease and progressive dementia. *Neurology*, **38**, 1520–8.

Burns, A., Luthert, P., Levy, R. et al. (1990). Accuracy of clinical diagnosis of Alzheimer's disease, *BMJ*, **301**, 1026.

Burns, A. (1991). Clinical diagnosis of Alzheimer's disease. *Dementia*, **2**, 186–94.

Byrne, E.J. (1995). Cortical Lewy body disease: an alternative view. In *Developments in Dementia and Functional Disorders in the Elderly*, ed. R. Levy & R. Howard, pp. 21–30. London: Wrightson Biomedical Publishing Ltd.

Byrne, E.J., Lennox, G., Louin, J. & Godwin Austen, R.B. (1989). Diffuse Lewy body disease: clinical features in 15 cases. *J. Neurol. Neurosurg. Psychiatry.*, **52**, 709–17.

Byrne, E.J., Lennox, G.G., Godwin-Austen, R.B. et al. (1991). Dementia associated with cortical Lewy bodies: proposed clinical diagnostic criteria. *Dementia*, **2**, 283–4.

Crystal, H.A., Dickson, D.W., Lizardi, J.E. et al. (1990). Antemortem diagnosis of diffuse Lewy body disease. *Neurology*, **40**, 1523–8.

Daniel, S.E. & Lees, A.J. (1991). Neuropathological features of Alzheimer's disease in non-demented parkinsonian patients. *J. Neurol. Neurosurg. Psychiatry*, **54**, 972–5.

Förstl, H., Burns, A., Luthert, P. et al. (1993). The Lewy-body variant of Alzheimer's disease: clinical and pathological findings. *Br. J. Psychiatry*, **162**, 385–92.

Galasko, D., Saitoh, T., Xia, Y. et al. (1994). The apolipoprotein E allele $\epsilon 4$ is overrepresented in patients with the Lewy body variant of Alzheimer's disease. *Neurology*, **44**, 1950–1.

Hansen, L., Salmon, D., Galasko, D., Masliah, E., Katzman, R. & De Teresa, R. (1990). The Lewy body variant of Alzheimer's disease: a clinical and pathologic entity. *Neurology*, **40**, 1–8.

Hughes, A.J., Daniel, S.E., Kilford, L. & Lees, A.J. (1992). The accuracy of clinical diagnosis of idiopathic Parkinson's disease: a clinicopathological study. *J. Neurol. Neurosurg. Psychiatry*, **55**, 181–4.

Hughes, A.J., Daniel, S.E., Blankson, S. & Lees, A.J. (1993). A clinicopathologic study of 100 cases of Parkinson's disease. *Arch. Neurol.*, **50**, 140–8.

Khachaturian, Z.S. (1985). Diagnosis of Alzheimer's disease. *Arch. Neurol.*, **42**, 1097–105.

McKeith, G., Perry, R.H., Fairbairn, A.F. et al. (1992). Operational criteria for senile dementia of Lewy body type (SDLT). *Psychol. Med.*, **22**, 911–22.

McKeith, I.G., Fairbairn, A.F., Bothwell, R.A. et al. (1994). An evaluation of the predictive validity and inter-rater reliability of clinical diagnostic criteria for senile dementia of the Lewy body type. *Neurology*, **44**, 872–7.

Morris, J.C., McKeel, D.W., Fulling, K. et al. (1988). Validation of clinical diagnostic criteria for Alzheimer's disease. *Ann. Neurol.*, **24**, 17–22.

Perry, R.H., Irving, D., Blessed, G., Fairbairn, A.F. & Perry, E. (1990). Senile dementia of Lewy body type: a clinically and neuropathologically distinct form of Lewy body dementia in the elderly. *J. Neurol. Sci.*, **95**, 119–35.

Rajput, A.H., Rozdilky, B. & Rajput, A. (1991). Accuracy of clinical diagnosis in parkinsonism – a prospective study. *Can. J. Neurol. Sci.*, **18**, 275–8.

Rempfer, R., Crook, R., Houlden, H. et al. (1994). Parkinson's disease, but not Alzheimer's disease Lewy body variant associated with mutant alleles at cytochrome P450 gene. *Lancet*, **344**, 815.

Shergill, S., Mullan, E., D'Atn, P. & Katona, C. (1994). What is the clinical prevalence of Lewy body dementia? *Int. J. Geriatr. Psychiatry*, **9**, 907–12.

Tierney, M., Fisher, R., Lewis, A. et al. (1988). The NINCDS–ADRDA workgroup criteria for the clinical diagnosis of probable Alzheimer's disease. A clinicopathological study of 57 cases. *Neurology*, **38**, 359–64.

Williams, S.W., Byrne, E.J., Stokes, P. (1993). The treatment of diffuse Lewy body disease: a pilot study of five cases. *Int. J. Geriatr. Psychiatry*, **8**, 731–9.

2

The nosological status of Lewy body dementia

D. GALASKO, D.P. SALMON, and L. J. THAL

Summary

Lewy bodies (LB), the pathological hallmark of Parkinson's disease, occur in cortical as well as subcortical areas in the brains of about 10–30% of patients with dementia clinically consistent with Alzheimer's disease (AD). Lewy body dementia (LBD) overlaps with AD both at autopsy, where most demented patients with cortical LB also have senile and neuritic plaques and to a lesser extent the neurofibrillary tangles typical of AD, and clinically, where patients with LBD generally meet clinical criteria for probable or possible AD. The nosology of LBD and proposed diagnostic criteria therefore need to take cognizance of AD.

A major pathological problem is how many plaques, tangles, or both are required to diagnose AD in the presence of LB. Similarly, since nondemented PD patients also show cortical LB, should LBD be defined pathologically by a threshold cortical LB count? A descriptive and quantitative approach to pathology in well-characterized patients with dementia (AD and LBD), and PD (with and without dementia) is needed.

Clinical criteria for LBD have been proposed and validated in studies that retrospectively reviewed entire case records. Key features are parkinsonian signs, cognitive fluctuations, hallucinations, and a 'frontal-subcortical' dementia profile. There are problems in reliably assessing and documenting each of these elements. We suggest a flexible approach that is compatible with published criteria and studies, and includes categories of probable and possible LBD, to help determine which combination of features optimally discriminates LBD from 'pure' AD and other dementias.

2.1 Introduction

The orthodox view of Lewy bodies (LB) as the signature lesion of Parkinson's disease (PD), a condition associated with a characteristic movement disorder that spared the intellect, has been challenged by the finding of neocortical LB in the brains of demented elderly patients. This suggests a cause and effect, and has spawned a large – and confusing – nomenclature that highlights important problems in the field. Kosaka first coined the term diffuse Lewy body disease (DLBD) for patients who had LB in the hippocampus, temporal lobe, cingulate and neocortex in addition to their classical sites of predilection in Parkinson's disease, namely the substantia nigra and other subcortical areas. He proposed that five or more cortical LB per 100 × field should be present to define DLBD. Since senile plaques (SP) and to a lesser extent neurofibrillary tangles (NFT) typical of Alzheimer's disease (AD) often coexisted with DLBD, Kosaka later modified the definition of DLBD to include two subgroups: a common form, with LB accompanied by AD lesions, and a pure form with absent or scanty AD change (Kosaka, 1990). The pure form comprised mainly younger patients who presented with juvenile onset parkinsonism, while dementia or psychosis was the usual presenting symptom in elderly patients, most of whom developed parkinsonism during the course of dementia.

Anti-ubiquitin immunostaining has facilitated the detection of cortical LB, and many centers have now reported their experience in autopsy series of demented patients, adopting names such as senile dementia of the Lewy body type (Perry et al., 1990b), Lewy body variant of Alzheimer's disease (Hansen et al., 1990), and diffuse cortical Lewy body disease (Gibb et al., 1987). In several large autopsy series of demented patients who were generally clinically diagnosed with progressive dementia consistent with AD, diffusely distributed LB were found in 10–30% of brains (Bergeron et al., 1989; Jellinger et al., 1990; Perry et al., 1990a; Mendez et al., 1992; Galasko et al., 1994). These studies suggest that LB dementia may be the second most common form of degenerative dementia in the elderly.

Since cortical LB have a slightly different appearance than classical nigral LB, it seemed plausible that diffuse LB could account for dementia, while LB restricted to subcortical areas were a marker of Parkinson's disease (PD). Additional pathological findings in LB dementia, including vacuolation in the temporal lobe, and dystrophic neuritic change in the CA2/CA3 regions of the hippocampus, could also contribute to cognitive changes.

It is now recognized that many patients with PD eventually develop dementia. In autopsy studies, demented PD patients usually show diffusely distributed LB, with or without concomitant AD pathology (Hughes et al., 1992). However, even in nondemented PD patients, in addition to the expected subcortical LB, cortical LB are usually present. The spectrum of dementia associated with LB thus includes PD, where the relationship between cortical LB load, additional pathology such as AD, and cognitive impairment needs further exploration.

We shall discuss some of the nosological problems that Lewy body dementia poses for neuropathologists and clinicians, and offer suggestions to aid in their resolution. For consistency we shall use Lewy body dementia (LBD) as a generic term that describes either the clinician's expectation of predicting LB, or the pathological finding of diffusely distributed LB, regardless of whether AD lesions are also present.

2.2 The pathological classification of LBD

2.2.1 Key questions and problems

Is LBD a separate condition from AD? At autopsy, most LBD patients have senile plaques (SP) and neurofibrillary tangles (NFT) characteristic of AD in addition to diffusely distributed LB. When the AD lesions are quantified, many patients with LBD have SP counts that meet NIA criteria, and neuritic plaque counts that meet CERAD criteria. For example, at the UCSD Alzheimer's Disease Research Center, we have found diffusely distributed LB (LBD) in the brains of 65 patients who initially presented with dementia – representing about 20% of autopsied cases of dementia that was consistent with AD; only seven of these had 'pure' DLBD with scanty AD lesions, while the other 58 met the above criteria for AD. Similar admixtures of LBD and AD are documented in series from other centers. Compared with patients having 'pure' AD, our LBD patients have similar numbers of SP, markedly fewer NFT in the neocortex and fewer – but appreciable – NFT in regions that are important in memory especially the hippocampus and temporal cortex (Hansen et al., 1993). It seems extreme to attribute the scanty NFT to aging alone, discounting their potential contribution to dementia, or to ignore the extensive amyloid deposition in LBD–AD. If the effects of AD lesions and LB on cognition are additive or synergistic, then to reach comparable stages of severity of dementia, patients with LBD–AD are likely to need somewhat less AD pathology than are patients with 'pure' AD.

How many cortical LB constitute LBD? Although lesion counts in AD have been correlated with agonal mental status scores, such studies are uncommon in LBD. There are several plausible reasons for this oversight. LB are found in deeper cortical layers, in neurons whose synaptic connections are not well understood, therefore it is not clear what cognitive effects to expect. The natural history of LB is not known, but it is likely that neurons that develop LB and later die can be lost completely without leaving a remnant or marker of the LB. For example, in the substantia nigra in PD, the density of LB greatly underestimates the degree of loss of pigmented dopaminergic neurons. Thus cortical LB, even when scanty, may be qualitative rather than quantitative markers of a disease process. In spite of these reservations, a 1989 study reported a strong correlation between LB counts in several cortical areas and a global rating of dementia severity close to the time of death (Lennox et al., 1989). We have recently replicated this study in patients with the LB variant of AD, and found significant correlations between Mini-Mental State Examination (MMSE) scores obtained within 18 months before death and LB counts in the superior temporal, frontal, cingulate and inferior parietal regions, with LB explaining 25% of the variance of the MMSE (Samuel et al., 1996). This suggests that the cortical LB burden is a meaningful measure. Similar studies in groups of patients with PD with and without dementia will help to establish whether a critical number of cortical LB is necessary for dementia. Other pathological changes, including subcortical neuron loss in areas such as the substantia nigra or ventral tegmental area, temporal lobe vacuolization, and CA2/CA3 neuritic change may also contribute to dementia in LB disorders, as may markers such as abnormal cytoskeletal proteins, levels of neurotransmitters and the densities of their receptors.

2.2.2 Suggestions to improve pathological nosology of LBD

Standards for tissue processing, immunostaining with anti-ubiquitin antibodies, and which brain areas and how many fields to examine for LB are discussed elsewhere in this volume.

Unless the concept that a threshold cortical LB burden defines LBD is proven, definitions of LB disorders need to be qualitative (LB present/absent) as well as quantitative. Semi-quantitative approaches to estimating LB density may be more reliable than attempts at exact counts, by analogy with the CERAD approach to AD lesions (Mirra et al., 1993).

The two approaches, either classifying cases discretely as entities such as LBD or LBD–AD, or describing findings by collecting semi-quantitative or quantitative information about lesion burden and distribution are complementary and both are valuable.

Ideally the pathological diagnosis should be descriptive and independent of the clinical diagnosis. Descriptive terms such as 'Lewy body disease' or 'diffuse Lewy body disease', that can be combined with other findings such as AD, have the virtue of being easily interpretable. Concomitant pathology, such as AD, infarcts, hippocampal sclerosis and other relevant findings should be reported if present. When a pathologist diagnoses combined LBD–AD, which is a descriptive term regardless of the clinical diagnoses that were made, the criteria that were used for AD, for example, NINCDS–ADRDA, CERAD, etc. should be specified. In this formulation, the LBD–AD combination may occur in a patient with dementia who may have developed parkinsonism, or in a patient with PD who later became demented due to superimposed AD. When needed for clinical–pathological studies, LBD–AD can be divided into subgroups according to the primary clinical presentation.

2.3 Clinical taxonomy in LBD and AD with parkinsonism

2.3.1 Clinical criteria: successes and unresolved questions

Is LBD a syndrome distinct from AD, or a clinical variant of AD? From our autopsy-verified series, the two conditions show substantial clinical overlap. For example, both LBD and AD present at a similar range of ages, with the insidious onset of dementia, usually and primarily affecting memory. As the dementia progresses, other cognitive areas become impaired. Survival from the onset of dementia until death is shorter in LBD than in AD in our autopsy series (Galasko et al., 1994) and in other reports (Perry et al., 1990b), and the annual rate of change of scores of cognitive tests such as the Mini-Mental State Examination is significantly faster in LBD than in AD. In clinical studies, patients with AD who develop parkinsonism (or extrapyramidal signs, EPS) or psychotic symptoms consistently have faster progression of dementia (see Chapter 3). Unfortunately, the rate of dementia progression varies too widely for it to be useful in differential diagnosis.

Attempts to identify LBD and to construct clinical criteria for this condition have drawn on findings in three areas: parkinsonian findings on the neurological examination, psychiatric or behavioral symptoms (notably confusional episodes, hallucinations and delusions), and patterns of neuropsychological deficits. When retrospectively applied to detailed case records that covered the entire course of dementia, each of the clinical features proposed by McKeith et al. (1992) had markedly higher frequencies in autopsied patients with LBD compared with AD. In a subsequent study, several clinicians applied the same diagnostic criteria to comprehensive case records of LBD, AD and vascular dementia patients evaluated at a psychogeriatric center (McKeith et al., 1994). Inter-rater reliability was very good, and the sensitivity for diagnosing LBD ranged from 55–90%, with specificity of over 90%. We have used a similar approach in a cohort of demented patients who met clinical criteria for probable or possible AD, received a standardized comprehensive research evaluation while at a mild to moderate stage of dementia severity, and were followed annually. We could not operationally define fluctuating cognitive impairment, the central feature of the criteria of McKeith et al. (1992), to our satisfaction from available structured interviews or rating scales. Nevertheless, we found significant clinical differences between a group of autopsy-verified LBD patients and a group of 'pure' AD patients matched for age and dementia severity at first evaluation, using the features of parkinsonism, psychotic symptoms and a 'frontal-subcortical' profile on neuropsychological testing. By combining these findings we could distinguish about 70% of LBD patients from AD, even relatively early in the course of dementia. Some of the problems that we have encountered are highlighted below.

2.3.2 Parkinsonian signs in LBD and AD

To what extent does LBD account for the parkinsonian signs that are found in many patients who otherwise appear to have AD? Varying frequencies of parkinsonian signs have been reported in AD, depending on which signs were rated, the type of rating scale used and the stage of AD. Many studies have shown that as AD progresses, parkinsonism becomes more prevalent, and may affect 50% or more of patients with advanced AD, even in the absence of neuroleptic exposure. Since at most 20–30% of AD patients have LB at autopsy, parkinsonism associated with AD must be multifactorial. There are pitfalls in deciding whether neurological findings in demented patients indicate parkinsonism; for instance, AD patients may show slowing of movement due to difficulty comprehending commands, loss of facial animation and a softening of the voice due to general apathy often associated with dementia, and nonspecific slowing of gait with a tendency to shuffle may be due to aging or to orthopedic problems. Patients with advanced AD lose the ability to walk and eventually develop paraplegia in flexion; rigidity, bradykinesia and other 'parkinsonian' findings lose their meaning at that stage. In elderly patients, medications with anti-dopaminergic actions such as neuroleptics, even when used at low doses, may produce parkinsonism that can persist for months after withdrawal. Recent exposure to such drugs in a demented patient may confound the diagnosis of LBD.

Traditional clinical criteria for idiopathic PD require at least two of the three major or cardinal signs, namely resting tremor, rigidity and bradykinesia. Impairment of postural reflexes, also called postural instability, is sometimes also listed as a major sign, but is less specific. Other signs such as hypophonic speech, parkinsonian gait, stooped posture, and masked facies are not accorded primary diagnostic significance. In our experience, the parkinsonian features in LBD appear to be clinically milder than in idiopathic PD, and resting tremor is rare. Although asymmetrical parkinsonian signs and a positive response to dopaminergic treatment are predictive of LB in clinically diagnosed PD, these features are unusual in LBD. In our series, over 60% of patients with autopsy proven LBD who were examined during the early to middle stages of dementia, without prior exposures to neuroleptics, showed two or more parkinsonian signs, at least one of which was a major sign. The most frequent signs were bradykinesia, masked facies and rigidity, each present in about 40–50% of patients; then shuffling gait, stooped posture, postural or action tremor, and hypophonic speech (20–30%); and least often postural instability and resting tremor (10% or less). Very few patients had a beneficial motor response to levodopa treatment, echoing the largely negative results of studies of levodopa, and more recently, of apomorphine treatment of patients with AD-EPS (Merello et al., 1994). Regardless of how they are defined, extrapyramidal signs in AD patients are markers of a faster rate of progression. An argument can thus be made to describe parkinsonian findings in demented patients as a continuum, calling the condition AD with parkinsonism or AD with EPS. Instruments such as the Unified Parkinson's Disease Rating Scale (UPDRS) are being applied to studies of AD and may help, when combined with autopsy follow-up, to define criteria for identifying specific parkinsonian signs, or combinations of signs that meet a given level of severity, that are predictive of LBD.

2.4 Does LBD produce a recognizable neuropsychiatric syndrome?

Psychiatric and behavioral symptoms are common in patients with LBD, and are consistent with the location of LB in limbic brain areas. Of these, delusions, usually paranoid in nature, hallucinations, and depression have been best described. Before inferring that these symptoms are markers of LBD, we need to consider how frequently they occur in AD. In our series, when autopsy confirmed patients with LBD and 'pure' AD were matched for age at presentation, sex and the level of cognitive severity when first seen, the rates of depression did not differ between the two patient groups, while delusions were slightly more frequent in LBD, and hallucinations were strikingly increased in LBD compared with pure AD (32% vs. 11%). In our few 'pure' LBD patients, who had rare AD lesions, hallucinations and delusions were again the most frequent psychiatric symptoms (Galasko et al., 1995). Consistent with the studies of the Newcastle group (Perry et al., 1990a; McKeith et al., 1994), we noted that hallucinations usually arose spontaneously, were most often visual, with formed – and often vivid – images of people, animals or objects, and lasted for days to months. In a few patients, hallucinations were part of delirium due to another disease process, most often an infection. Unprovoked hallucinations thus serve as useful pointers to LBD, while depression or delusions do not appear to be specific.

Why do fluctuations in cognition and alertness, as emphasized by the Newcastle group (McKeith et al., 1992, 1994), not appear in all reports of LBD, or in clinical descriptions of AD with parkinsonism? At our center, the assessment routinely includes the Hachinski Ischemic Index, which contains a question about a fluctuating course of dementia, a detailed structured history from a caregiver, and review of outside medical records. Of our autopsied LBD patients, about 30% had episodes of decreased responsiveness during the mild to moderate stages of dementia, that sometimes were striking enough to raise the question of a transient ischemic attack or a seizure, and represent large fluctuations of cognition. We have noticed several grey areas when determining a history of fluctuating condition. First, the borderline between sundowning, which is common in the middle and later stages of AD, and fluctuating confusion is unclear. Second, it is difficult to distinguish transient cognitive changes from delirium, especially when patients have concomitant medical conditions, are on several medications, or develop infections. It is also possible that the patients assessed at an Alzheimer's Disease Research Center may differ from those evaluated at a psychogeriatric unit. We therefore place less weight on fluctuation being a mandatory diagnostic feature of LBD.

Can we attribute a cognitive profile to LBD? Since cortical LB have a different laminar and regional distribution to the neurofibrillary changes of AD, they are likely to produce cognitive deficits distinct from those of AD. Several studies have examined neuropsychological profiles in autopsy-defined LBD, LBD-AD, and in clinical AD with parkinsonism. It is important to compare patients with these syndromes with AD patients who were tested when at a similar level of cognitive impairment and to control for variables such as age and education that can influence psychometric test scores. In our original series of 'Lewy body variant' (Hansen et al., 1990) we noted that AD and LBD patients showed a similar degree of impairment on tests of language, recent and remote memory and praxis. However LBD patients were more severely impaired in areas such as constructional ability, psychomotor speed, problem-solving and verbal fluency. This pattern of relatively severe deficits of visuospatial function and of tests of executive function is suggestive of frontal-subcortical dementia (Brown & Marsden, 1988). More recently in our clinical–pathological series we have extended our findings to LBD–AD patients at relatively mild stages of dementia (Galasko et al., 1995) and to patients with 'pure' LBD at autopsy (Salmon et al., 1996), using a more detailed neuropsychological test battery, and have found that discriminant function analysis places AD patients into a 'cortical' dementia profile, almost all of the 'pure' LBD patients into a 'frontal-subcortical' profile, and patients with LBD and AD between these two. Similar patterns of deficits on 'frontal-subcortical' tests have been found in patients with AD-EPS (Richards et al., 1993; Merello et al., 1994). Even nondemented PD patients show mild deficits on tests of visuospatial and of executive function when compared with age-matched controls. This converging body of evidence indicates that LB disorders – despite different clinical appellations – have relatively selective effects on cognitive function, that may be incorporated into the diagnostic approach to these disorders.

2.4.1 Suggestions for clinical criteria and nosology

In approaching 'LBD', criteria and nomenclature need to be flexible to accommodate different clinical and research questions. As a start, the relative merits of clinical and psychometric approaches to the diagnosis of dementia itself in conditions such as LBD, AD with parkinsonism, and PD-dementia need further exploration. The DSM-IV and NINCDS–ADRDA approaches to dementia contain as integral elements the insidious onset of cognitive decline of sufficient magnitude to affect social and, if appropriate, occupational function, the documentation of cognitive impairment on mental status testing, and the exclusion of metabolic, vascular and other neurodegenerative causes of dementia. For AD, many diagnostic criteria require impairment of memory and at least one other area of cognitive function. If primacy is similarly given to memory difficulty in LBD, then patients with visuospatial and executive deficits severe enough to impair intellectual function, whose memory performance lies in a normal or minimally impaired range, will not be called demented. As a possible remedy, we suggest also testing the approach initially developed by Cummings and Benson that defines dementia as significant dysfunction in three or more areas of cognition (not necessarily memory) using psychometric tests with age-standardized normative data.

A nosological scheme must incorporate two clinical syndromes: (1) variant syndromes of AD, such as AD with parkinsonism or with psychosis, which as mentioned earlier may have several different underlying causes and (2) LB dementia, a syndrome with high predictive value for underlying LB, defined in a more restricted way using various clinical features and neurological examination findings. Regarding AD with parkinsonism, important considerations are whether to use a formal rating scale or clinical judgement and what threshold of parkinsonian signs is necessary or significant. Similar considerations enter into LBD, but affect far more variables. The criteria proposed by McKeith et al. (1992) and Byrne et al. (1991) represent early and promising steps. In essence both approaches are similar, but do not incorporate neuropsychological test profiles. From the discussion of our own and other studies, we suggest that clinical guidelines for LBD should contain the key elements listed below. This formulation is compatible with both sets of proposed criteria for LBD, and would not change the classification of most of the patients in the McKeith et al. (1994) study.

2.4.2 Mandatory feature of LBD

Dementia by history, confirmed on mental status testing, and unexplained by metabolic, vascular, or degenerative conditions. If the diagnosis of idiopathic PD clearly preceded dementia, the terminology of PD-dementia is preferable to LBD. Further studies are needed to define whether memory impairment is essential to LBD.

2.4.3 Probable LBD

Parkinsonian signs: At least two physical signs, both of which are major signs, namely bradykinesia, rigidity, or resting tremor, in the absence of neuroleptics or other causes such as basal ganglia stroke or progressive supranuclear palsy.

2.4.4 Possible LBD

At least two of the following:

1. Less clear *parkinsonism*: only one major sign, with at least one or more minor signs. Minor signs that may be useful are masked facies, parkinsonian (shuffling) gait, stooped posture, postural instability, hypophonic speech.
2. Marked *cognitive fluctuations* occurring in the absence of an identified cause of delirium.
3. *Hallucinations* in the absence of an identified cause.
4. A *neuropsychological profile* of disproportionately severe deficits on psychometric tests of executive function and visuospatial performance.

2.5 Conclusions

The clinical and pathological boundaries of LB disorders are still being surveyed. It should be evident from the terminology that our research group has adopted, 'Lewy body variant of Alzheimer's disease', that we have been struck by the overlap between these two processes in demented patients. The aim of the above suggestions is to try and establish a flexible framework of definitions so that investigators can achieve early clinical diagnosis and consensus when comparing groups of patients, to advance our understanding of what we think will prove to be a spectrum of LB disorders. Prospective studies of well-characterized patients, with autopsy validation, will provide a framework to optimize diagnostic criteria for clinicians interested in these conditions.

References

Bergeron, C. & Pollanen, M. (1989). Lewy bodies in Alzheimer's disease – one or two diseases? *Alzheimer Dis. Assoc. Disord.*, **3**, 197–204.

Brown, R.G. & Marsden, C.D. (1988). Subcortical dementia: the neuropsychological evidence. *Neuroscience*, **25**, 363–87.

Byrne, E.J., Lennox, G.G., Godwin-Austen, R.B. et al. (1991). Dementia associated with cortical Lewy bodies: proposed clinical diagnostic criteria. *Dementia*, **2**, 283–4.

Galasko, D., Hansen, L.A., Katzman, R. et al. (1994). Clinical-neuropathological correlations in Alzheimer's disease and related dementias. *Arch. Neurol.*, **51**, 888–95.

Galasko, D., Katzman, R., Salmon, D.P. & Thal, L.J. (1996). Clinical and neuropathological findings in Lewy body dementias. *Brain and Cognition*, in press.

Gibb, W.R.G., Esiri, M.M. & Lees, A.J. (1985). Clinical and pathological features of diffuse cortical Lewy body disease (Lewy body dementia). *Brain*, **110**, 1131–53.

Hansen, L., Salmon, D.P., Galasko, D. et al. (1990). The Lewy body variant of Alzheimer's disease: a clinical and pathological entity. *Neurology*, **40**, 1–8.

Hansen, L., Masliah, E., Galasko, D. & Terry, R.D. (1993). Plaque-only Alzheimer disease is usually the Lewy body variant, and vice versa. *J. Neuropathol. Exp. Neurol.*, **52**, 648–54.

Hughes, D., Daniel, S., Blankson, S. & Lees, A. (1992): A clinicopathologic study of 100 cases of Parkinson's disease. *Arch. Neurol.*, **50**, 140–8.

Jellinger, K., Danielczyk, W., Fischer, P. & Gabriel, E. (1990). Clinicopathological analysis of dementia disorders in the elderly. *J. Neurol. Sci.*, **95**, 239–58.

Kosaka, K. (1990). Diffuse Lewy body disease in Japan. *J. Neurol.*, **237**, 197–204.

Lennox, G., Lowe, J., Morell, K. et al. (1989). Diffuse Lewy body disease: correlative neuropathology using anti-ubiquitin immunocytochemistry. *J. Neurol. Neurosurg. Psychiatry*, **52**, 1236–47.

McKeith, I.G., Perry, R.H., Fairbairn, A.F., Jabeen, S. & Perry, E.K. (1992). Operational criteria for senile dementia of Lewy body type (SDLT). *Psychol. Med.*, **22**, 911–22.

McKeith, I.G., Fairbairn, A.F., Bothwell, R.A. et al. (1994). An evaluation of the predictive validity and inter-rater reliability of clinical diagnostic criteria for senile dementia of the Lewy body type. *Neurology*, **44**, 872–7.

Mendez, M., Mastri, A.R., Sung, J.H. & Frey, W.H. (1992). Clinically diagnosed Alzheimer's disease: Neuropathologic findings in 650 cases. *Alzheimer Dis. Assoc. Disord.*, **6**, 35–43.

Merello, M., Sabe, S., Teson, A. et al. (1994). Extrapyramidalism in Alzheimer's disease: prevalence, psychiatric, and neuropsychological consequences. *J. Neurol. Neurosurg. Psychiatry*, **57**, 1503–9.

Mirra, S.S., Hart, M.N. & Terry, R.D. (1993). Making the diagnosis of Alzheimer's disease. *Arch. Pathol. Lab. Med.*, **117**, 132–44.

Perry, R., Irving, D. & Tomlinson, B. (1990a). Lewy body prevalence in the aging brain: relationship to neuropsychiatric disorders, Alzheimer-type pathology and catecholaminergic nuclei. *J. Neurol. Sci.*, **100**, 223–33.

Perry, R.H., Irving, D., Blessed, G., Fairbairn, A. & Perry, E.K. (1990b). Senile dementia of Lewy body type: a clinically and neuropathologically distinct form of Lewy body dementia in the elderly. *J. Neurol. Sci.*, **95**, 119–39.

Richards, M., Bell, K., Dooneief, G. et al. (1993). Patterns of neuropsychological performance in Alzheimer's disease patients with and without extrapyramidal signs. *Neurology*, **43**, 1708–11.

Salmon, D.P., Galasko, D., Hansen, L.A., Masliah, E., Butters, N. Thal, L.J., Katzman, R. (1996). Neuropsychological deficits associated with diffuse Lewy body disease. *Brain and Cognition*, in press.

Samuel, W., Galasko, D., Masliah, E., Hansen, L.A. (1996). Neocortical Lewy body counts correlate with dementia in the Lewy body variant of Alzheimer's disease. *J. Neuropathol. Exp. Neurol.*, **55**, 44–52.

3

Putative clinical and genetic antecedents of dementia associated with Parkinson's disease

R. MAYEUX and K. MARDER

Summary

Dementia is a constant manifestation of Parkinson's disease; it is the third most common cause of dementia after Alzheimer's disease and stroke. The clinical manifestations are similar to those seen in other degenerative disorders that cause dementia with some minimal differences; some specific disturbances such as depression and a decline in verbal fluency may identify individuals who are in the early stages of dementia. While patients advanced in age seem to be at higher risk of dementia with Parkinson's disease, the risk is uniform throughout the duration of disease. There are no known environmental risk factors specific for dementia, though many putative factors have been identified for Parkinson's disease. There is a strong evidence to suggest a genetic etiology, but more work is essential because of the unusual relationship between Alzheimer's disease, Lewy body dementia and the dementia of Parkinson's disease.

3.1 Introduction

Nearly all of the therapeutic success in Parkinson's disease during the last three decades have been dampened by the presence of dementia which occurs as a regular manifestation. There is general agreement that dementia is most common in older patients with Parkinson's disease and that it is the single most important factor limiting treatment. Most also agree that there is a considerable overlap in clinical manifestations with Alzheimer's disease and dementia of the Lewy body type. The frequency of dementia in Parkinson's disease is even higher than appreciated (Girotti et al., 1988; Mayeux et al., 1990) and it increases the mortality rate by at least twofold compared with nondemented persons of the same age with and without Parkinson's disease (Marder et al., 1991). While there is evidence to suggest that the pathological and biochemical bases for dementia in Parkinson's disease are similar to that in Alzheimer's disease, it is clear that parkinsonian dementia may result from a number of unique processes (Jellinger & Paulus, 1992). For example, the Lewy body, a pathological hallmark for the idiopathic form of Parkinson's disease when seen in the brainstem, has been associated with another form of dementia with and without parkinsonian features when the inclusion is found in the cerebral cortex (Hansen et al., 1990).

3.2 Definitions of dementia in Parkinson's disease

Dementia is a syndrome defined by a constellation of signs and symptoms. *The Diagnostic and Statistical Manual of Mental Disorders*, Third revised edition (American Psychiatric Association, 1987), provides criteria for the diagnosis of dementia in degenerative disorders. An abbreviated version of these criteria are seen in Table 3.1. The diagnosis of dementia in Parkinson's disease can pose some problems because there are well-documented changes in intellectual function associated with the disease even before dementia is apparent. Moreover, the motor manifestations may be the initial focus of attention. Jacobs and her colleagues (Jacobs et al., 1995) described a particular cognitive profile which may identify patients who will later develop dementia. Impaired performance in verbal fluency, memory and a language task were each associated with a significant increase in the probability of dementia over a three year period. Thus, while the features of dementia in patients with Parkinson's disease are generally similar to those of any other disease causing dementia, the cognitive manifestations prior to the onset of overt dementia may differ.

A 'Lewy body variant' of Alzheimer's disease characterized by a greater degree of impairment in attention, verbal fluency and visuospatial function than typically seen in Alzheimer's disease has also been described (Hansen et al., 1990). While these studies have been retrospective as they are based on postmortem investigations, others (Crystal et al., 1990) indicated that antemortem diagnosis was possible by the presence of an abnormal electroencephalogram and parkinsonism. Although criteria for dementia associated with cortical Lewy bodies has been proposed by the Nottingham Group for the Study of Neurodegenerative Diseases (Byrne et al., 1991), they require the presence of parkinsonism

Table 3.1. *Criteria for primary degenerative dementia.* (*Modified from the* Diagnostic and Statistical Manual of Mental Disorders, *Third edition, revised*)

1. Impaired memory
2. Impairment in at least one of the following:
   (a) abstract thinking
   (b) judgement
   (c) language
   (d) emotional expression
3. Impairment must interfere with work or usual activity
4. No evidence for delirium
5. Not accounted for by other major psychiatric problems

which is an inconsistent finding (Dickson et al., 1987). Some patients with cortical Lewy bodies and dementia have no history or clinical evidence for rigidity, tremor, bradykinesia or postural change. A fluctuating decline in cognitive function, characterized by episodes of confusion and lucid intervals is believed by some (McKeith et al., 1992) to distinguish between senile dementia of the Lewy body type and Alzheimer's disease. Depression, complex visual hallucinations and delusions are also part of the clinical spectrum. Yet none of these clinical manifestations are specific to any single form of dementia. Thus, at the present time the clinical diagnosis of parkinsonian dementia as well as dementia of the Lewy body type remain uncertain and rest on subjective or judgemental criteria of the clinician or investigator.

3.3 Epidemiology of dementia in Parkinson's disease

To estimate the frequency of a disease or syndrome within a disease such as dementia, investigators usually rely on measures of disease frequency such as prevalence (the proportion of a population affected by the disease or symptom at any given time) and incidence rate (the number of disease- or syndrome-free individuals who become affected during a specified time period in a population). Most estimates of the frequency of dementia in the idiopathic form of Parkinson's disease have been in terms of prevalence as noted in Table 3.2.

Dementia has been consistently found in 10% to 30% of patients with prevalent Parkinson's disease (Celesia & Wanamaker 1972; Marttila & Rinne 1976; Lieberman et al., 1979; Sutcliffe 1985; Rajput et al., 1987; Girotti et al., 1988; Mayeux et al., 1988; Mayeux et al., 1990). Mayeux

Table 3.2. *Prevalence of dementia in Parkinson's disease*

Investigators	Year	Percent
Celesia and Wanamaker	1972	39%
Marttila and Rinne[*]	1976	18%
Lieberman et al.	1979	32%
Sutcliffe et al.[*]	1985	12%
Rajput et al.[*]	1987	9%
Mayeux et al.	1988	16%
Girotti et al.	1988	14%
Mayeux *et al.*[*]	1990	41%

[*]Population-based.

and his associates (Mayeux et al., 1988) found a similar prevalence rate for dementia in a hospital-based investigation; their initial estimate was 11.9% which was later corrected to 15.9% in a subsequent study (Mayeux et al., 1990). The age-specific prevalence rate in the hospital-based study was 21% for patients with motor manifestations beginning after age 70. These investigators completed a New York-based community study of Parkinson's disease with and without dementia and found 41.3% of the 179 prevalent cases to be demented (Mayeux et al., 1992). The overall crude prevalence of Parkinson's disease with dementia was 41.1 per 100,000 persons (over age 35: 90.8 per 100,000). The age-specific prevalence of Parkinson's disease-dementia also increased with age, parallel to the increase in Parkinson's disease overall, from 0.5 per 100,000 below age 50 to 787.1 per 100,000 above age 80. The prevalence standardized to the estimated distribution of the 1988 USA population, ranged from 5.3 per 100,000 between age 35 and 64 to 62.5 per 100,000 over age 75.

Taking all studies into consideration, the proportion of patients with Parkinson's disease who are demented depends on the population from which the sample is identified. In clinics or hospitals the proportion of demented patients with Parkinson's disease is likely to be about 12–20%, while the prevalence of dementia in community-dwelling individuals is probably much closer to 40%. The population-based figure also indicates the dramatic risk in prevalence of dementia with advanced age.

Incidence rates for dementia have also been estimated in a cohort of patients with idiopathic Parkinson's disease after nearly five years of follow-up (Mayeux et al., 1990). There were 65 new cases of dementia from the 249 patients followed leading to an estimated incidence rate of 6.9% per year. As age increased, the cumulative incidence, or cumulative risk, of dementia in the cohort also increased. By age 85, the cumulative incidence of dementia in this cohort had reached over 65%.

In a community-based study by the same group of investigators the annual incidence rate for dementia in that cohort was 11.3% per year (Marder et al., 1995). This was twice the frequency reported among the healthy elderly comparison group who resided in the same community.

Marder and her associates (Marder et al., 1991) have also examined the frequency of death among demented and nondemented patients matched for duration of disease. They found that the presence of dementia was associated with increased mortality among patients with Parkinson's disease, even when their advanced age is taken into consideration, suggesting that the frequency of dementia is much higher than reported in prevalence estimates. Incidence rates provide a more stable estimate of the frequency of dementia because they are not affected by mortality. In terms of the individual patient, this study also indicated that the cumulative risk of dementia was as high as 65% by 85 years of age.

3.4 Antecedent clinical manifestations associated with dementia in Parkinson's disease

Dementia in Parkinson's disease has most often been found in patients with advanced age. However, aging is a confounder being related both to dementia and Parkinson's disease. In a prospective study (Stern et al., 1993a) of clinical features related to dementia in Parkinson's disease, not only were advanced age and the severity of Parkinson's disease important as predictors (Table 3.3), but episodes of depression and a history of confusion while on levodopa were also strongly associated with dementia independent of age and disease severity. This study was based on a cohort

Table 3.3. *Antecedent factors associated with dementia in patients with Parkinson's disease*

1. Over age 70
2. United Parkinson's Disease Rating Scale score over 25
3. Prior history of depression
4. Prior history of confusion on levodopa
5. Akinesia as a presenting clinical sign

of patients identified in a movement disorder treatment center in New York City. In a community-based cohort study, however, similar predictors were found by Marder et al. (1995) in their study of incident dementia in patients with Parkinson's disease. The risk of dementia with Parkinson's disease was higher for individuals with an extrapyramidal score from the United Parkinson's Disease Rating Scale greater than 25 (relative risk 3.6 95% C1 = 1.4–8.9) and when the Hamilton Depression Rating Scale score exceeded 10 (relative risk 3.6 95% C1 = 1.6–7.9). In their discussion, they noted that others have previously reported an association between dementia and the severity of parkinsonism (Richards et al., 1993; Stern et al., 1993b). These features may be best characterized as early or antecedent manifestations of dementia in patients with Parkinson's disease rather than as risk factors. The authors of these studies surmise that dopamine deficiency alone might explain both the cognitive and motor manifestations because dementia has been found to be accompanied by neuronal loss in the media substantia nigra, which projects to the caudate and frontal association area (Rinne et al., 1989). The classic motor manifestations of Parkinson's disease are associated with loss of dopaminergic neurons in the lateral substantia nigra that project to the putamen and then premotor areas. The relationship between severity of extrapyramidal signs and dementia could imply a parallel decline of these two dopaminergic pathways. The serotonergic neurotransmitter system may also be involved as suggested by the association between depression and dementia in Parkinson's disease (Sano et al., 1989; Starkstein et al., 1990).

A search for environmental risk factors associated with dementia in patients with Parkinson's disease has not been revealing. Clearly, not all factors associated with Parkinson's disease have been explored. For example, Parkinson's disease appears to be more prevalent in industrialized nations and death records of the USA between 1959 and 1961 indicate a higher mortality from Parkinson's disease in the North where industrialization is more common than in the South. Pesticide and chemical exposure have been found in some areas with higher prevalence of Parkinson's disease. Two studies, one in Saskatchewan (Lux, 1987) and one in Chicago (Li, 1985), found that patients were more likely than controls to have been born and raised in rural environment and to have used well water as the primary drinking source, but no specific metal or toxin was implicated. Aging alone might promote the effects of an environmental toxin, but evidence to suggest such an interaction is lacking; reactive gliosis is still in progress and areas of the substantia nigra not typically affected in Parkinson's disease remain well populated at death.

Patients with Parkinson's disease, with and without dementia, have a significantly higher caloric intake which was attributed to increased intake of animal fat (Logroscino et al., 1996). This association was strongest among patients with PD and dementia, but it was also present in patients without dementia. Intake of vitamin E, vitamin C, carotenoids and retinol were not associated with PD.

3.5 Family history and genetic susceptibility

No specific gene or genetic risk factor has been reported in demented patients with Parkinson's disease, though evidence for genetic susceptibility is accumulating (Table 3.4). Familial aggregation of dementia, presumably Alzheimer's disease, in families of patients with Parkinson's disease (some of whom may have been demented) has been suggested in three studies. Marder et al. (1990) reported a sixfold increase in risk for first-degree relatives, mostly siblings, of demented patients with Parkinson's disease compared with relatives of nondemented patients with Parkinson's disease. A similar investigation found that first-degree relatives of patients with Alzheimer's disease were three times more likely to develop Parkinson's disease than relatives of controls (Hofman et al., 1989), and others (Majoor-Krakauer et al., 1994) observed that amyotrophic lateral sclerosis, Parkinson's disease and dementia may all cosegregate in families. Lewy body parkinsonism has been described as an autosomal dominant disorder in which 'memory loss' was an inconsistent feature (Golbe et al., 1993; Waters, 1994), and Lewy bodies have been observed in two family members with the 717 (val→Ile) mutation in the amyloid precursor protein (Lantos et al., 1994). These reports, though anecdotal, suggest a genetic component to dementia in patients with various forms of Parkinson's disease or parkinsonism. Thus, familial aggregation of Alzheimer's disease and Parkinson's disease with and without dementia implies at least the possibility of a shared genetic etiology.

Because of the pathological, biochemical and clinical similarities between dementia of Parkinson's disease and that of Alzheimer's disease, several investigators have examined the relationship of dementia in Parkinson's disease to polymorphisms of apolipoprotein E (APO E) on chromosome 19. At least three investigations (Benjamin et al., 1994; Marder et al., 1995; Koller et al., 1995) involving over 100 patients and

Table 3.4. *Evidence favoring a genetic etiology for dementia in patients with Parkinson's disease*

1. Familial accumulation of dementia among first-degree relatives in patients with Parkinson's disease.
2. 'Lewy body parkinsonism' with cortical Lewy bodies may be accompanied by dementia in an autosomal dominant form.
3. The Lewy body variant of Alzheimer's disease and possibly patients with parkinsonian dementia share an increased frequency of the CYP2D6 variant 'B' allele.
4. The Lewy body variant of Alzheimer's disease may be associated with a higher than expected frequency of the APOE-ϵ allele.
5. Parkinsonism associated with other familial dementias.

controls indicate that, unlike Alzheimer's disease, the ϵ4 variant of APO E is not associated with the dementia of Parkinson's disease. However, one study in a Japanese population found a higher frequency of the APO E ϵ4 allele in patients with Parkinson's disease and dementia (Arai et al., 1994), though other postmortem studies have confirmed the lack of an association between APO E ϵ4 and dementia in Parkinson's disease (Schneider et al., 1995).

A higher than expected frequency of the ϵ4 variant of APO E has been reported (St. Clair et al., 1994), among patients with the Lewy body variant of Alzheimer's disease, but not in patients with diffuse Lewy body disease (Galasko et al., 1994). However, when patients with Alzheimer's disease, with and without Lewy bodies, were compared with patients having Parkinson's disease and healthy elderly controls, the APO E ϵ4 frequency was found to be highest among patients with AD without Lewy bodies and lowest among patients with Parkinson's disease regardless of the presence or absence of dementia (Hardy et al., 1994). Patients with Lewy bodies and dementia were intermediate leading the authors to infer that the overlap represented a 'co-occurrence of the two syndromes': Alzheimer's disease and dementia of the Lewy body type. Excess accumulations of β-amyloid but not phosphorylated tau or tau in the form of paired helical filaments have been observed in Alzheimer's disease and dementia of the Lewy body type when compared with that found in patients with Parkinson's disease or controls (Harrington et al., 1994). However, the abnormal accumulations of these proteins were significantly higher in Alzheimer's disease. Other APO E genotypic pathology has been identified in Lewy body disease (Lippa et al., 1995). Thus, while the frequency of APO E ϵ4 may be increased over that in controls, there is no clear biological explanation for this observation in dementia of the Lewy body type. Furthermore, it is unlikely that APO E ε4 has a role in the dementia of Parkinson's disease.

The presence of an APO E ε4 allele is neither 'necessary nor sufficient' to cause Alzheimer's disease, rather it appears to influence the age-at-onset of disease (Roses, 1995). Whether APO E ε4 similarly influences age-at-onset in patients with dementia of the Lewy body type has not been established. There is no evidence that the presence of APO E ε4 accounts for any variation in the age-at-onset of dementia in patients with Parkinson's disease.

Specific alleles of CYP2D6, one of the cytochrome P450 mono-oxygenases, have been reported to be increased in patients with Parkinson's disease compared with controls. It has been proposed that variants of CYP2D6 either abnormally metabolize environmental toxins reducing the capacity to remove neurotoxins or interact with neurotransmitter antagonists. The CYP2D6 locus has several common alleles (Daly et al., 1991). The most common (wild type) allele is present in most individuals and in all ethnic groups. The 'A' and 'B' variant alleles of CYP2D6 are associated with a reduced debrisoquine hydroxylase activity due to multiple sequence differences that result in both missense and nonsense mutations without a gross rearrangement of the locus (Gough et al., 1990; Heim, 1990). An association between the 'B' allele of CYP2D6 and Parkinson's disease has been reported (Armstrong et al., 1992). The CYP2D6 B allele frequency is about 10% in the normal population. A larger series did not confirm that association, but found that the rarer 'A' allele to be 1.8 times more common in Parkinson's disease than in controls (Smith et al., 1992). Most significantly, the investigators found that having two mutant alleles (they only looked at A and B alleles) was 2.4 times more frequent in Parkinson's disease (Kondo, 1991). Curiously, an increased frequency of the 'B' allele of CYP2D6 has been observed in patients with dementia of the Lewy body type (Saitoh et al., 1995). We observed an increase in the odds ratio for parkinsonian dementia associated with CYP2D6 'B' allele when confined to the homozygous configuration compared with controls and to patients with Parkinson's disease who were not demented (OR 4.0; 95% c.i. 1.1–25.5). However, Plante-Bordeneuve et al. (1994) reported no evidence for genetic linkage in Parkinson's disease using a sib-pair analysis at the ch22q13.1 site, but did find an increased frequency of the 'B' allele among 'older' patients with sporadic disease. The presence or absence of dementia in these patients was not described.

These results are somewhat contradictory suggesting that the CYP2D6 gene product may have no causal relationship with Parkinson's disease but it may suggest that it is in linkage disequilibrium with a nearby genetic locus.

Other forms of dementia with parkinsonism have been described and linked to a region on chromosome 17q21-22 (Lynch et al., 1994; Wilhelmsen et al., 1994). The clinical features include dementia, loss of inhibition, parkinsonism and amyotrophy. Nigral degeneration is present, but Lewy body formation is not a consistent finding. Thus, this form of 'frontal-lobe' dementia is quite distinct from the dementia of Parkinson's disease and from the dementias associated with Lewy body formation.

The relationship between Parkinson's disease with dementia and dementia of the Lewy body type has not been elaborated. They may share clinical and pathological features as well as a similar etiology.

Acknowledgements

This work was supported by Federal Grants AG07232, AG10963, NS32527, RR00645 and The Parkinson's Disease Foundation.

References

American Psychiatric Association (1987). *Diagnostic and Statistical Manual of Mental Disorders* (Third revised edition), Washington, DC.

Arai, H., Muramatsu, T., Higuchi, S., Sasaki, H. & Trojanowski, J.Q. (1994). Apolipoprotein E gene in Parkinson's disease with or without dementia. *Lancet*, **344**, 889.

Armstrong, M., Daly, A.K., Cholerton, S. et al. (1992). Mutant debrisoquine hydroxylation genes in Parkinson's disease. *Lancet*, **339**, 1017–18.

Benjamin, R., Leake, A., Edwardson, J.A. et al. (1994). Apolipoprotein E genes in Lewy body and Parkinson's disease. *Lancet*, **343**, 1565.

Byrne, E.J., Lennox, G.G., Godwin-Austen, R. B. et al. (1991). Dementia associated with cortical Lewy bodies: proposed clinical diagnostic criteria. *Dementia*, **2**, 283–4.

Celesia, G.G. & Wanamaker, W.M. (1972). Psychiatric disturbances in Parkinson's disease. *Diseases of the Nervous System*, **33**, 577–83.

Crystal, H.A., Dickson, D.A., Lizardi, J.E., Davis, P. & Wolfson, L.I. (1990). Antemortem diagnosis of diffuse Lewy body disease. *Neurology*, **40**, 1523–8.

Daly, A.K., Armstrong, M., Monkman, S.C. et al. (1991). Genetic and metabolic criteria for the assignment of debrisoquine 4-hydroxylation (cytochrome P4502D6) phenotypes. *Pharmacogenetics*, **1**, 33–41.

Dickson, D.W., Davies, P., Mayeux, R. et al. (1987). Diffuse Lewy Body Disease, neuropathological and biochemical studies of six patients. *Acta Neuropathol. (Berl.)*, **75**, 8–15.

Galasko, D., Saitoh, T., Xia, Y. et al. (1994). The apolipoprotein E allele epsilon 4 is over represented in patients with the Lewy body variant of Alzheimer's disease. *Neurology*, **44**, 1950–1.

Girotti, F., Soliveri, P., Carella, F. et al. (1988). Dementia and cognitive impairment in Parkinson's disease. *J. Neurol. Neurosurg. Psychiatry*, **51**, 1498–502.

Golbe, L.I., Lassarini, A.M., Schwartz, K.O. et al. (1993). Autosomal dominant parkinsonism with benign course and typical Lewy-body pathology. *Neurology*, **43**, 2222–7.

Gough, A.C., Miles, J.S., Spurr, N.K. et al. (1990). Identification of the primary defect at the cytochrome P450 CYP2D locus. *Nature*, **347**, 773–6.

Heim, M. & Meyer, U.A. (1990). Genotyping of poor metabolizers of debrisoquine by allele-specific PCR amplification. *Lancet*, **336**, 529–32.

Hansen, L., Salmon, D., Galasko, D. et al. (1990). The Lewy body variant of Alzheimer's disease: A clinical and pathologic entity. *Neurology*, **40**, 1–7.

Hardy, J., Crook, R., Prihar, G. et al. (1994). Senile dementia of the Lewy body type has an apolipoprotein E epsilon 4 frequency intermediate between controls and Alzheimer's disease. *Neurosci. Lett.*, **182**, 1–2.

Harrington, C.R., Louwagie, J., Rossau, R. et al. (1994). Influence of apolipoprotein E genotype on senile dementia of the Alzheimer and Lewy body types. Significance for etiological theories of Alzheimer's disease. *Am. J. Path.*, **145**, 1472–82.

Hofman, A., Schulte, W., Tanja, T.A. et al. (1989). History of dementia and Parkinson's disease in 1st-degree relative of patients with Alzheimer's disease. *Neurology*, **39**, 1589–92.

Jacobs, D.M., Marder, K., Cote, L.J., Sano, M., Stern, Y. & Mayeux, R. (1995). Neuropsychological characteristics of preclinical dementia in Parkinson's disease. *Neurology*, **45**, 1691–6.

Jellinger, K.A. & Paulus, W. (1992). Clinico-pathological correlations in Parkinson's disease. *Clin. Neurol. Neurosurg* (suppl), **94**, S86–8.

Koller, W.C., Glatt, S.L., Hubble, J.P. et al. (1995). Apolipoprotein E genotypes in Parkinson's disease with and without dementia. *Ann. Neurol.*, **37**, 242–5.

Kondo, I. & Kanazawa, I. (1991). Association of Xba I allele (Xba I 44kb) of the human cytochrome P-450dbl (CYP2D6) gene in Japanese patients with idiopathic Parkinson's disease. In *Parkinson's disease: From Clinical Aspects to Molecular Basis*, ed. T. Nagatsu, H. Naabayashi & M. Yoshida, pp. 111–17. New York: Springer-Verlag.

Lantos, P.L., Ovenstone, I.M., Johnson, J. et al. (1994). Lewy bodies in the brain of two members of a family with 717 (val to Ile) mutation of the amyloid precursor protein gene. *Neurosci. Lett.*, **172**, 77–9.

Li, S., Schoenberg, B., Wang, C. et al. (1985). A prevalence survey of Parkinson's disease and other movement disorders in the People's Republic of China. *Arch. Neurol.*, **42**, 655–7.

Lieberman, A., Dziatolowski, M., Coopersmith, M. et al. (1979). Dementia in Parkinson's disease. *Ann. Neurol.*, **6**, 355–9.

Lippa, C.F., Smith, T.W., Saunders, A.M. et al. (1995). Apolipoprotein E genotype and Lewy body disease. *Neurology*, **45**, 97–103.

Logroscino, G., Marder, K., Cote, L.J., Tang, M-X & Mayeux, R. (1996).
    Dietary lipids and antioxidants in Parkinson's disease: a population-based,
    case-control study. *Ann. Neurol.*
Lux, W. & Kirtzke, J. (1987). Is Parkinson's disease acquired? *Neurology*, **37**,
    467.
Lynch, T., Sano, M., Marder, K.S. et al. (1994). Clinical characteristics of a
    family with chromosome 17-linked disinhibition-dementia-parkinsonism-
    amyotrophy complex. *Neurology*, **44**, 1878–84.
Majoor-Krakauer, D., Ottman, R., Johnson, W.G. & Rowland, L.P. (1994).
    Familial aggregation of amyotrophic lateral sclerosis, dementia, and
    Parkinson's disease: evidence of shared genetic susceptibility. *Neurology*,
    44, 1872–7.
Marder, K., Flood, P., Cote, L. & Mayeux, R. (1990). A pilot study of risk
    factors for dementia in Parkinson's disease. *Mov. Disord.*, **5**, 156–61.
Marder, K., Leung, D., Tang, M. et al. (1991). Are demented patients with
    Parkinson's disease accurately reflected in prevalence surveys? A survival
    analysis. *Neurology*, **41**, 1240–1224.
Marder, K., Maestre, G., Cote, L.J. et al. (1994). The apolipoprotein-ε4 allele
    in Parkinson's disease with and without dementia. *Neurology*, **44**, 1330–1.
Marder, K., Tang, M-X, Cote, L.J., Stern, Y. & Mayeux, R. (1995). The
    frequency and associated risk factors for dementia in patients with
    Parkinson's disease. *Arch. Neurol.*, **52**, 695–701.
Marttila, R.J. & Rinne, U.K. (1976). Dementia in Parkinson's disease. *Acta
    Neur. Scand.*, **54**, 431–41.
Mayeux, R., Stern, Y., Rosenstein, R. et al. (1988). An estimate of the
    prevalence of dementia in idiopathic Parkinson's disease. *Arch. Neurol.*, **45**,
    260–3.
Mayeux, R., Chen, J., Mirabello, E. et al. (1990). An estimate of the incidence
    of dementia in patients with idiopathic Parkinson's disease. *Neurology*, **40**,
    1513–17.
Mayeux, R., Denaro, J., Hemenegildo, N. et al. (1992). A population-based
    investigation of Parkinson's disease with and without dementia:
    relationship to age and gender. *Arch. Neurol.*, **49**, 492–7.
McKeith, I.G., Perry, R.H., Fairbairn, A.F., Jabeen, S. & Perry, E.K. (1992).
    Operational criteria for senile dementia of the Lewy body type (SDLT).
    Psychol. Med., **22**, 673–8.
Plante-Bordeneuve, V., Davis, M.B., Maraganore, D.M., Marsden, C.D. &
    Harding, A.E. (1994). Debrisoquine hydroxylase gene polymorphism in
    familial Parkinson's disease. *J. Neurol. Neurosurg. Psychiatry*, **57**, 911–13.
Rajput, A.H., Offord, K.P., Beard, C.M. & Kurland, L.T. (1987). A case-
    control study of smoking habits, dementia, and other illnesses in
    idiopathic Parkinson's disease. *Neurology*, **37**, 226–32.
Richards, M., Stern, Y. & Mayeux, R. (1993). Subtle extrapyramidal signs can
    predict the development of dementia in elderly individuals. *Neurology*, **43**,
    2184–8.
Rinne, J.O., Rummukainen, J., Paljarvi, L. & Rinne, U.K. (1989). Dementia in
    Parkinson's disease is related to neuronal loss in the medial substantia
    nigra. *Ann. Neurol.*, **26**, 47–50.
Roses, A.D. (1995). Apolipoprotein E genotyping in the differential diagnosis,
    not prediction of Alzheimer's disease. *Ann. Neurol.*, **38**, 6–14.

Saitoh, T., Xia, Y., Chen, X. et al. (1995). The CYP2D6B allele is overrepresented in the Lewy body variant of Alzheimer's disease. *Ann. Neurol.*, **37**, 110–12.

Sano, M., Stern, Y., Williams, J., Cote, L., Rosenstein, R. & Mayeux, R. (1989). Co-existing dementia and depression in Parkinson's disease. *Arch. Neurol.*, **46**, 1284–7.

Schneider, J.A., Gearing, M., Robbins, R.S., de l'Aune, W. & Mirra, S.S. (1995). Apolipoprotein E genotype in diverse neurodegenerative disorders. *Ann Neurol.*, **38**, 131–5.

Smith, C.A., Gough, A.C., Leigh, P.N. et al. (1992). Debrisoquine hydroxylase gene polymorphism and susceptibility to Parkinson's disease. *Lancet*, **339**, 1375–7.

St. Clair, D., Norman, J., Perry, R. et al. (1994). Apolipoprotein E epsilon 4 allele frequency in patients with Lewy body dementia, Alzheimer's disease and age-matched controls. *Neurosci. Lett.*, **176**, 45–6.

Starkstein, S.E., Bolduc, P.L., Mayberg, H.S., Preziosi, T.J. & Robinson, R.G. (1990). Cognitive impairments and depression in Parkinson's disease: a follow-up study. *J. Neurol. Neurosurg. Psychiatry*, **53**, 597–602.

Stern, Y., Marder, K., Tang, M-X. & Mayeux, R. (1993a). Antecedent clinical features associated with dementia in Parkinson's disease. *Neurology*, **46**, 1690–3.

Stern, Y., Richards, M., Sano, M. & Mayeux, R. (1993b). Comparison of cognitive changes in patients with Alzheimer's and Parkinson's disease. *Arch. Neurol.*, **50**, 1040–5.

Sutcliffe, R.L.G. (1985). Parkinson's disease in the district of the Northampton Health Authority, United Kingdom. A study of prevalence and disability. *Acta Neurol. Scand.*, **72**, 363–79.

Waters, Ch. & Miller, C.A. (1994). Autosomal dominant Lewy body parkinsonism in a four-generation family. *Ann. Neurol.*, **35**, 59–64.

Wilhelmsen, K.C., Lynch, T., Pavlou, E., Higgins, M. & Nygaard, T.G. (1994). Localization of disinhibition-dementia-parkinsonism-amyotrophy complex to 17q21-22. *Am. J. Hum. Gen.*, **55**, 1159–65.

4

Clinical features of patients with Alzheimer's disease and Lewy bodies

A. BURNS

Summary

There have been a number of reports detailing the occurrence of pathology sufficient for the diagnosis of Alzheimer's disease and Lewy body dementia in the same patient, leading to the term 'Lewy body variant of Alzheimer's disease' (LBV). The data available emphasize the difficulty in differentiating patients with pure Alzheimer's disease from those with the Lewy body variant but clinical features such as extrapyramidal signs or psychotic phenomena may be helpful. Patients with LBV can present with progressive memory loss and so, at least in the early stages of the disease, they are indistinguishable from patients with pure Alzheimer's disease and it is likely that such patients will be found in groups of patients with Alzheimer's disease. Generally, neuropsychological tests are disappointing in differentiating the two groups although there is a suggestion that frontal lobe dysfunction (as evidenced by atrophy on Computed Tomography scanning and neuropsychological tests) is more common in patients with Lewy bodies than those without. It is traditional to view such a clinical dilemma in terms of a spectrum disorder. One would postulate that the presence of Lewy bodies along with Alzheimer's disease pathology edges patients towards a presentation more clearly associated with diffuse Lewy body disease (confusional states, psychotic features, extrapyramidal signs). This is confirmed by clinical observations and supported by biological marker studies (such as apolipoprotein $\epsilon4$) in which patients with Lewy bodies take up an intermediate position between pure Lewy body disease and pure Alzheimer's disease. The exact contribution of Lewy bodies to the clinical syndrome of dementia needs to be more fully evaluated.

4.1 Introduction

This review will examine the clinical features of patients who have been diagnosed histologically as having both the pathological changes of Alzheimer's disease and the presence of Lewy bodies, the so-called Lewy body variant (LBV) of Alzheimer's disease (Hansen et al., 1990; Förstl et al., 1993). The clinical manifestations of Alzheimer's disease have been documented elsewhere and a description of these will be confined to areas where direct comparisons are available between patients with Alzheimer's disease alone and patients with both Alzheimer changes and Lewy bodies. The number of published cases of LBV is small and so invariably the conclusions drawn will be speculative. The complex relationship between Lewy bodies in the brain and the clinical manifestations of their presence is currently being appreciated in terms of other characteristic presentations of the disorder, such as those seen in dementia of the Lewy body type without Alzheimer changes, which have been codified in diagnostic criteria appearing elsewhere in this compendium (Byrne et al., 1991; McKeith et al., 1992). The presence of dual pathology confounds the already complex relationship between histological changes and clinical features, making any explanation of the association more problematic.

4.2 Diagnosis of the Lewy body variant of Alzheimer's disease

One of the first descriptions of the LBV was by Hansen et al. (1990), who classified patients on the basis of the coexistence of subcortical Lewy bodies and Alzheimer changes. Clearly, the pathological diagnosis of LBV depends on the detection of Lewy bodies, but also by the histological criteria by which Alzheimer's disease pathology is diagnosed (Lippa et al., 1994). Hansen et al. (1990) examined 36 patients with clinically and pathologically diagnosed Alzheimer's disease of whom 13 had additional Lewy bodies. Pathologically this group was characterized by gross pallor of the substantia nigra, and greater (when compared with patients having Alzheimer's disease alone) neuronal loss in the locus coeruleus, substantia nigra and substantia innominata, lower neocortical choline acetyltransferase levels and fewer tangles in the mid-frontal region. Spongiform vacuolization in the medial temporal lobe was also seen in the LBV group. The justification for the dual diagnosis rested on the presence of widespread neocortical neuritic plaques and neurofibrillary tangles satisfying Khachaturian criteria for Alzheimer's disease (Khachaturian,

1985). The pathological hallmark of Parkinson's disease, degeneration in the substantia nigra, was absent in 4 of 13 LBV cases, suggesting that they were not merely cases representing a chance association between Parkinson's disease and Alzheimer's disease. Gibb (1989) examined this putative association in a separate pathological study of 273 control patients without Parkinson's disease and 121 cases of Alzheimer's disease. Patients with both Alzheimer changes and Lewy bodies, compared with those having Alzheimer changes alone, had lower tangle and plaque counts in the hippocampus, frontal and temporal cortex but similar levels of choline acetyltransferase suggesting that nucleus basalis Lewy body degeneration contributes to cortical choline acetyltransferase loss but not to cortical Alzheimer pathology. The additive effects of Lewy body and tangle pathology were thought to be aetiologically significant in the causation of the dementia syndrome. The less severe Alzheimer pathology in patients with additional Lewy bodies, has also been found by Hansen et al. (1989) and Bergeron and Pollanen (1989) but seems to be related to tangle and not plaque pathology. In patients diagnosed as having Parkinson's disease, Lewy bodies in the substantia nigra were invariably associated with their presence in the neocortex (Hughes et al., 1992). Burkhardt et al. (1988) reported four cases of Lewy body disease and round plaques and tangles in the subiculum, hippocampus, parahippocampal gyrus and temporal cortex but not of a sufficient number to merit a diagnosis of Alzheimer's disease.

4.3 Lewy body variant case – pathological findings

The present review is based on 34 cases presented in six studies (Gibb et al., 1985; Byrne et al., 1989; Crystal et al., 1990; Hansen et al., 1990; Förstl et al., 1993 and Lippa et al., 1994). Seventeen patients have been directly compared with age and sex matched patients with pure Alzheimer's disease drawn from the same clinico-pathological studies (Hansen et al., 1990; Förstl et al., 1993). These comparisons are particularly important in trying to untangle the essential clinical question, i.e. how can patients with Alzheimer's disease and Lewy bodies be differentiated in vivo. The results are summarized in Tables 4.1 through 4.4.

Gibb et al. (1985) described four cases with severe dementia and a parkinsonian syndrome with associated cortical signs and psychotic features. Three had Alzheimer pathology (hippocampal tangles in one, and hippocampal and occipital plaques in the other two), with the Alzheimer pathology not colocalized with the presence of Lewy bodies which were particularly numerous in the temporal and parietal lobes. Byrne et al. (1989), reported 15 cases of whom 4 had 'sufficient numbers of neurofibrillary tangles in the hippocampus and temporal cortex, to suggest a second diagnosis of Alzheimer's disease'. Lewy bodies were present in the substantia nigra and small neurones in the temporal, anterior cingulate, insular, entorhinal and frontal cortices. Hansen et al. (1990) compared nine patients with Lewy body and Alzheimer pathology with nine demonstrating pure Alzheimer changes. This was part of a larger group of 36 patients, 13 of whom had both pathologies, the remaining 23 having pure Alzheimer's disease, diagnosed according to the Khachaturian (1985) criteria. Twelve of the LBV cases (nine of whom were matched for overall severity of dementia with the pure Alzheimer group) had Lewy bodies in more than one sub-cortical location – locus coeruleus, substantia nigra or substantia innominata. Two of the 23 pure Alzheimer cases had subcortical Lewy bodies but none had cortical Lewy bodies.

Crystal et al. (1990) described three of six patients with diffuse Lewy body disease who had sufficient cortical neurofibrillary tangles (according to Khachaturian criteria) to warrant a diagnosis of Alzheimer's disease. Förstl et al. (1993) reported a prospectively studied clinical population of 178 patients satisfying NINCDS–ADRDA criteria for Alzheimer's disease (McKhann et al., 1984). Of 65 consecutive postmortems, eight patients had both cortical and sub-cortical Lewy bodies in addition to Alzheimer pathology. Finally, Lippa et al. (1994) found seven patients with both Lewy bodies and Alzheimer's disease in a study detailing clinical and pathological data on five normal controls, five patients with Lewy body disease alone and six patients with pure Alzheimer's disease.

4.4 Clinical findings

These are reviewed in Tables 4.1–4.4. Inevitably, it is difficult to draw comparisons between studies where the number of patients is small and the amount of clinical information presented is variable.

4.4.1 Initial symptoms

In the 22 cases where early signs were described (Tables 4.1 and 4.3) memory loss was the commonest in 16 (plus one who had topographic amnesia and one who had mental slowing as a marked feature in addition to memory loss). Two patients presented with confusional states, one with Parkinson's disease and one with depression. Presenting signs of

Table 4.1. *Summary of the clinical features of series of patients discussed in the text. (Gibb et al., 1985; Byrne et al., 1989; Förstl et al., 1993)*

	Sex	Age at death	Duration (years)	Initial symptoms	Delusions	Hallucinations	Falls	EPS*
Gibb et al. (1985)								
Case 2	F	38	5	Depression	Yes	Yes	Yes	PS
Case 3	M	60	5	Topographic amnesia	No	No	No	PS
Case 4	M	73	3	ML Aggression	No	Yes	No	PS
Byrne et al. (1989)								
Case 2	F	80	6	PD	No	No	Yes	PD
Case 3	F	77	6	ML	No	Yes	No	PS
Case 4	F	77	6	ML	No	Yes	No	PS
Case 5	M	86	3	ML	No	No	Yes	PS
Förstl et al. (1993)								
Case 1	M	78	12	ML	Yes	No	No	PS
Case 2	M	75	?6	ML/Slowing	Yes	Yes	No	PS
Case 3	F	77	7	Confusion	No	No	No	PS
Case 4	F	80	7	ML	No	No	No	PS
Case 5	M	82	8	ML	No	No	No	–
Case 6	M	77	0.3	Confusion	Yes	Yes	No	–
Case 7	F	82	5	ML/Depression	No	No	No	–
Case 8	F	88	6	ML Misidentification	No	No	No	–

*Key: ML = Memory Loss, EPS = Extrapyramidal symptoms, PD = Parkinson's disease, PS = Parkinsonian syndrome

Table 4.2. *Summary of the clinical features of series of patients discussed in the text (after Hansen et al., 1990)*

9 patients with AD, 9 with Lewy body variant (LBV) of AD
Neurological signs

	LBV	AD	Difference
Masked facies	5	0	p = 0.012
Essential tremor	5	1	p = 0.048
Neuropsychological tests			
Attention			
Digit span sub-test	10.00	14.00	p = 0.02
Language/semantic memory			
Letter fluency test	6.0	17.00	p = 0.02
Errors in writing to dictation	5/9	0/8	p = 0.02
Visuospatial processing			
Block design subtest	0.00	15.00	p = 0.02
Copy-a-cross test	4.0	1.50	p = 0.03
Conceptualization/problem solving			
Similarities subtest	2.00	9.00	p = 0.04

Table 4.3. *Summary of the clinical features of series of patients discussed in the text (after Lippa et al., 1994)*

Case	Sex	Age	Duration of illness (years)	Initial symptom	Clinical diagnosis
11	M	78	4	Cognitive	AD/PD
12	M	79	4	Cognitive	Dementia
13	F	88	4	Cognitive	Dementia/ PD
14	M	79	10	Cognitive	AD/PD
15	M	75	5	Cognitive	AD
16	F	85	–	Cognitive	AD
17	F	56	10	Cognitive	AD

Table 4.4. *Summary of the clinical features of series of patients discussed in the text (after Crystal et al., 1990)*

Case	Sex	Age of onset	Duration (years)	Gait abnormality	Resting tremor	Tone ability
30	M	74	14	Yes	No	Yes
31	F	?66	12	Yes[*]	No	No
33	M	78	6	Yes	No	Yes

[*]only in final stages

noncognitive features included depression, misidentification and aggression, which were generally accompaniments to memory loss.

4.4.2 Neurological signs

Parkinsonian features were almost universal, Parkinson's disease being the clinical diagnosis in four of the 22 cases. Hansen et al. (1990) examined a number of neurological signs and found only two to be significantly associated with Lewy bodies (masked facies and essential tremor, Table 4.2) but nuchal rigidity, bradykinesia and a parkinsonian gait were completely absent in the pure Alzheimer group, the small sample size presumably contributing to the lack of statistical significance. Crystal et al. (1990) (Table 4.4) followed patients longitudinally and examined the development of neurological signs. Gait abnormalities (assessed on a 5-point scale) were found in patients in all groups (Parkinson's disease, diffuse Lewy body disease, pure Alzheimer's disease and LBV) developing later in the illness in one case in each group. Resting tremor was absent in all LBV cases but present in two of three Alzheimer and two of three diffuse Lewy body patients. Abnormalities of tone (which included both cogwheel rigidity and gegenhalten) were seen in two of three LBV patients and in all Alzheimer subjects. Parkinsonian symptoms were seen in all the patients reported by Gibb et al. (1985) and Byrne et al. (1989) but only in half of the NINCDS–ADRDA patients reported by Förstl et al. (1993). Falls were also described but no comparative data are available to assess whether their presence is related to the presence of Lewy bodies (if so, they may be related to extrapyramidal signs). Förstl et al. (1993) found that five of the eight patients with LBV, developed rigidity with only one of the eight with pure Alzheimer's disease. In a corroborating study, Förstl et al. (1992) found rigidity to be related to the presence of Lewy bodies in the substantia nigra and neocortex.

4.4.3 Psychiatric symptoms

These are not always reported by studies but the high proportion of delusions and hallucinations can be seen from Table 4.1. Six of the nine patients presenting with memory loss also had psychiatric symptoms with hallucinations being slightly more common than delusions. Förstl et al. (1993) found that there was no difference in the proportion of patients with hallucinations in either the LBV or pure Alzheimer group. Hansen et al. (1990) found two patients in each of their groups to have been depressed.

4.4.4 Neuropsychological profile

Hansen et al. (1990) examined neuropsychological performance in each of their two groups of nine subjects who were matched for degree of dementia. There were greater deficits in attention, fluency and visuospatial processing in the LBV group. Förstl et al. (1993) age and sex matched two groups of eight patients and found no differences in cognitive function but the instruments used were not as detailed as those reported by Hansen et al. (1990).

4.4.5 Ancillary investigations

Förstl et al. (1993) found that patients with LBV had significantly greater atrophy of the frontal lobes compared with pure Alzheimer's disease yet lateral ventricular volume was the same in the two groups. Crystal et al. (1993) reported EEG changes, finding in the combined group one normal tracing and another with 6–7 Hz activity in the posterior region. The EEG was unhelpful in differentiating between diffuse Lewy body disease alone and Alzheimer's disease.

4.5 Apolipoprotein E

The presence of the apolipoprotein $\epsilon4$ is a significant risk factor for patients with familial or sporadic Alzheimer's disease. Three studies have examined this in relation to Lewy body disease. Both Pickering-

Brown et al. (1994) and Benjamin et al. (1994) found an increased rate
of ϵ4 in relation to the normal population (41.6 cf 14.3 and 31.4 cf 14.5,
respectively). Galasko and colleagues (1994) further subdivided patients
with Lewy body disease into those with LBV and those without Alzheimer changes and found that the increased risk was only for the LBV
group (frequencies in controls, Alzheimer's disease, LBV and Lewy
body disease – 14.2, 39.6, 29.0 and 6.25 respectively). This emphasizes
the common pathophysiological mechanism underlying the changes in
the Lewy body variant of Alzheimer's disease and pure Alzheimer's
disease.

4.6 Conclusion

1. A small number of patients with both Alzheimer and Lewy body
   pathology have been adequately described in terms of their clinical
   presentation. Clinico-pathological studies are needed to tease out specific clinical features, which can distinguish the Lewy body variant
   from pure Alzheimer's disease. It is likely that such patients will be
   found with Alzheimer populations and revisiting groups of patients
   with clinically diagnosed Alzheimer's disease will be helpful.
2. Available clinical information shows the difficulty in differentiating
   patients with pure AD and those with LBV, although some features
   such as extrapyramidal signs or psychotic phenomena may be helpful.
   Many patients with LBV present with progressive memory loss and so,
   at least in the early stages of the disease, they are indistinguishable
   from patients with pure Alzheimer's disease. In view of the considerable clinical overlap between dementias of apparently different origin
   (such as vascular dementia and Alzheimer's disease), this is an opti-
   mistic proposal.
3. The Lewy body variant of Alzheimer's disease represents more than
   merely a chance association between Parkinson's disease and Alzheimer's disease.
4. Neuropsychological tests are disappointing in differentiating the two
   groups although there is a suggestion that frontal lobe dysfunction (as
   evidenced by atrophy on Computed Tomography scanning and neuropsychological tests) is more a feature of the LBV than pure Alzheimer's disease.
5. It is traditional to view such a clinical dilemma in terms of a spectrum
   disorder. One would postulate that the presence of Lewy bodies along
   with Alzheimer's disease pathology edges patients towards a presenta-

tion more clearly associated with diffuse Lewy body disease (confusional states, psychotic features, extrapyramidal signs). This is confirmed by clinical observations and supported by biological marker studies (such as apolipoprotein ε4) with the LBV taking up an intermediate position between Lewy body disease and Alzheimer's disease. The exact contribution of the additional Lewy bodies to the clinical syndrome needs to be more fully evaluated.

References

Benjamin, R., Leake, A., Edwardson, J.A., McKeith, I.G. et al. (1994). Apolipoprotein E genes in Lewy body and Parkinson's disease. *Lancet*, **343**, 1565.

Bergeron, C. & Pollanen, M. (1989). Lewy bodies in Alzheimer's disease – One or Two Diseases? *Alzheimer Dis. Assoc. Disord.*, **3**, 4, 197–204.

Burkhardt, C.R., Filley, C.M., Kleinschmidt-DeMasters, B.K., de la Monte, S., Norenberg, M.D. & Schneck, S.A. (1988). Diffuse Lewy body disease and progressive dementia. *Neurology*, **38**, 1520–8.

Byrne, E.J., Lennox, G., Lowe, J. & Godwin-Austen, R.B. (1989). Diffuse Lewy body disease: Clinical features in 15 cases. *J. Neurol. Neurosurg. Psychiatry*, **52**, 709–17.

Byrne, E.J., Lennox, G., Godwin-Austen, R.B., Jefferson, D. et al. (1991). Dementia associated with cortical Lewy bodies: Proposed clinical diagnostic criteria. *Dementia*, **2**, 283–4.

Crystal, H.A., Dickson, D.W., Lizardi, J.E., Davies, P. & Wolfson, L.I. (1990). Antemortem diagnosis of diffuse Lewy body disease. *Neurology*, **40**, 1523–8.

Förstl, H., Burns, A., Levy, R., Cairns, N., Luthert, P. & Lantos, P. (1992). Neurologic signs in Alzheimer's disease: results of a prospective clinical and neuropathologic study. *Arch. Neurol.*, **49**, 1038–42.

Förstl, H., Burns, A., Luthert, P., Cairns, N. & Levy, R. (1993). The Lewy-body variant of Alzheimer's disease: Clinical and pathological findings. *Br. J. Psychiatry*, **162**, 385–92.

Galasko, D., Saitch, T., Xia, Y., Thal, L.J. et al. (1994). The apolipoprotein E allele ε4 is over-represented in patients with the Lewy body variant of Alzheimer's disease. *Neurology*, **44**, 1950–1.

Gibb, W.R.G., Esiri, M.M. & Lees, A.J. (1985). Clinical and pathological features of diffuse cortical Lewy body disease (Lewy body dementia). *Brain*, **110**, 1131–53.

Gibb, W.R.G., Mountjoy, C.Q., Mann, D.M.A. & Lees, A.J. (1989). A pathological study of the association between Lewy body disease and Alzheimer's disease. *J. Neurol., Neurosurg. Psychiatry*, **52**, 701–8.

Hansen, L.A., Masliah, E., Terry, R.D. & Mirra, S.S. (1989). A neuropathological subset of Alzheimer's disease with concomitant Lewy body disease and spongiform change. *Acta Neuropathol.*, **78**, 194–201.

Hansen, L., Salmon, D., Galasko, D., Masliah, E. et al. (1990). The Lewy
    body variant of Alzheimer's disease: a clinical and pathologic entity.
    Neurology, **40**, 1–8.
Hughes, A.J., Daniel, S.E., Kilford, L. & Lees, A.J. (1992). Accuracy of clinical
    diagnosis of idiopathic Parkinson's disease: A clinico-pathological study of
    100 cases. *J. Neurol., Neurosurg. Psychiatry*, **55**, 181–4.
Khachaturian, Z. (1985). Diagnosis of Alzheimer's disease. *Arch. Neurol.*, **42**,
    1097–105.
Lippa, C.F., Smith, T.W. & Swearer, J.M. (1994). Alzheimer's disease and
    Lewy body disease: a comparative clinicopathological study. *Ann. Neurol.*,
    35, 1, 81–8.
McKeith, I. G., Perry, R.H., Fairbairn, A.F., Jabeen, S. & Perry, E.K. (1992).
    Operational criteria for senile dementia of Lewy body type (SDLT).
    Psychol. Med., **22**, 911–22.
McKhann, G., Drachmann, D., Folstein, M., Katzman, R., Pryce, D. &
    Stadlan, E. (1984). Clinical diagnosis of Alzheimer's disease: Report of the
    NINCDS/ADRDA workgroup. *Neurology*, **34**, 939–44.
Pickering-Brown, S.M., Mann, D.M.A., Bourke, J.P. et al. (1994).
    Apolipoprotein E4 and Alzheimer's disease pathology in Lewy body
    disease and in other β-amyloid-forming diseases. *Lancet*, **343**, 1155.

5

The nature of the cognitive decline in Lewy body dementia

E.J. BYRNE

Summary

That cognitive decline is a feature of LBD is not disputed. The dispute arises about the type of cognitive decline, whether it has characteristic features that distinguish it from other forms of dementia, its severity and its course. Early case reports include descriptions of a variability of cognition, usually of arousal, in LBD confirmed by larger retrospective clinico-pathological series. Fluctuation in cognitive state either in the form of episodic confusional states resembling delirium or transient periods of reduced or loss of consciousness, superimposed on a background variability is described in 80% of patients in some series. This fluctuation of cognition may be less marked in those LBD cases who most resemble AD.

Some suggest that cognitive abnormality in LBD is milder at onset, and has characteristic features (especially deficits of attention). Others do not confirm these observations. The course of the cognitive decline is variable, a few cases have a rapid onset and decline, the mean durations of illness in most series are between five and seven years. EEG findings, which resemble those of experimental delirium, and neurochemistry in LBD suggest the most likely candidate for the variability in cognition in AD is the relative involvement of the cholinergic and dopaminergic systems. The contribution of cortical Lewy bodies themselves to the cognitive decline is as yet unknown.

Much of the controversy about Lewy body dementia (LBD) arises from the relatively small database and disparity of samples. The same consideration applies to a discussion of cognitive decline in LBD. From the first case reports (Okazaki et al., 1961) dementia has been described in the majority of cases. The dispute arises about the type of cognitive decline, whether it has characteristic features that distinguish it from other forms of dementia, its severity and its course.

5.1 A different dementia?

The earliest reports of LBD (reviewed by Kosaka et al., 1984 and Gibb et al., 1987) make reference to the severity of cognitive change in LBD, sometimes in a semi-quantitative form. Specific profiles of cognitive dysfunction are not described, although an indication of initial symptomatology is usually given. The majority of these early cases presented with dementia, with or without parkinsonism symptoms. It is of interest that all but one of these first cases was 70 years or less at the onset of symptoms. Series of case reports in the 1970s and 1980s gave more detail of the cognitive changes. All describe some patients with transient or episodic confusional states, usually early in the course of illness (Forno et al., 1978; Ikeda et al., 1978; Clark et al., 1986; Gibb et al., 1987; Burkhardt et al., 1988).

Some of these reports also suggest a variability in cognition, usually of arousal, as a continuous feature of LBD, typical comments included 'his level of alertness and agitation fluctuated wildly' (Burkhardt et al. – Case 4), 'At times she sat with her eyes closed and was apparently difficult to rouse, on other occasions she was affable and responded to commands' (Gibb et al., 1987).

5.2 Fluctuation in cognition

The Nottingham (Byrne et al., 1989) and Newcastle (Perry et al., 1990a) series found fluctuation in cognitive states in 80% and 86% respectively, both groups suggesting that this was a characteristic feature of LBD. Both groups comment on the frequent and early episodes of confusional state which resemble delirium but for which no apparent cause was found. That they are truly idiopathic is supported by the observation that they occurred in drug naive patients (Byrne et al., 1989). The duration of the episodic confusional states is not given in any reports. That idiopathic clouding of consciousness (ICC) is a distinguishing feature of LBD is also suggested by the findings of Ballard et al. (1993). In this study, 16 out of of 58 patients assessed for dementia in a day hospital had ICC, 14 of these (87.50%) fulfilled one set of diagnostic criteria for LBD (McKeith et al., 1992). McKeith et al. (1992) also describe 'transient periods of reduced or entire loss of consciousness'. These episodes were short lived (few minutes) usually recovering to the previous state and seemed unconnected to the use of neuroleptics or other psychotropics and were often diagnosed as transient ischaemic attacks. The misdiagnosis of LBD as vascular dementia is not infrequent (Byrne et al., 1987; McKeith et al., 1994).

In clinically diagnosed patients (using Byrne et al., 1991 criteria) the background variability in cognitive state has been longitudinally observed by Williams et al. (1993). Prior to commencing an open treatment trial of levodopa, measurements of cognitive function were performed over a period of weeks. Only one of the five cases showed no variability in cognitive test scores using the Mini-Mental State Examination (MMSE) (Folstein et al., 1975), three showed variability between 3 to 5 points and one case had a 17 point variability. This variation could not be accounted for on the basis of a practice effect as the highest scores were not always at the end of the pretreatment observation period.

One recent study in which LBD was found in eight patients who had fulfilled the NINCDS–ADRDA criteria (McKhann et al., 1984) for Alzheimer's disease (AD), did not find fluctuation in cognitive state to be a feature and only one case had a florid confusional state (Förstl et al., 1993).

In a similar sample (NINCDS–ADRDA positive cases) Hansen et al. (1990) made no reference to fluctuation in cognitive state as a distinguishing feature of LBD. They did, however, compare LBD cases with age-matched AD cases on a variety of psychometric tests, and found that LBD cases had a more severe attention disorder (digit span) and were more impaired in some aspects of verbal fluency and visuospatial function. Other specific cognitive deficits have been examined by Sahgal et al. (1992) who found that clinically diagnosed patients (using McKeith et al., 1992 criteria) with LBD were more impaired in delayed visual recognition memory than patients with AD.

5.3 Severity of the cognitive change

The Japanese cases reviewed by Kosaka (1990) using a semi-quantitative measure of dementia severity fall in to two groups; the 'common' form of LBD in which memory disturbance is a prominent early symptom and is associated with less prominent parkinsonism and a late age of onset and death; and the 'pure' form in which parkinsonism is the prominent presenting symptom with memory impairment developing in most cases later in the course. An overall assessment of dementia severity is given by the authors. Omitting cases where there is a question mark beside the rating (two in the common form and one in the pure form) gives a mean rating of 2.77 for the common group and 2.4 for the pure group (0 = no dementia, 3 + = severe dementia).

Lennox et al. (1989) used a similar semi-quantitative measure of dementia severity (the five point scale of Strub & Black (1981)). In 15 pathologically confirmed cases of LBD dementia, severity was mild in one case, moderate in one case, severe in six cases and very severe in seven cases. The least cognitively impaired individuals in this study both presented with parkinsonism.

Others have suggested that at presentation (i.e. the initial assessment) the dementia of LBD is less severe than that of Alzheimer's disease (AD). Perry et al. (1990a) compared initial Mental Test Scores (MTS) (Blessed et al., 1968) in 14 cases of LBD and 14 cases of AD (autopsy confirmed) who were matched for age. They found the LBD cases had significantly higher MTS scores than the AD cases. Crystal et al. (1990) data suggests a similar trend but from a very small number. Three cases of 'pure' LBD had a mean (initial assessment) cognitive test score (Blessed et al., 1968) of 11, compared with a mean of 22 for three 'common' LBD cases and 19.6 for three AD cases. Förstl et al. (1993) and Galasko et al. (1994), however, found no difference between pathologically diagnosed LBD and AD cases in their initial cognitive test scores, using the CAMCOG (the cognitive assessment scale from the CAMDEX) (Roth et al., 1986) and the Mini-Mental State Examination (MMSE) (Folstein et al., 1975) respectively.

5.4 Course of the cognitive decline

A summary of the age of onset (or death) and duration of disease, in pathologically confirmed cases of LBD, is given in Table 5.1. The majority of these mean durations are between 5 and 7 years.

There is a great variability in the mode of onset of LBD (see above) but within that variability there may be a trend towards an inverse relationship between age of onset and cognitive change as an initial symptom. This may be because young LBD cases are more likely to have the 'pure' form. Prospective studies need to evaluate this further.

Cognitive change in LBD may also be related to the severity of the cholinergic deficit and the presence or absence of hallucinations. Perry et al. (1990a) found that in pathologically confirmed cases of LBD, those with hallucinations tended to have a greater rate of cognitive decline than

Table 5.1. *Duration of illness in LBD: data from pathologically confirmed cases*

Study	n	Mean age of onset (years) (range)	Mean age at death (years) (range)	Mean duration of illness (years) (range)
Sima et al. (1986)	3	–	71.6 (71–72)	5.75 (1.25–10)
Gibb et al. (1987)	4	46.5 (27–70)	–	4.25 (3–5.5)
Burkhardt[*]et al. (1988)	3	68.6 (65–71)	–	4.6 (4–5)
Lennox et al. (1989)	15	72 (58–83)	–	5.5 (2–19)
Kosaka et al. (1990)	37			
Pure = 9		32.8 (12–64)	41.6 (15–69)	8.7 (2.5–14)
Common = 28		69.2 (55–87)	75.6 (59–87)	6.4 (1.5–24)
Perry et al. (1990a)	18	–	81 (–)	5.6 (–)
Crystal et al. (1990)				
Pure = 3		74.6 (67–80)	79.3 (72–85)	4.6 (4–5)
Common = 3		72.6 (66–78)	83.3 (78–88)	10 (6–12)
Förstl et al. (1993)	8	73.3 (65–92)	–	6.6 (<1–13)
Galasko et al. (1994)	38	71 (–)	–	7.5 (–)
Lippa et al. (1994)				
Pure = 5		70 (–)	76 (61–84)	5 (0–10)
Common = 7		70 (–)	77 (56–88)	6 (4–10)

[*]Incomplete data on one patient

those without hallucinations, although this did not reach statistical significance. The hallucinators did have statistically significantly lower levels of choline acetyl transferase levels in the cortex than nonhallucinators.

In many cases the symptoms of LBD, including cognitive change, mimic those of AD, as may its course (Philpot et al., 1986; Hansen et al., 1990; Förstl et al., 1993). In such cases current diagnostic criteria have low sensitivity (Byrne, 1995).

There is some evidence for a 'subset' of LBD cases with very rapid onset of symptoms and relatively rapid courses (total duration of illness three years or less). Hansen et al. (1989) describe one such case amongst five LBD cases with spongiform change in the neuropil, none of whom showed evidence of prion proteins. Other rapidly progressive cases have been described (Sima et al., 1986; Burkhardt et al., 1988; Byrne et al., 1989) most of whom share the neuropathological features of the 'subset' described by Hansen et al. (1989).

5.5 Electrophysiological correlates of cognitive change

Crystal et al. (1990) suggest that electroencephalographic (EEG) changes occur early in the course of LBD, and together with clinical features may help in diagnosis. They describe frontal bursts of slow wave activity on a generally slow recording. Other groups have reported similar findings (Gibb et al., 1987; Burkhardt et al., 1988; Yamamoto & Imai, 1988; Byrne et al., 1989). Whilst these abnormalities are non-specific they are similar to findings in late AD and also in delirium. The EEG may prove to be a useful and widely available tool for further study of cognitive changes in LBD. Quantitative EEG (QEEG) or brain electrical activity mapping (BEAM) may be even more helpful, particularly in longitudinal assessment and in comparisons with other forms of dementia and delirium.

5.6 Cortical or chemical basis for cognitive decline?

There is conflicting data on the relationship between cortical Lewy bodies (CLB) and cognitive decline in LBD (Gibb & Luthert, 1994). One study found a significant relationship between numbers of CLB and the severity of cognitive impairment (Lennox et al., 1989). Most groups comment on the occurrence of coexisting Alzheimer pathology (plaques and tangles) in varying degrees in the majority of cases of LBD.

The topographical distribution of CLB reported by many groups is consistent. They are found in layers 5 and 6 of the cerebral cortex, in frontal, temporal, and parietal cortex, and in the insula. Anterior cingulate cortex is often most severely affected (Forno, 1969; Yoshimura, 1983; Sima et al., 1986; Gibb et al., 1987; Lennox et al., 1989). Sima et al. (1986) suggest that this distribution 'correlates well with the proposed mesocortical dopaminergic projections to the cerebral cortex'.

Confusional states may arise from other pathologies in these areas. Several groups report either acute florid delirium or chronic confusional states arising from strokes in the territory of the right middle cerebral artery (Mullaly et al., 1982; Schmidley & Messing, 1984; Mori & Yamadouri, 1987). It is therefore possible that the *site* of the lesions in LBD is related to the nature of cognitive change. It is likely, however, that more diffuse mechanisms are involved. The most likely candidate on the basis of the published data is the relative involvement of the cholinergic and dopaminergic systems in LBD. The cholinergic system is more severely depleted in LBD than in AD (Dickson et al., 1987; Perry et al., 1990b) and correlates with the degree of cognitive impairment (Perry et al., 1990b).

Furthermore Perry et al. (1990b) suggest that the relative levels of ChAT and dopamine are important in the genesis of noncognitive features in LBD – hallucinators having significantly lower ChAT levels than nonhallucinators and nonhallucinating PD cases with equally low ChAT levels having lower dopamine levels than LBD cases.

These findings are strikingly echoed in the work on experimental delirium correlating EEG findings with various anticholinergic agents (Lipowski, 1990). For example Ital and Fink (1966) observed the behavioural and EEG changes at different dose levels of Ditran, a synthetic anticholinergic agent. At low doses, slight changes in attention and consciousness were observed together with increased slow wave activity on the EEG. Fluctuation of awareness, increased slow wave activity and reduction of alpha activity wave were seen with high doses of Ditran. In some cases, at an intermediate dose, stupor occurred. Dopamine blockade (using chlorpromazine) restored both the mental state and the EEG towards normality. Lipowski's extensive review (Lipowski, 1990) includes other fascinating observations from this experimental work, including those that even the most severely delirious subjects have lucid intervals, and that Ditran in particular (but also other anticholinergic agents) reduces REM sleep. Sleep disturbance in LBD has not been extensively studied. Clinical observations on my own patients currently being studied suggests that disturbance of the sleep–wake cycle is common during the episodic confusional states. The vivid psychotic phenomena are often worse at night and patients frequently report feeling as if they were 'having a dream' during the day, or report an increase in dreaming at night. Lipowski (1990) concludes that this experimental work suggests 'an imbalance of central cholinergic and adrenergic neurotransmitters . . . represented a major pathogenic mechanism in delirium'.

5.7 Conclusion

The nature of the cognitive decline in LBD is still not fully elucidated. In some cases cognitive change analogous to delirium is observed, in others the cognitive profile may more closely resemble that of AD, possibly with differences in specific cognitive functions. The course of the decline is likewise variable. Definitive clinico-pathological correlations await the collection of large prospective data sets. The electro-physiological correlates of the cognitive changes in LBD offers a fruitful area for future research.

References

Ballard, C.G., Mohan, R.N.C., Patel, A. et al. (1993). Idiopathic clouding of consciousness – do the patients have cortical Lewy body disease? *Int. J. Geriatr. Psychiatry*, **9**, 571–6.

Blessed, G., Tomlinson, B.E. & Roth, M. (1968). The association between quantitative measures of dementia and senile change in the cerebral grey matter of elderly subjects. *Br. J. Psychiatry*, **114**, 797–811.

Burkhardt, C.R., Filley, C.M., Kleinschmidt-DeMasters, B.K., de la Monte, S., Norenberg, M.D. & Schneck, S.A. (1988). Diffuse Lewy body disease and progressive dementia. *Neurology*, **38**, 1520–8.

Byrne, E.J. (1995). Cortical Lewy body disease: an alternative view. In *Developments in Dementia and Functional Disorders in the Elderly*. ed. R. Levy & R. Howard, pp. 21–30. Petersfield, UK: Wrightson.

Byrne, E.J., Lowe, J. & Godwin-Austen, R.B., Arie, T. & Jones, R. (1987). Dementia and Parkinson's disease associated with diffuse cortical Lewy bodies. *Lancet*, **i**, 57.

Byrne, E.J., Lennox, G., Lowe, J. & Godwin-Austen, R.B. (1989). Diffuse Lewy body disease: clinical features in 15 cases. *J. Neurol. Neurosurg. Psychiatry*, **52**, 709–17.

Byrne, E.J., Lennox, G., Lowe, J., Godwin-Austen, R.B., Jefferson, D., Mayer, R.J., Landon, M. & Doherty, F.J. (Nottingham Group of the Study of Neurodegenerative Disorders) (1991). Diagnostic criteria for dementia associated with cortical Lewy bodies. *Dementia*, **2**, 283–4.

Clark, B., Whitehouse, P.J., Lehmann, J. & Coyle, J.T. (1986). Primary degenerative dementia without Alzheimer pathology. *Can. J. Neurol. Sci.*, **13**, 462–70.

Crystal, H.A., Dickson, D.W., Lizardi, J.E., Davies, P. & Wolfson, L.I. (1990). Antemortem diagnosis of diffuse Lewy body disease. *Neurology*, **40**, 1523–8.

Dickson, D.A., Davies, P., Mayeux, R. et al. (1987). Diffuse Lewy body disease. Neuropathological and biochemical studies of six cases. *Acta Neuropathol. (Berl.)*, **75**, 8–15.

Folstein, M.R., Folstein, S.E. & McHugh, P.Z. (1975). Mini-Mental State: A practical method for grading the cognitive state of patients for the clinician. *J. Psychiatric Res.*, **12**, 189–98.

Forno, L.A. (1969). Concentric hyalin intraneuronal inclusions of Lewy type in the brains of elderly persons (50 incidental cases). Relationship to Parkinsonism. *J. Am. Geriatr. Soc.*, **17**, 557–75.

Forno, L.A., Barbour, P.J. & Norville, R.L. (1978). Presenile dementia with Lewy bodies and neurofibrillary tangles. *Arch. Neurol.,* **35**, 818–22.

Förstl, H., Burns, A., Luthert, P., Cairns, N. & Levy, R. (1993). The Lewy body variant of Alzheimer's disease – clinical and neuropathological findings. *Br. J. Psychiatry,* **162**, 385–92.

Galasko, D., Hansen, L.A., Katzman, R. et al. (1994). Clinical-neuropathological correlations in Alzheimer's disease and related dementias. *Arch. Neurol.,* **51**, 88–95.

Gibb, W.R.G. & Luthert, P.J. (1994). Dementia in Parkinson's disease and Lewy body disease. In *Dementia,* ed. A. Burns & R. Levy, pp. 719–37. London: Chapman & Hall.

Gibb, W.R.G., Esiri, M.M. & Lees, A.J. (1987). Clinical and pathological features of diffuse cortical Lewy body disease (Lewy body dementia). *Brain,* **110**, 1131–53.

Hansen, L.A., Masliah, E., Terry, R.D. et al. (1989). A neuropathological subset of Alzheimer's disease with concomitant Lewy body disease and spongiform change. *Acta Neuropathol. (Berl.),* **78**, 194–201.

Hansen, L., Salmon, D., Galasko, D. et al. (1990). The Lewy body variant of Alzheimer's disease: a clinical pathological entity. *Neurology,* **40**, 108.

Ikeda, K., Ikeda, S., Yoshimura, T., Kato, H. & Namba, M. (1978). Idiopathic parkinsonism with Lewy-type inclusions in cerebral cortex. A case report. *Acta Neuropathol. (Berl.),* **41**, 165–8.

Ital, T. & Fink, M. (1966). Anticholinergic drug-induced delirium: experimental modification, quantitative EEG and behavioural correlations. *J. Nerv. Ment. Dis.,* **143**, 492–507.

Kosaka, K. (1990). Diffuse Lewy body disease in Japan. *J. Neurol,* **237**, 197–204.

Kosaka, K., Yoshimura, M., Ikeda, K. & Budha, H. (1984). Diffuse type of Lewy body disease: progressive dementia with abundant cortical Lewy bodies and senile changes of varying degree – a new disease? *J. Neurol. Neurosurg. Psychiatry,* **3**, 185–92.

Lennox, G., Lowe, J., Landon, M., Byrne, E.J., Mayer, R.J. & Godwin-Austen, R.B. (1989). Diffuse Lewy body disease, correlative neuropathology using anti-ubiquitin immunocytochemistry. *J. Neurol. Neurosurg. Psychiatry,* **52**, 1236–47.

Lipowski, Z.J. (1990). *Delirium: Acute Confusional States,* pp. 141–69. Oxford: Oxford University Press.

Lippa, C.F., Smith, T.W. & Swearer, J.M. (1994). Alzheimer's disease and Lewy body disease. A comparative clinicopathological study. *Ann. Neurol.,* **35**, 81–8.

McKeith, I.G., Perry, R.H., Fairbairn, A.F., Jabeen, S. & Perry, E.K. (1992). Operational criteria for senile dementia of Lewy body type (SDLT). *Psychol. Med.,* **22**, 911–22.

McKeith, I.G., Fairbairn, A.F., Perry, R. & Thompson, P. (1994). The clinical diagnosis and misdiagnosis of senile dementia of Lewy body type (SDLT) – do the diagnostic systems for dementia need to be revised? *Br. J. Psychiatry,* **165**, 324–332.

McKhann, G., Drachman, D., Folstein, M., Katzman, R., Price, D. & Stadlan, E.M. (1984). Clinical diagnosis of Alzheimer's disease: report of the NINCDS–ADRDA work group under the auspices of Department of Health and Human Service Task Force on Alzheimer's disease. *Neurology,* **34**, 939–44.

Mori, E. & Yamadouri, A. (1987). Acute confusional state and acute agitated delirium. *Arch. Neurol.,* **44**, 1139–43.

Mullaly, W., Huff, K., Ranthol, M. et al. (1982). Frequency of acute confusional states in patients with lesions in the right hemisphere. *Arch. Neurol.,* **12**, 113.

Okazaki, H., Lipkin, L.E. & Aronson, S.M. (1961). Diffuse intracytoplasmic ganglionic inclusions (Lewy type) associated with progressive dementia and quadriparesis in flexion. *J. Neuropathol. Exp. Neurol.,* **20**, 237–44.

Perry, R.H., Irving, D., Blessed, G., Perry, E.K. & Fairbairn, A.F. (1990a). Senile dementia of Lewy body type. A clinically and neuropathologically distinct type of Lewy body dementia in the elderly. *J. Neurol. Sci.,* **95**, 119–39.

Perry, E.K., Marshall, E., Perry, R.H. et al. (1990b). Cholinergic and dopaminergic activities in senile dementia of the Lewy body type. *Alzheimer Dis. Assoc. Disord.,* **4**, 87–95.

Philpot, M., Colgan, J., Janota, I. & Levy, R. (1986). Dementia without Alzheimer pathology. *Neurology,* **36**, 133.

Roth, M., Tym, E., Mountjoy, C. et al. (1986). CAMDEX: a standardised instrument for the diagnosis of mental disorder in the elderly with special reference to the early detection of dementia. *Br. J. Psychiatry,* **149**, 698–709.

Sahgal, A., Galloway, P.H., McKeith, I.G. et al. (1992). Matching-to-sample deficits in patients with senile dementias of the Alzheimer and Lewy body types. *Arch. Neurol.,* **49**, 1043–6.

Schmidley, N.W. & Messing, R.O. (1984). Acute confusional states in patients with right hemisphere infarctions. *Stroke,* **15**, 883–5.

Sima, A.A.F., Clark, A.W., Stemberger, N.A. & Stemberger, L.A. (1986). Lewy body dementia without Alzheimer changes. *Can. J. Neurol. Sci.,* **13**, 490–7.

Strub, R.K. & Black, F.W. (1981). *Organic Brain Syndromes*, pp. 119–164. Philadelphia: F.A Davies,.

Williams, S.W., Byrne, E.J. & Stokes, P. (1993). The treatment of diffuse Lewy body disease: a pilot study of five cases. *Int. J. Geriatr. Psychiatry,* **8**, 731–5.

Yamamoto, T. & Imai, T. (1988). A case of diffuse Lewy body and Alzheimer's disease with periodic synchronous discharges. *J. Neuropathol. Exp. Neurol.,* **47**, 536–48.

Yoshimura, M. (1983). Cortical changes in the Parkinsonian brain: a contribution to the delineation of 'diffuse Lewy body disease'. *J. Neurol.,* **229**, 17–32.

6

Noncognitive symptoms in Lewy body dementia

C. BALLARD, K. LOWERY, R. HARRISON
and I.G. McKEITH

Summary

Information regarding non-cognitive symptoms in patients with senile dementia of Lewy body type (SDLT) was abstracted from a number of sources including postmortem, clinical and prospective studies. Psychotic symptoms occur in more than 80% of patients with SDLT. Visual hallucinations are especially common. Visual hallucinations, auditory hallucinations and delusional misidentification occur significantly more often in SDLT than Alzheimer's disease. Major depression occurs in 15% of patients with SDLT and Alzheimer's disease. Falls are common in SDLT occurring in 50% or more of patients, but not all studies find them to be significantly more common in SDLT than Alzheimer's disease. Little is known about the association of psychotic symptoms, depression or falls in SDLT and no effective treatment strategies are established.

Other important symptoms such as anxiety, aggression, wandering and inappropriate sexual activity have not been systematically studied.

6.1 Introduction

It is necessary to set the scene by considering the prevalence rates and the importance of noncognitive features in patients with Alzheimer's disease as there is only rudimentary information available concerning these symptoms in Lewy body dementia (LBD). Fifteen to 30% of patients with Alzheimer's disease in contact with clinical services suffer from concurrent depression and the prevalence rate of psychotic symptoms in clinical samples exceeds 60%. Psychotic symptoms cause distress to carers and to the patients themselves. They reduce the likelihood of

67

people continuing to live in their own homes (Steele et al., 1990), are associated with increased family discord and there is accumulating evidence to suggest that the presence of psychotic symptoms predicts a more rapid rate of cognitive decline (Rosen & Zubenko, 1991). Depression is also distressing for carers and patients themselves, as well as causing excess disability by further impairing cognitive function and instrumental activities of daily living. Life expectancy is reduced in dementia patients with concurrent depression (Burns, 1991).

Other noncognitive symptoms have received less attention. Wandering has been described in 25% to 63% of dementia suffers in contact with clinical services (Burns et al., 1990). Wandering too is perceived to be stressful by carers (Rabins et al., 1982) and is associated with an increased risk of falls (Buchner & Larson, 1987). Violent behaviour has been reported amongst 20% of dementia sufferers in contact with clinical services (Burns et al., 1990). Violence is poorly tolerated by carers and frequently results in admission to residential or nursing home care (Burns et al., 1990).

It is likely that noncognitive symptoms are important in patients with LBD for many of the same reasons. Certain symptoms assume an even greater importance in LBD as they may help discriminate between LBD and other dementias. Visual hallucinations, auditory hallucinations and frequent falls are included in the McKeith et al. (1992a) criteria for senile dementia of Lewy body type (SDLT).

Published data pertaining to noncognitive symptoms in LBD comes from several main sources. Between the early 1960s and the mid-1980s a number of single cases and small case series were described. The cases were initially identified by postmortem examination and clinical histories determined from case note review. Single cases are subject to a number of publishing biases and only series containing three or more patients are described in this chapter. In the late 1980s and early 1990s, several larger case series were described. Again the patients were first identified at postmortem examination and the clinical history obtained from case notes. Although these were extremely important studies, the retrospective design is likely to have underestimated noncognitive symptoms. More recently several clinical studies have been reported. These have the advantage of more detailed clinical assessments but are disadvantaged by the absence of neuropathological diagnosis. Some of these studies, such as Ballard et al. (1993), did not make use of schedules specifically designed to measure noncognitive symptoms in dementia sufferers and may still have underestimated the prevalence rates of some symptoms.

Information is also presented about two as yet unpublished pieces of work. Galasko et al., reported in more detail in Chapter 2, describe a research sample of 44 LBD patients in contact with a neurology service who were prospectively assessed using the Diagnostic Interview Schedule (DIS) for the DSM-IIIR. Diagnosis was made at postmortem. Although the DIS is a psychiatric interview, it was not designed to evaluate psychiatric symptoms in dementia sufferers and may again have underestimated prevalence rates.

Finally, there is a prospective study of SDLT in progress in Newcastle upon Tyne, funded by the UK Medical Research Council. The study involves a detailed assessment of noncognitive symptoms using a standardized schedule designed specifically for use in dementia patients and their carers. The assessment of psychotic symptoms is based upon the definitions of Burns et al. (1990). Symptoms also have to occur on two occasions more than one week apart (Ballard, 1995). Depression is diagnosed according to DSM-IIIR criteria. Falls are also assessed according to standardized criteria. The study will provide neuropathological diagnosis, although these data are not yet available. Preliminary data pertaining to the first 73 subjects clinically assessed are presented here for the first time.

A number of diagnostic issues could potentially confound comparisons between different studies. Several neuropathological categorizations of Lewy body disease have been proposed. One method has been to segregate Lewy body disease into diffuse cortical Lewy bodies, transitional Lewy body disease (with Lewy bodies mainly in the brainstem but with some evident in the cortex) and brainstem only Lewy body disease. In practice, all of the patients with diffuse cortical Lewy bodies and half of the transitional cases but none of the brainstem cases have dementia. Patients with dementia in this classification are therefore similar to patients diagnosed neuropathologically to have LBD in other studies. A further classification has been proposed to segregate patients with Lewy bodies alone, from those who have Lewy bodies together with senile plaques and neurofibrillary tangles (Chapter 2). Only very limited information is available regarding the pure type and it is too early to judge whether this is a useful distinction.

Clinically, two major sets of diagnostic criteria have been proposed. McKeith et al. (1992a) proposed criteria for senile dementia of Lewy body type (SDLT) and Byrne et al. (1991) proposed criteria for dementia associated with cortical Lewy bodies (DLB). The McKeith et al. (1992a) criteria, but not the Byrne et al. (1991) criteria, place an emphasis on noncognitive symptoms, including visual hallucinations, auditory hallu-cinations and falls. As a result, the use of different diagnostic criteria for entry into clinical studies, could influence the prevalence rates of some categories of noncognitive symptoms.

The data pertaining to psychotic symptoms, mood disorders, wander-ing, falls and aggression will be presented in separate sections for each of the respective categories of symptom.

6.2 Psychotic symptoms

6.2.1 Visual hallucinations

Fifty-six patients with LBD have been described in 10 small postmortem series, each including between 3 and 10 patients. These are shown in Table 6.1. Nine (16.1%) patients experienced visual hallucinations. Four larger series including 10 or more patients have also been reported (McKeith et al., 1992a, 1994; Byrne et al., 1989 and Chapter 2).

The prevalence rates of visual hallucinations have varied from 13.3% (Byrne et al., 1989) to 80% (McKeith et al., 1994). Lower prevalence rates were found in neurological samples (27.1%) than psychiatric sam-ples (63.4%). Galasko et al. (Chapter 2) divided their patients into pure LBD and LBD associated with Alzheimer type changes. Unfortunately there were only six patients in the latter category which precluded any meaningful comparisons. Galasko and his colleagues (Chapter 2) and McKeith et al. (1992a, 1994) both found visual hallucinations to be sig-nificantly more common in LBD than Alzheimer's disease.

Ballard et al. (1993) described a clinical sample of dementia sufferers in contact with a psychiatric day hospital. Sixteen patients suffered from SDLT, diagnosed according to the Newcastle criteria, of whom four had visual hallucinations (25%). Visual hallucinations were again sig-nificantly more common in SDLT than Alzheimer's disease. Ballard (1995) reported a further series of 12 patients with SDLT in contact with psychiatric services of whom 10 (83.3%) had experienced visual hallucinations in the month prior to the assessment. A standardized interview schedule, the Burn's Symptom Check List, was used to iden-tify psychotic symptoms. Again, patients with SDLT were significantly more likely to harbour these symptoms than patients with Alzheimer's disease. The study also examined some of the symptom characteristics, finding that patients with SDLT experienced hallucinatory episodes sig-nificantly more often than patients with Alzheimer's disease and their

Table 6.1. *Postmortem studies of Lewy body dementia including 3–10 patients*

Authors	Number of subjects
Hughes et al. (1993)	8
Burkhardt et al. (1988)	3
Woodard (1962)	6
Gibb et al. (1989)	4
Gibb, Esiri & Lees (1985)	7
Hansen et al. (1990)	9
Förstl et al. (1993)	8
Kuzuhara & Yoshimira (1993)	8
Sima et al. (1986)	3

hallucinations were significantly more likely to persist during one year of follow-up.

Data are available from the first 73 patients enrolled in the Newcastle prospective study of SDLT. The cohort includes 42 patients with SDLT, of whom 24 are female and 18 male. The mean age of patients at the time of first assessment was 73.6 and the mean Mini-Mental State Examination score was 14.9. A further 30 patients had Alzheimer's disease and one patient was excluded because of diagnostic uncertainty. During the course of the illness up to the time of assessment, 39 (92.9%) had experienced at least one type of visual hallucination (Table 6.2), and 22 (56.4%) experienced two or more. The most common themes were people, animals, objects, children and insects. Individual patients experienced visual hallucinations of fire and birds. Forty-six percent of patients with visual hallucinations of people had accompanying phantom border delusions. Visual hallucinations were of complete forms in 87% of individuals, 76% saw their hallucinations move and 51% heard their hallucinations speak or make a noise. Hallucinations were detailed in 89% of cases and 84% were of normal size. Four patients had Lilliputian visual hallucinations and one patient saw an enlarged figure. A further patient saw small and normal size images concurrently. Twenty per cent of patients saw their hallucinations predominantly in the afternoon or evening whereas 20% saw them predominantly at night. No diurnal pattern was evident in two-thirds of the patients. Visual hallucinations were found to be highly persistent amongst 44% of these patients. Again, compared with patients having Alzheimer's disease, patients with SDLT were significantly more likely to experience visual hallucinations. The themes of the visual hallucinations were, however, very similar to the

Table 6.2. *The prevalence rate of noncognitive symptoms in patients with SDLT from the Newcastle prospective study*

	Number of people with each symptom
Visual hallucinations	39 (92.9%)
Delusions	25 (59.5%)
Delusional misidentification	14 (33.3%)
DSM IIIR major depression	5 (11.9%)
DSM IIIR dysthymia	3 (7.1%)
Frequent falls	21 (50%)

themes experienced by patients with Alzheimer's disease, mirroring the findings of Ballard (1995). The characteristics of the visual hallucinations were generally similar in the two dementias, although all visual hallucinations in patients with Alzheimer's disease were mute (Fisher's exact test $p = 0.007$). There was no significant association between visual hallucinations and taking anticholinergic or anti-parkinsonian drugs in patients with SDLT. All 14 patients with concurrent visual impairment experienced visual hallucinations but in view of the high prevalence rate of visual hallucinations in patients with SDLT, a much larger sample would be needed to determine whether a significant association exists. Patients with visual impairment were significantly more likely to experience vague as opposed to detailed images (Fisher's exact test $p = 0.007$). Thirty-five patients fulfilled the Byrne et al. (1991) criteria for DLB, 31 (88.6%) of whom had visual hallucinations. Differences in diagnostic criteria per se do not account for dramatic differences in the prevalence rates of these symptoms.

Summarizing, patients with LBD in contact with psychiatric services have a prevalence rate of visual hallucinations in excess of 80%. The prevalence rate may be lower amongst patients in contact with neurology services, although these patients have not been assessed with an instrument specifically designed to evaluate psychotic symptoms in dementia sufferers. Patients with LBD are significantly more likely to experience visual hallucinations than patients with Alzheimer's disease. They also experience the hallucinations more frequently and the hallucinations are more likely to be persistent.

Charles Bonnet described the case of his grandfather Charles Lullin, who at the age of 78 experienced highly organized visions of men, women, birds and complex scenes following cataract surgery. He saw a mixture of normal size and small images which could be differentiated from real images. These themes are said to be typical of the Charles Bonnet syndrome and are similar to the themes of visual hallucinations in SDLT. Howard and Levy (1994) described a recent series of 18 cases fulfilling the criteria for the Charles Bonnet syndrome. Fifty per cent of the visions were accompanied by auditory hallucinations and two thirds were of normal size. Beck and Harris (1994) summarized 117 case reports of visual hallucinations in the elderly. The images seen tended to be detailed and complete, except when vascular lesions were identified. In these patients the images were often bizarre and distorted. The characteristics of visual hallucinations in the elderly without dementia (excluding hallucinations related to vascular lesions), are hence similar to those seen in LBD. Beck and Harris (1994) also found that visual hallucinations may occur in specific visual fields and may disappear when the eyes are closed. These characteristics are often very difficult to examine in dementia sufferers.

Visual hallucinations are reported as common in patients with Parkinson's disease (Cummings, 1992). Generally these symptoms are attributed to the effects of anti-parkinsonian drugs, although this is unproven. Visual hallucinations might be more common amongst parkinsonian patients with concurrent dementia (Cummings, 1992). The most common themes are people and animals. Three quarters are nonthreatening, a third are experienced with concurrent auditory hallucinations and the majority occur at night (Cummings, 1992). The reported prevalence rates of visual hallucinations in patients with Parkinson's disease vary enormously (Cummings, 1992) and have not been reported for parkinsonian patients with dementia. The themes and characteristics of visual hallucinations are again similar to those seen in patients with SDLT, although the diurnal pattern may be different.

6.2.2 *Delusions*

Delusions were identified in 7 out of 56 (12.5%) cases from small post-mortem series. In the larger neuropathological studies, the prevalence rate of delusions varied from 20% (Byrne et al., 1989) to 80% (McKeith et al., 1994). The trend was once more for higher rates to be reported in samples from psychiatric services, with 68.3% of psychiatric patients and 39.0% of neurology patients experiencing delusions. McKeith et al. (1992a, 1994) found delusions to be more common in patients with LBD than amongst patients with Alzheimer's disease, although this finding was not supported by either Galasko et al. (Chapter 2) or Byrne et al. (1989).

In the clinical studies, Ballard et al. (1993) found 7 of 16 patients (43.8%) with SDLT to have delusions. They were significantly more common in SDLT than Alzheimer's disease. Ballard (1995) found 9 out of 12 (75%) patients with SDLT to experience delusions, although this was not significantly higher than the prevalence rate of delusions in patients with Alzheimer's disease. The most commonly described delusions were delusions of reference, persecutory delusions, delusions of theft and delusions of abandonment. These were similar to the type of delusions experienced by patients with other dementias. Six patients with delusions in the context of SDLT were followed up for one year. The beliefs were highly persistent in three patients but resolved within three months in the others. A similar pattern was seen in Alzheimer's disease. In the prospective Newcastle sample, delusions occurred in 25 out of 42 (59.5%) patients with SDLT (Table 6.2) and 21 of 35 (60.0%) of the patients with DLB. Patients with SDLT were significantly more likely to have delusions than patients with Alzheimer's disease. The most common individual symptoms were persecutory delusions, delusions of abandonment and delusions of unfaithfulness. Again they were similar in SDLT and Alzheimer's disease. There was a significant association between the presence of delusions and pharmacotherapy with levodopa. Levodopa is associated with delusions in patients with Parkinson's disease (Cummings, 1992), although the majority occur in the context of an acute confusional state. Dopamine excess is of course also central to the main explanatory hypothesis of functional psychosis.

Delusions are highly prevalent amongst patients with LBD, particularly amongst patients in contact with psychiatric services. The type of delusions experienced and their course appear to be similar to those seen in Alzheimer's disease but dissimilar to delusions in Parkinson's disease which are less complex and tend to be associated with acute confusional states. There is also little overlap with the types of delusions described in late paraphrenia where complex delusional systems involving delusions of partition and associated with auditory hallucinations, predominate. Although there is some evidence to suggest that delusions are more prevalent in LBD than Alzheimer's disease, the case is unproven, and delusions are probably not a good discriminator between the two conditions. The prevalence rate of delusions in clinical samples is similar amongst patients diagnosed according to the Newcastle SDLT and the Nottingham DLB criteria.

The neuropathological and neurochemical associations of delusions have not been studied in LBD. In patients with Alzheimer's disease, an association has been found between psychotic symptoms and the severity of the disease process in the prosubiculum. There is a need to explore hypotheses such as this in patients with LBD.

6.2.3 Other hallucinations

Auditory hallucinations were described in 6 out of 56 (10.7%) patients with LBD from small neuropathological series, 13 out 56 LBD patients in larger post-mortem series (26.8%) and 5 out of 12 (41.7%) SDLT patients in Ballard's (1995) clinical series. McKeith et al. (1992a, 1994) found auditory hallucinations to be significantly more common in patients with LBD than patients with Alzheimer's disease. Provisional data from the Newcastle prospective study suggests a prevalence of 57.1% (27/42) in patients with SDLT and 51.4% (18/35) in patients with DLB. Auditory hallucinations were persistent in a quarter of cases. The majority of auditory hallucinations were experienced concurrently with visual hallucinations and were perceived as the visual hallucinations talking or making a noise. Auditory hallucinations were significantly more common in SDLT than in Alzheimer's disease.

Auditory hallucinations have been generally less well studied than visual hallucinations and little comparative data are available. The type of hallucinations experienced is very different from late paraphrenia where they are rarely accompaniments of visual hallucinations. Auditory hallucinations are again highly prevalent in patients with LBD and probably have a greater frequency than they do in Alzheimer's disease.

Other forms of hallucinations have been poorly studied in LBD. The provisional data from the prospective Newcastle study suggests that olfactory hallucinations occur in 11.9% of patients. No tactile or gustatory hallucinations were identified.

6.2.4 Delusional misidentification

Burns et al. (1990) suggested that psychotic symptoms in dementia sufferers should be divided into three categories, hallucinations, delusions and delusional misidentification. The latter category includes the Capgras syndrome, the belief that images on television or in photographs occur in real space, the belief that one's mirror image is somebody else and delusional misidentification of one's house. Ballard (1995) confirmed this categorization with a principal components analysis. As the category of delusional misidentification has only recently been clarified, little data are available regarding these symptoms in LBD. Ballard (1995) found 6 out of 12 (50%) patients with SDLT to have one or more misidentification symptom and they occurred significantly more often in SDLT than in Alzheimer's disease. Fourteen (33.3%) cases of delusional misidentification were identified amongst patients with SDLT in the prospective Newcastle study (Table 6.2), the symptoms were transient in 85% of patients. Ten per cent of patients had the Capgras syndrome, television misidentification occurred in 19% of patients, delusional misidentification of a mirror image occurred in 9.5% of patients and delusional misidentification of one's house occurred in 2.4% of patients. Delusional misidentification was significantly more common in SDLT than Alzheimer's disease. Twenty-six per cent of patients with DLB had symptoms of delusional misidentification.

6.2.5 *Psychotic symptoms overall*

Unfortunately much of the available data is not presented in a manner from which the number of people who have at least one different form of psychotic symptom can be calculated. In the clinical studies, 11 out of 12 (91.7%) SDLT patients in Ballard (1995) study had at least one psychotic symptom as did 41 of the 42 (97.6%) patients with SDLT in the prospective Newcastle study. Ballard (1995) found that none of these 11 patients had any insight into their beliefs or hallucinations and five acted upon them. Six of the 11 patients experienced some distress as a result of their symptoms. Five out of 7 patients with SDLT followed up for one year did not experience symptom resolution.

Each category of psychotic symptoms is significantly more prevalent in patients with LBD than patients with Alzheimer's disease. This is consistent with Ballard's (1995) finding that psychotic patients with SDLT experience a mean of 4.4 different symptoms whereas psychotic patients with Alzheimer's disease experience a mean of only 2.6 symptoms. This was confirmed in the prospective Newcastle sample where psychotic patients with SDLT had a mean of 4.1 symptoms compared with a mean of 2.2 in psychotic patients with Alzheimer's disease. This is rather a curious finding as each of the three major categories of psychotic symptom has a different basis. Visual hallucinations are associated with cholinergic deficits and the presence of eye disease, delusions are associated with lesions of the prosubiculum and delusional misidentification require the misperception of images with delusional misinterpretation. Frith (1992) has emphasized the role of error monitoring and the failure of error monitoring systems in the development of psychosis. Error monitoring impairments could explain the increased occurrence of all three discreet categories of psychotic symptoms in patients with LBD. It is also consistent with the available data which suggests that these patients have prominent frontal lobe deficits (Sahgal et al., 1992).

Further work is required to tease out in greater detail the characteristics and associations of psychotic symptoms in LBD, to examine the course of these symptoms and to try and develop effective treatment strategies. The latter is a particularly difficult area given the marked neuroleptic sensitivity reactions in some patients (McKeith et al., 1992b). Case reports of successful treatment interventions with low doses of risperidone have appeared in the literature, although the information is highly provisional and neuroleptic sensitivity reactions to risperidone do occur. Very low doses of risperidone in the region of 0.6 mg daily have successfully treated psychotic symptoms in patients with Parkinson's disease, although other authors have reported severe worsening of parkinsonian symptoms with marginally higher doses. There is an accumulating literature describing the successful treatment of psychotic symptoms in patients with Parkinson's disease using clozapine. More than 100 cases treated with this regime have now been published, 75% of whom had a good outcome (Auzou et al., 1995). Clozapine is not licensed for the treatment of psychosis in dementia sufferers, although may form the basis of a useful treatment regime in the future. Neuroleptics, despite being widely used, have only limited efficacy in treating psychotic symptoms in dementia. There is, therefore, a need to look at alternative treatment regimes based upon empirical neurochemical evidence. One could for example postulate that cholinesterase inhibitors may be an effective treatment for visual hallucinations in patients with LBD (Perry et al., 1990). Further work is required to generate hypothesis which could be the basis of novel treatment approaches for delusions and delusional misidentification. Treatment issues are discussed in more detail in Chapter 29.

6.3 Mood disorders

Depression is the only mood disorder which has been systematically studied in patients with LBD. Of the 56 patients described in small post-mortem series, eight (14.3%) suffered from depression. No standardized criteria were used. There is a remarkable similarity between this figure and the prevalence rate of DSM-IIIR major depression reported in the four larger neuropathological series, where prevalence rates of between 13.3% and 16% were found. Although in McKeith et al.'s (1992a) study only 13.3% of the LBD patients suffered from major depression, a further 23.8% of patients were judged to have significant depressive symptoms. None of these groups reported prevalence rates in LBD patients that were significantly different from the rates found in patients with Alzheimer's disease. In clinical series Ballard et al. (1993) found 7 out of 16 (43.8%) patients with SDLT to fulfil the CAMDEX criteria for depression. Ballard (1995) found 4 out 12 (33.3%) patients with SDLT to fulfil Research Diagnostic Criteria for major depression, a further four (33.3%) fulfilled the criteria for RDC minor depression. The prospective Newcastle data included five (11.9%) SDLT patients with DSM-IIIR major depression and a further three (7.1%) patients suffering from DSM-IIIR dysthymia (Table 6.2). Major depression or dysthymia in SDLT patients was significantly associated with concurrent Parkinson's disease (Fisher's exact test $p = 0.02$) and with taking levodopa (Fisher's exact test $p = 0.03$). These are interesting findings, but only small numbers of patients are so far involved. Depression is of course extremely common amongst patients with Parkinson's disease, occurring in up to 50% of sufferers (Cummings, 1992), although the relationship with dementia in these patients is unclear. Only Ballard et al. (1993) found a significantly higher prevalence rate of depression in SDLT than in Alzheimer's disease. Twenty per cent of patients with DLB suffered from DSM-IIIR major depression or dysthymia in the prospective Newcastle study.

There is a great deal of consistency between the different neuropathological studies which all found prevalence rates of DSM-IIIR major depression to be approximately 15%. Clearly there are a number of patients with significant symptoms of depression who do not meet the DSM-IIIR criteria for major depression. Reflecting this, clinical studies which have used less-restrictive criteria have found higher prevalence rates. The true prevalence rate of depression in LBD can only be determined when a satisfactory definition of depression is available. Longitudinal data regarding the course of these symptoms and the degree to which they cause excess disability is required if this is to be achieved. Standardized assessment instruments may help to clarify the situation to some degree. Although depressive symptoms occur in a substantial number of patients with LBD, they are equally prevalent in patients with Alzheimer's disease and hence do not help distinguish between the two dementias. Ballard (1995) found the symptom profiles of depression to be highly correlated, further emphasizing the similarity.

There is a paucity of longitudinal data. Ballard (1995) followed up seven depressed patients with SDLT for one year, four (57.1%) of whom experienced resolution of their depression within three months, but the depression persisted for six months or longer in the other three. Although the numbers are small, a duration of three months may be a suitable cut off to recommend treatment interventions.

In patients with depression in the context of Alzheimer's disease, an exciting literature is emerging suggesting an association between depression and the severity of the Alzheimer's disease process in the locus coeruleus. The regional distribution of senile plaques, neurofibrillary tangles and Lewy bodies in patients with and without depression in the context of LBD is an important area for investigation, particularly focusing on the locus coeruleus as a region of interest (Förstl et al., 1992).

Not much attention has been paid to mood disorders other than depression in patients with LBD. Provisional data from the prospective Newcastle study identified two (4.8%) cases of DSM-IIIR Generalised Anxiety Disorder. The DSM-IIIR criteria are highly restrictive and may have excluded some patients with significant anxiety symptoms. What little literature is available pertaining to patients with Alzheimer's disease suggests a prevalence rate in the region of 30% (Ballard et al., 1994). Anxiety symptoms are also reported as occurring in between 8 and 20% of patients with Parkinson's disease (Cummings, 1992), although again the relationship with dementia is unclear. Anxiety symptoms are hence common in related disorders and require further study in patients with LBD.

None of the 42 patients with SDLT in the prospective Newcastle sample had a bipolar affective disorder as part of their dementia. Burns et al. (1990) suggested a prevalence rate of 2 to 3% in patients with Alzheimer's disease, the prevalence rate in patients with LBD is currently unknown.

6.4 Falls

Falls are an important cause of morbidity and mortality amongst dementia sufferers. During the three-year follow-up study (Buchner & Larson 1987) 50% of patients with Alzheimer's disease experienced falls and 15% suffered fractures, most commonly of the hip. Falls are a frequent reason for admission to residential or nursing home care. Falls assume an even greater importance in patients with LBD as they are probably more common in these patients and are included amongst the Newcastle diagnostic criteria for SDLT.

Frequent falls were described in 8 of the 56 (14.3%) patients with LBD described in small neuropathological series and were identified in between 26.7% (Byrne et al., 1989) and 50% (McKeith et al., 1994) of patients in the larger postmortem series. In clinical series, falls occurred in 15 out of 16 (93.8%) patients in Ballard et al.'s (1993) study, 9 out of 30 (30%) patients in Shergill et al.'s (1994) series and 4 out of 12 (33.3%) patients in Ballard's (1995) series. The prospective Newcastle study identified 21 (50%) SDLT patients with two or more falls (Table 6.2), of whom five (23.8%) experienced at least five falls. Sixty per cent of patients with DLB had two or more falls, suggesting that the choice of clinical criteria does not markedly affect frequency estimates. A clustering of prevalence estimates in the 25% to 50% range is evident for frequent falls in patients with LBD. In addition, 10% of patients with Lewy body dementia have extremely frequent falls and are at very high risk of injury. Falls occurred significantly more frequently in patients with Lewy body dementia than patients with Alzheimer's disease in the McKeith et al. (1992a) study, the Ballard et al. (1993) study and the prospective Newcastle study but not the McKeith et al. (1994) study or the Ballard (1995) study.

The causes of falls in patients with LBD are unknown. The prospective Newcastle study provides descriptive data. Balance problems were felt to be the cause of the falls in 38.5% of patients, trips were said to account for 19.2% of falls and postural hypotension was thought to be responsible in 7.7% of patients. No causes were determined for the other 34.6%. There was no association between falls and taking neuroleptic medication or between falls and the presence of concurrent Parkinson's disease.

Falls occur commonly in patients with LBD, although it is unclear whether they help discriminate between LBD and Alzheimer's disease. Research in this area is rather still in the provisional stages and a lot more information is required. Factors such as muscle weakness, restlessness, wandering, the number of psychotropic drugs taken, vulnerability to adverse drug reactions, superimposed acute confusional state and poor balance have all been reported as significant association of falls in patients with Alzheimer's disease (Buchner & Larson, 1987). A significant association has also been reported between falls and Parkinson's disease (Traubm et al., 1980). It is not surprising that falls are highly prevalent in patients with LBD, given the frequent occurrence of many of these risk factors. Nevertheless it is important to tease out the relative importance of these different factors. In particular it is important to study the group of patients with very frequent falls in greater detail. Investigations of this kind may offer treatment alternatives either in terms of the type of drug treatments used, physiotherapy aimed to build up muscle strength or techniques which could improve balance. It is also important to determine the number of patients who sustain serious injuries as a result of their falls.

6.5 Wandering

Amongst patients with Alzheimer's disease 25% to 40% of patients (Burns et al., 1990) will leave or try to leave their homes. If other behaviours such as restless pacing, overactivity and following the carer around the home are included the prevalence rate increases to over 60%. These symptoms are distressing to carers (Rabins et al., 1982) and are associated with an increased risk of falls (Buchner & Larson, 1987). If patients leave the house unaccompanied they may be vulnerable to a number of other injury risks.

Unfortunately there is only very sparse information about wandering repeated in the LBD literature. Out of the 56 cases reported in small neuropathological series, five (8.9%) were considered to wander. Of the larger postmortem series, only Byrne et al.'s (1989) group describe wandering which was reported in 1 of the 15 patients. The retrospective designs are likely to have seriously underestimated the prevalence rates of wandering, but no prospective data are available.

Wandering is an important and common problem in patients with Alzheimer's disease. Although some patients with LBD may have their mobility limited by symptoms of Parkinson's disease, wandering is likely to be far more common than reported in the retrospective series.

6.6 Aggression

Violent behaviour has been reported consistently in 20% of patients with Alzheimer's disease (Burns et al., 1990). When other aggressive behaviours such as verbal outbursts are included there is a marked increase in prevalence. Aggression is one of the symptoms found to be intolerable by carers (Burns et al., 1990) and frequently leads to residential or nursing home placement. The subject has received only very sparse consideration in patients with LBD. Three of the 56 (5.4%) patients included in small postmortem series were described as aggressive. This is likely to be a marked underestimate of the true prevalence rate.

6.7 Other noncognitive symptoms

Agitation is a concept often used in clinical practice and has been defined to encompass a spectrum of behaviours including restlessness, irritability and aggression. It is probably best to consider the component behaviours in separate categories and avoid vague terminology as far as possible.

Sexual overactivity occurs frequently in frontal lobe dementias and occasionally Alzheimer's disease and Parkinson's disease. No information is available pertaining to sexual overactivity in patients with LBD.

6.8 Conclusion

There are far more questions raised than answers provided from the work so far completed. Nevertheless considering that it is only in the last decade that LBD has been identified as a common condition, knowledge has accumulated at an impressive rate. There is, however, no room for complacency. With the possible exception of visual hallucinations, little is known about the underlying neurochemical basis of the psychiatric symptoms occurring in patients with LBD and there is only a very rudimentary understanding of why these patients are liable to frequent falls. Although the vast majority of patients with LBD experience a number of unpleasant or troublesome noncognitive symptoms, no safe or effective treatment regimes have been established. Several large prospective studies are now in progress. Hopefully important information pertaining to noncognitive symptoms will emerge from these studies clarifying the answers to some of these questions.

References

Auzou, P., Cote, L. & Fahn, S. (1995). Clozapine in Parkinson's disease. *Lancet*, **345**, 516–17.

Ballard, C.G. (1995). Depression and Psychotic Symptoms in Dementia Sufferers. MD thesis, University of Leicester, UK.

Ballard, C.G., Mohan, R.N.C., Patel, A. & Bannister, C. (1993). Idiopathic clouding of consciousness – Do the patients have cortical Lewy body disease? *Int. J. Geriatr. Psychiatry*, **8**, 571–6.

Ballard, C.G., Mohan, R.N.G., Patel, A. & Graham, C. (1994). Anxiety disorders in dementia. *Irish J. Psychol. Med.*, **11**, 108–9.

Beck, J. & Harris, J. (1994). Visual hallucinations in non-delusional elderly. *Int. J. Geriatr. Psychiatry*, **9**, 531–6.

Buchner, D.M. & Larson, E.R. (1987). Falls and fractures in patients with Alzheimer's type dementia. *J. Am. Med. Ass.*, **257**, 1492–5.

Burns, A. (1991). Affective symptoms in Alzheimer's disease. *Int. J. Geriatr. Psychiatry*, **6**, 371–6.

Burns, A., Jacoby, R. & Levy, R. (1990). Psychiatric phenomena in Alzheimer's disease. I. Disorders of thought content and II: Disorders of perception. *Br. J. Psychiatry*, **157**, 72–81.

Byrne, E.J., Lennox, G., Lowe, J. & Godwin-Austen, R.B. (1989). Lewy body disease, clinical features in 15 cases. *J. Neurol., Neurosurg. Psychiatry*, **52**, 709–17.

Byrne, E.J., Lennox, G. & Godwin-Austen, L.B. (1991). Dementia associated with cortical Lewy bodies: Proposed diagnostic criteria. *Dementia*, **2**, 283–4.

Cummings, J.L. (1992). Neuropsychiatric Complications of Drug Treatment of Parkinson's Disease. In *Parkinson's Disease, Neurobehavioural Aspects*, ed. S.J. Huber & J.L. Cummings, pp. 313–27. Oxford: Oxford University Press.

Förstl, H., Burns, A., Luthert, P. et al. (1992). Clinical and neuropathological correlations of depression in Alzheimer's disease. *Psychol. Med.*, **22**, 877–84.

Frith, C. (1992). *The Cognitive Neuropsychology of Schizophrenia*. Hove: Lawrence Erlbaum Associates.

Howard, R. & Levy, R. (1994). Charles-Bonnet syndrome plus complex visual hallucinations of Charles Bonnet type in late paraphrenia. *Int. J. Geriatr. Psychiatry*, **9**, 399–404.

McKeith, I.G., Perry, R.H., Fairbairn, A.F., Jabeen, S. & Perry, E.K. (1992a). Operational criteria for senile dementia of Lewy body type. *Psychol Med.*, **22**, 911–22.

McKeith, I.G., Fairbairn, A.F., Perry, R., Thompson, P. & Perry, E.K. (1992b). Neuroleptic sensitivity in patients with senile dementia of Lewy body type. *BMJ*, **305**, 673–8.

McKeith, I.G., Fairbairn, A.F., Bothwall, R.A. et al. (1994). An evaluation of the predictive validity and inter-rater reliability of clinical diagnostic criteria for SDLT. *Neurology*, **44**, 872–7.

Perry, E.K., Marshall, E., Kerwin, J. et al. (1990). Evidence of a monoaminergic-cholinergic imbalance related to visual hallucinations in Lewy body dementia. *J. Neurochem.*, **55**, 1454–6.

Rabins, P.V., Mace, N.L. & Lucas, M.J. (1982). The impact of dementia on the family. *J. Am. Med. Ass.*, **248**, 333–5.

Rosen, J. & Zubenko, G.S. (1991). Emergence of psychosis and depression in the longitudinal evaluation of Alzheimer's disease. *Biol. Psychiatry*, **29**, 2224–32.

Sahgal, A., Galloway, P.H., McKeith, I.G., Edwardson, J.A. & Lloyd, S. (1992). A comparative study of attentional deficits in senile dementia of Alzheimer and Lewy body types. *Dementia*, **3**, 350–4.

Shergill, S., Mullen, E., D'Ath, P. & Katona, C. (1994). What is the clinical prevalence of Lewy body dementia? *Int. J. Geriatr. Psychiatry*, **9**, 907–12.

Steele, C., Rovner, B., Chase, G.A. & Folstein, M. (1990). Psychiatric symptoms and nursing home placement of patients with Alzheimer's disease. *Am. J. Psychiatry*, **147**, 1049–51.

Traubm, M., Rothwell, J.G. & Marsden, D. (1980). Anticipating postural reflexes in Parkinson's disease and other akinetic rigid syndrome and cerebellar ataxia. *Brain*, **103**, 393–412.

7

Hallucinations, cortical Lewy body pathology, cognitive function and neuroleptic use in dementia

R. McSHANE, J. KEENE, K. GEDLING
and T. HOPE

Summary

Hallucinations are one of the defining features of the clinical syndrome associated with cortical Lewy body pathology. However, it is not clear whether the time course of hallucinations in Lewy body dementia is different from that in other dementias. We therefore studied the natural history of hallucinations in dementia. Since neuroleptics may be used to treat hallucinations and may have deleterious effects, we also examined the impact of neuroleptic use on cognitive decline. Ninety-eight patients with dementia were assessed every 4 months on a median of eight occasions. Fifty-one patients came to autopsy. Our longitudinal study shows that hallucinations beginning within the first three years of dementia are associated with cortical Lewy body pathology and reduced life expectancy. Patients with cortical Lewy body pathology were more likely to have persistent as opposed to fleeting hallucinations. This information could be incorporated into operational clinical criteria for Lewy body dementia. We did not find an increased mortality amongst those with cortical Lewy body pathology who took neuroleptics. However, men who took neuroleptics had a more rapid rate of cognitive decline than those who did not. This association was not apparent in women. We did not find evidence of increased fluctuation in cognitive ability in the Lewy body group.

7.1 Introduction

The appearance of hallucinations in the context of dementia has implications for diagnosis, prognosis and management. The possibility that hallucinations occur as part of a clinical syndrome is suggested by the findings that hallucinations co-occur more commonly than would be expected with fluctuating cognitive impairment (Ballard et al., 1993) and with extrapyramidal symptoms in patients having a clinical diagnosis of Alzheimer's disease (Mayeux et al., 1985). Several retrospective, case note studies have shown that the three elements of this syndrome are associated with cortical Lewy body pathology. One of the proposed sets of operational diagnostic criteria for the clinical diagnosis of Lewy body dementia includes 'visual or auditory hallucinations, which are usually accompanied by secondary paranoid delusions'. It is suggested that the hallucinations should persist over 'weeks or months' (McKeith et al., 1992a). Other sets of clinical criteria have also made reference to hallucinations (Crystal et al., 1990; Byrne et al., 1991). However, little is known of the natural history of the symptom in patients with dementia. Are they generally persistent, or do they come and go? Are hallucinations of early and late onset associated with different neuropathological diagnoses?

It is known that the occurrence of psychosis in dementia is associated with a poorer prognosis, in terms of cognitive decline. Studies using cross-sectional data have shown that demented patients who had psychotic symptoms in life were more demented at death than those who did not (Flynn et al., 1991; Gilley et al., 1991). This might be explained if it was shown that there was an increased prevalence of hallucinations in those surviving into severe dementia. More recently, however, several groups have shown that patients with psychosis (Mayeux et al., 1985; Drevets & Rubin, 1989; Rosen & Zubenko, 1991; Stern et al., 1994) or hallucinations (Burns et al., 1990; Förstl et al., 1993a; Chui et al., 1994; Mortimer et al., 1992) have a faster rate of cognitive decline. The mechanism underlying this link is not known. The use of neuroleptics, the presence of cortical Lewy bodies or alterations in biogenic amine systems have all been advanced as possible explanations (Chui et al., 1994).

As well as the diagnostic and prognostic implications of psychosis, such symptoms have implications for the management of patients with dementia. For example, decisions about their pharmacotherapy are complicated by the possibility that they may be at risk of developing severe extrapyramidal reactions to neuroleptics (McKeith et al., 1992b). Hallucinations are also associated with increased aggression (Deutsch et al., 1991) and risk of institutionalization (Steele et al., 1990).

In this chapter we discuss these issues in more detail, drawing on unpublished data from a longitudinal study of behaviour in 98 patients with dementia of whom 51 had autopsies.

7.2 Subjects and methods

A sample of 104 subjects fulfilling DSM-IIIR criteria for dementia (American Psychiatric Association, 1987) and with a diagnosis of either probable Alzheimer's disease (McKhann et al., 1984) or vascular dementia was recruited through local general practitioners, community psychiatric nurses and consultant psychogeriatricians. All subjects were initially living at home with a carer. Ninety eight subjects completed the study, of whom 86 were followed until death. Autopsy results are available on 51 cases. The median age at study entry was 78 years (range 61–95). Fifty two cases were male.

The behaviour of the subjects prior to entry into the study was assessed using the 'Past Behavioural History Interview (PBHI)' which is based on the Present Behavioural Examination (PBE) (Hope & Fairburn, 1992) and includes the question 'Since the onset of the memory problems/dementia do you think there have been periods when he or she has heard or seen things that aren't really there? For example, heard imaginary voices or seen imaginary things?' Carers were also asked how long prior to the interview the hallucinations had started and when they had stopped.

After entry into the study each subject was assessed every 4 months over a period of up to 6 years until death. The median number of interviews before death was 8 (range 1–17). The cognitive function of subjects was examined using an expanded version of the Mini-Mental State Examination (MMSE) (Wilcock et al., 1989). This includes items relating to verbal fluency and abstract thinking in addition to all the items of the MMSE (Folstein et al., 1975). The behaviour and mental health of subjects was assessed using the PBE. This is a semi-structured interview, which is administered to carers. It includes an item rating hallucinations on a 7-point frequency scale, relating to the number of days on which the symptom occurred over the four week period prior to the interview. Hallucinations were defined as 'persistent' if they occurred on more than 5 of the previous 28 days at two consecutive interviews (spaced 4 months apart) (McShane et al., 1995). Symptoms which could have been related to temporary physical illness or to changes in medication were related as 'missing' throughout the prospective study. The subject's medication was recorded at each interview.

The degree of cortical Lewy body pathology was determined quantitatively in four cortical areas as described previously (McShane et al., 1995). Nine of the 51 autopsy cases had cortical Lewy bodies in at least two cortical areas. This pathology was assessed blind to nigral pathology, pathology in the other areas and clinical data.

7.3 Incidence and prevalence of hallucinations

The incidence and prevalence of hallucinations in each of the years after study entry is shown in Table 7.1. The one year period prevalence over the first year was 25.5%. There was no increase in the prevalence or incidence with increasing severity of dementia. The annual incidence in the three interviews of the first year was 9.9%. Over the four years of the study, the overall incidence was 26.8%. Hallucinators did not differ from other subjects in age, age at onset of dementia or sex.

These incidence figures are considerably higher than that in retrospective (Cummings et al., 1987; Burns et al., 1990; Jeste et al., 1992) but not other prospective (Ballard et al., 1995) studies. Our data do not support the claims that hallucinations appear as a manifestation of a stage of late dementia (Reisberg et al., 1981).

7.4 Time course of hallucinations

The time of onset of hallucinations was unimodally distributed: they most commonly began in the fourth year of dementia. A potentially important finding was that if the hallucinations started within the first three years of dementia the subsequent time course of hallucinations and dementia was different (Table 7.2). Specifically, the length of the episode of hallucinations was almost twice as great in those whose hallucinations began early compared with those with late onset hallucinations. However, patients with early onset hallucinations had a shorter overall duration of dementia than those with late onset hallucinations or those without any hallucinations.

There have been very few studies of the extent to which hallucinations come and go. Our frequent, regular and prolonged follow-up using standardized instruments allowed detailed information about the onset and offset, and hence persistence, of hallucinations to be collected. Only 15% of all subjects (38.5% of those who had hallucinations at any point in the prospective study) had 'persistent' hallucinations, as defined above. Once established, the hallucinations tend to be a stable phenomena which persisted into the year before death in 71% of cases. No subject had more than one episode of persistent hallucinations. Furthermore, when hallucinations were persistent, they tended to be severe. During such an

Table 7.1. *Incidence and prevalence of hallucinations in 98 demented patients studied over 3 years*

Year of study	Incidence[*]	% per year	Prevalence	%	Mean cognitive score ($\pm$SD)[‡]	
					MMSE	eMMS
1	7/71	9.9	25/98	25.5	14.8 ± 7.7	31.9 ± 1.4
2	8/53	15.1	22/81	27.2	10.6 ± 8.1	23.7 ± 1.8
3	2/38	5.3	14/69	20.3	8.9 ± 8.1	20.2 ± 2.1

[*]Excludes cases who hallucinated before study entry, or where data was missing. Cases who began hallucinating in each year, or who died, were excluded from analysis in subsequent years, hence the variable denominator.
‡ Cognitive scores at interviews 1, 4 and 7.

Table 7.2. *Relationship between time of onset of hallucinations, duration of hallucinations, and duration of dementia before death*

	Onset of hallucinations in first 36 months of dementia $N = 15$	Onset of hallucinations after first 36 months of dementia $N = 26$	Student's t-test p
Mean overall duration of dementia before death (yr)	5.78 ± 0.47	9.68 ± 0.78	0.001
Mean duration of hallucinations (yr)	2.64 ± 0.45	1.49 ± 0.27	0.04

episode the hallucinations were present, on average, on at least half the days. Hallucinations which did not last long enough to be persistent are termed 'fleeting'.

Our results correspond closely with those of Ballard and colleagues (Chapter 6) who found that visual hallucinations persisted in only 43% of cases in whom the symptom was present at study entry. In contrast, Rosen and Zubenko (1991) found that psychosis remitted in only 2 of 15 (13%) patients with psychosis.

These findings are qualified by several methodological caveats. Many of the patients who hallucinated during the prospective study had also done so prior to study entry and the retrospective data about the time of onset in these cases will inevitably be less accurate than the prospective information. Nevertheless, it is possible that the time of onset of hallucinations may be more accurately datable than the more insidious memory loss. In any case, inaccuracies in the dating of symptom onset would have had the effect of obscuring any associations between the time of onset and prognosis. Indeed, it may be easier for carers to provide a clear data for the onset of psychotic symptoms than it is for clinicians to elicit reliable information about their exact phenomenology.

7.5 Cortical Lewy bodies and time course of hallucinations

These distinctions between early and late onset, and between fleeting and persistent hallucinations may be useful diagnostically as well as prognostically. Amongst the 24 cases who had hallucinations at any point and have come to autopsy, those with hallucinations of early onset were more likely to have cortical LBs than those with hallucinations of late onset (Fisher's exact test $p = 0.03$). We have previously demonstrated a link between the persistence and severity of hallucinations and the presence of cortical Lewy body pathology (McShane et al., 1995). Poor vision contributes to the severity of hallucinations but does not prolong them. We suggested an operational definition of 'persistent' hallucinations based on its capacity to predict cortical Lewy body pathology in a group of 41 of the current 51 cases. The association between persistent hallucinations and cortical LBs is also apparent in the larger group of 51: only 2 of 6 cases with persistent hallucinations did not have cortical LBs, whereas 4 of 9 cases with cortical LBs had persistent hallucinations; 40 cases had neither hallucinations nor cortical Lewy bodies. Those with fleeting hallucinations were no more likely to have cortical LBs than those without any hallucinations.

If our results are replicated, we suggest that the criterion of 'time of onset' be added to that of 'persistence' in operational criteria for Lewy body dementia. The diagnostic sensitivity of 'persistent' and 'early onset' hallucinations may not be as good as that for a more widely defined symptom. However, such information may help clinicians and researchers in deciding what weight to attach to the symptom in an individual patient.

7.6 Cortical Lewy bodies and cognitive decline

The importance of cortical Lewy bodies in determining cognitive decline is open to question. Only one group (Lennox et al., 1989) has found a correlation between the density of cortical Lewy bodies and the severity of dementia. We found that those with cortical Lewy bodies had worse cognitive function at death (eMMS $= 4.9 \pm 3.7$ vs 16.2 ± 2.5; $p = 0.04$) than those without, despite having had a shorter duration of dementia before death (6.4 ± 1.0 vs 9.1 ± 0.75 years; $p = 0.05$). We excluded other potential factors which might confound this association. For example, those with cortical Lewy body pathology did not have significantly worse cognitive function at study entry than those without (eMMS 25.9 ± 5.7 vs 32.4 ± 2.1; $p = 0.3$, 95% CI: -7.2 to 20.4), nor was there a significant difference in the age at death or in sex ratio. There was a nonsignificant trend for those with cortical LBs to be older at onset of dementia (76.4 ± 1.0 vs 72.0 ± 1.2 years; $p = 0.09$).

Interestingly, those with cortical Lewy bodies did not have a faster rate of cognitive decline over the first 20 months (difference in eMMS between first and sixth interviews: 11.6 ± 3.2 vs 10.1 ± 1.7; p-0.7, 95% CI: -9.5 to 6.5) than those without. At first sight there is apparently a paradox in the findings that cognitive function is worse at death and duration of dementia is shorter but the rate of cognitive decline is not different. Two possible explanations suggest themselves. First, there might be a type 2 error: there were only eight cases with cortical Lewy bodies which were followed for 20 months. Secondly, patients with cortical Lewy bodies may be prone to a late terminal dip in cognitive function. This may reflect the tempo at which Lewy bodies develop in cortical and/or basal forebrain neurones. If such pathology is indeed developing relatively late in the course of the illness, this might be a confounding factor in the assessment of neuroleptic sensitivity in those with cortical Lewy bodies.

7.7 Cortical Lewy bodies and neuroleptics

In contrast to the findings of McKeith and colleagues (1992b), in our sample, those with cortical Lewy bodies did not have an increased mortality over the year after starting neuroleptics. Of the nine patients with cortical Lewy bodies, five took neuroleptics at some point. Two patients (that is, 40%) died within a year of starting neuroleptics (one male and one female) and a male patient died after one interview in the study. He was taking neuroleptics at this point but we do not have information about how long he was taking it before study entry. Of the remaining patients who had autopsies, 23 took neuroleptics at some point and of these, nine died within a year of starting neuroleptics. In other words, 39% of those without Lewy body pathology also died soon after starting neuroleptics. When a shorter time frame (i.e. within 4 months of death) or when time from presentation (as opposed to time from starting neuroleptics) to death were examined, we similarly failed to find any association between mortality, cortical Lewy pathology and neuroleptics.

This difference in findings from McKeith and colleagues may be because, in contrast to their sample, our sample excluded those who presented with Parkinson's disease. The mean level of nigral cell loss and dopaminergic function – and hence susceptibility to neuroleptics – may have therefore been more severe in their sample of Lewy body cases. Against this possibility is the fact that only 3/7 of their cases with severe reactions had extrapyramidal features before starting neuroleptics.

7.8 Cortical Lewy bodies and fluctuation

The presence of fluctuating cognitive and functional ability has been found by the Newcastle group to be a good clinical discriminator of senile dementia of the Lewy body type (McKeith et al., 1994). The Nottingham group also commented on fluctuating cognitive state as feature in 80% of cases, suggesting that this resembled delirium (Byrne et al., 1989). Similarly, Hansen et al. (1990) found more severe attentional deficits as assessed by digit span. However, Förstl et al. (1993b) did not find any excess of fluctuation in the Lewy body group although one case had a striking confusional state.

We examined the issue of fluctuation by defining fluctuating cognitive ability in three ways: (1) as an increase in eMMS of at least 3 points between two consecutive four monthly interviews; (2) as an increase of at least 5 points between two consecutive interviews; and (3) as the standard deviation of the differences in eMMS between each successive interview. Definitions based on increases in cognitive scores were used because such increases are more likely to represent unexpected fluctuations than decreases in cognitive scores, which are to be expected.

Neither the presence of cortical Lewy bodies nor the occurrence of hallucinations were associated with fluctuating cognitive ability which was any greater than that in the rest of the sample of any of the definitions used.

It is possible that our definitions of fluctuation, since they were based on a 4 month time frame were insufficiently sensitive to detect relevant changes. It is not clear over what time frame 'fluctuation' is to be regarded as important. Using a CAMDEX item, Ballard et al. (1993) have shown that fluctuation with an episodicity of 'days or weeks' is associated with hallucinations, extrapyramidal symptoms and falls. There has only been one other prospective examination of fluctuation in Lewy body dementia in which Williams et al. (1993) followed five patients with clinically-defined Lewy body dementia monthly over a period of at least three months: three subjects had improvements in MMSE scores at successive interviews of 4, 3 and 1 points respectively. Such increases were, however, common in our neuropathologically characterized nonLewy body group.

The refutation of this clinical criterion for Lewy body dementia is going to be difficult. The extent of episodic fluctuations in attention, of 'good days and bad days' and of longer spells of delirium for which no physical cause can be found, needs to be carefully examined in other dementias before a convincing case can be made for excessive fluctuation in cortical Lewy body dementia.

7.9 Neuroleptics and cognitive decline

Given the frequency with which neuroleptics are prescribed for aggression, agitation, sleep disturbance and psychosis in dementia it is remarkable how little is known of the extent to which cognitive function in patients with dementia (of all types) is affected by neuroleptics. We know of only one previous study, reported as an abstract (Bennett et al., 1992), which has examined the question of cognitive decline and psychosis in dementia and that has also investigated the possible contribution of neuroleptics. Bennett et al. (1992) found that neuroleptics had a deleterious effect on cognitive function that was independent of psychosis. Burns et al. (1990) found that those who hallucinated were no more likely to take neuroleptics than those without (a finding which we have replicated in our sample), but do not report the rates of cognitive decline in the different subgroups.

In our study, amongst those who were followed for at least 20 months, the mean decline in eMMS over this period was 9.35 ± 1.3 in those who did not take neuroleptics and 20.7 ± 2.9 in those who took more than an average of 10 mg chlorpromazine daily ($p = 0.002$) (or its equivalent (Foster, 1989)). This effect of neuroleptics was even more marked in men (8.9 ± 2.0 vs 23.8 ± 3.2; $p = 0.001$) but the association was not apparent in women. The decline in eMMS scores in women taking neuroleptics was 15.5 ± 5.4 compared with 23.8 ± 3.2 in men. There was no difference between the sexes in the total dose of neuroleptics which was taken and neither was there any significant difference between the cognitive function of men and women at study entry.

This association of more rapid cognitive decline with neuroleptics may have been mediated by extrapyramidal effects. It has been shown that even amongst those who are not taking neuroleptics, extrapyramidal signs predict for subsequent more rapid cognitive decline (Stern et al., 1994). Indeed, the presence of extrapyramidal signs in the apparently healthy elderly predicts for the subsequent development of dementia (Richards et al., 1993). Further evidence for possible toxicity of neuroleptics in dementia has been advanced by Chen et al. (1996). In a subgroup of 20 cases in the current sample, they found neurochemical evidence to suggest that neuroleptics may reduce compensatory plasticity of the degenerating 5-HT system in Alzheimer's disease.

The finding of sex difference in the effect of neuroleptics on cognitive function in dementia is intriguing and is at present the subject of further analysis. We are not aware of previously documented sex differences in neuroleptic side-effects or responsiveness in which men deteriorate more rapidly.

7.10 Hallucinations and cognitive decline

We have referred above to our finding that the prevalence of hallucinations does not increase with worsening cognitive decline (Table 7.1), which would tend to refute the idea hallucinations were a manifestation of a stage of dementia which all patients would go through if they lived long enough. We also found that those with hallucinations declined more rapidly over the first 20 months of the study than those without hallucinations. (Difference in eMMS between first and sixth interviews: 16.0 ± 2.4 vs 9.4 ± 1.4; $p = 0.02$.) This association was apparent in those who had persistent hallucinations over this period, but not those in whom the symptom was fleeting. There was no difference in the rate of decline between those with late or early onset hallucinations. Cognitive function at death was also significantly worse in those who ever had hallucinations (7.9 ± 1.6 vs 18.1 ± 2.3; $p = 0.001$). This did not depend on whether the hallucinations were early, late, persistent or fleeting.

This finding of an increased rate of cognitive decline in those who hallucinate is not new (Chui et al., 1994). However, other studies have not been able to exclude the possibility that this association arises because hallucinators were already on a steeper trajectory of cognitive decline before the onset of the symptom. We therefore examined this question in 18 subjects who had not hallucinated prior to the prospective part of the study. We compared the eMMS scores of the 18 hallucinators in the year before and the year after the onset of hallucinations with eMMS scores of a group of non-hallucinators matched to within 4 points either side of the eMMS at the onset of hallucinations in the hallucinator. The worsening of cognitive function in those with hallucinations was not apparent a year before hallucinations started (paired Wilcoxon $p = 0.79$), but was apparent one year after the onset of hallucinations ($p = 0.01$).

This suggests that the point of onset of hallucinations is close to the time at which the cognitive function of hallucinators and nonhallucinators begins to differ. One possible explanation for this finding is that a pathological process associated with hallucinations is also responsible for worsening cognitive decline. Such a process could either be a sudden exacerbation of an existing condition such as Alzheimer's disease, or the development of a second pathology such as Lewy body involvement of brainstem or cortex. Only one of our de novo hallucinators was subsequently shown to have Lewy body pathology and the onset of hallucinations did not coincide with an obvious sudden deterioration in this case. A second possible explanation is that the hallucinations themselves interfered with the performance of cognitive testing. However, our interviewers report that patients were only very rarely observed to be hallucinating during the interview, consistent with the findings of Cummings et al. (1987).

A third explanation for the association between the onset of hallucinations and more rapid cognitive decline relates to the use of neuroleptics. In this sample of 'de novo' hallucinators, patients who went on to hallucinate were more likely to have taken neuroleptics in the year *prior* to the onset of hallucinations than the group matched for level of cognitive decline, but the trend in this direction did not reach significance in the year after the onset of hallucinations. These findings are preliminary, but raise the possibility that increased neuroleptic use in the year prior to the onset of hallucinations had a toxic effect on cognitive function which was delayed. This would be consistent with the association of neuroleptics with more rapid cognitive decline which was noted in the larger sample.

7.11 Conclusions

Cortical Lewy body pathology is associated with hallucinations which are more likely to be of early onset and to be persistent than are those in other causes of dementia. We did not find evidence of fluctuation or of increased mortality in those with cortical Lewy bodies in this small, but prospectively studied group. Our data support the previously identified associations of cortical LB pathology and hallucinations with severe cognitive decline in dementia. The more rapid cognitive decline seen in patients with hallucinations appears to start soon after the onset of hallucinations. We have also shown that neuroleptic treatment is associated with more rapid cognitive decline. Our data do not suggest that patients with cortical Lewy body dementia are more susceptible to the effects of neuroleptics than patients with other causes of dementia. Nevertheless, our findings highlight the need to find alternatives to neuroleptics for the treatment of behavioural problems in dementia as a whole.

References

American Psychiatric Association (1987). *Diagnostic and Statistical Manual of Mental Disorders (Third Edition–Revised) DSM-IIIR*. Washington DC: American Psychiatric Association.

Ballard, C., Mohan, R.N.C., Patel, A. & Bannister, C. (1993). Idiopathic clouding of consciousness – do the patients have cortical Lewy body disease? *Int. J. Geriatr. Psychiatry*, **8**, 571–6.

Ballard, C.G., Saad, K., Patel, A. et al. (1995). The prevalence and phenomenology of psychotic symptoms in dementia sufferers. *Int. J. Geriatr. Psychiatry*, **10**, 477–85.

Bennett, D.A., Gilley, D.W. & Wilson, R.S. (1992). Rate of cognitive decline and neuroleptic use in Alzheimer's disease (AD). *Neurology*, **42** (suppl 3), 276.

Burns, A., Jacoby, R. & Levy, R. (1990). Psychiatric phenomena in Alzheimer's disease. II: Disorders of perception. *Br. J. Psychiatry*, **157**, 76–81.

Byrne, E.J., Lennox, G., Lowe, J. & Godwin-Austen, R.B. (1989). Diffuse Lewy body disease: clinical features in 15 cases. *J. Neurol. Neurosurg. Psychiatry*, **52**, 709–17.

Byrne, E.J., Lennox, G.G., Godwin-Austen, R.B. et al. (1991). Dementia associated with cortical Lewy bodies: proposed clinical diagnostic criteria. *Dementia*, **2**, 283–4.

Chen, C.P.L., Adler, J.T., Bowen, D.M. et al. (1996). Presynaptic serotonergic markers in community-acquired cases of Alzheimer's disease: correlations with depression and neuroleptic medication. *J. Neurochem.*, **66**, 1592–98.

Chui, H.C., Lyness, S.A., Sobel, E. & Schneider, L.S. (1994). Extrapyramidal signs and psychiatric symptoms predict faster cognitive decline in Alzheimer's disease. *Arch. Neurol.*, **51**, 676–81.

Crystal, H.A., Dickson, D.W., Lizardi, J.E., Davies, P. & Wolfson, L.I. (1990). Antemortem diagnosis of diffuse Lewy body disease. *Neurology*, **40**, 1523–8.

Cummings, J.L., Miller, B., Hill, M.A. et al. (1987). Neuropsychiatric aspects of multi-infarct dementia and dementia of the Alzheimer type. *Arch. Neurol.*, **44**, 389–93.

Deutsch, L.H., Bylsma, F.W., Rovner, B.W., Steele, C. & Folstein, M.F. (1991). Psychosis and physical aggression in probable Alzheimer's disease. *Am. J. Psychiatry*, **148**, 1159–63.

Drevets, W.C. & Rubin, E.H. (1989). Psychotic symptoms and the longitudinal course of senile dementia of the Alzheimer type. *Biol. Psychiatry*, **25**, 39–48.

Flynn, F.G., Cummings, J.L. & Gornbein, J. (1991). Delusions in dementia syndromes: investigation of behavioral and neuropsychological correlates. *J. Neuropsychiatry. Clin. Neurosci.*, **3**, 364–70.

Folstein, M.F., Folstein, S.E. & McHugh, P.R. (1975). 'Mini-Mental State': A practical method for grading the cognitive state of patients for the clinician. *J. Psychiatr. Res.*, **12**, 189–98.

Förstl, H., Besthorn, C., Geiger-Kabisch, C., Sattel, H. & Scheiter-Gasser, U. (1993a). Psychotic features and the course of Alzheimer's disease: relationship to cognitive, electroencephalographic and computerised tomography findings. *Acta Psychiatr. Scand.*, **87**, 395–9.

Förstl, H., Burns, A., Luthert, P., Cairns, N. & Levy, R. (1993b). The Lewy-body variant of Alzheimer's disease. Clinical and pathological findings. *Br. J. Psychiatry*, **162**, 385–92.

Foster, P. (1989). Neuroleptic equivalence. *Pharmaceutical J.*, Sept. 30, 431–2.

Gilley, D.W., Whaler, M.E., Wilson, R.S. & Bennett, D.A. (1991). Hallucinations and associated factors in Alzheimer's disease. *J. Neuropsychiatry. Clin. Neurosci.*, **3**, 371–6.

Hansen, L., Salmon, D., Galasko, D. et al. (1990). The Lewy body variant of Alzheimer's disease: a clinical and pathologic entity. *Neurology*, **40**, 1–8.

Hope, T. & Fairburn, C.G. (1992). The Present Behavioural Examination (PBE): the development of an interview to measure current behavioural abnormalities. *Psychol. Med.*, **22**, 223–30.

Jeste, D.V., Wragg, R.E., Salmon, D.P., Harris, M.J. & Thal, L.J. (1992). Cognitive deficits of patients with Alzheimer's disease with and without delusions. *Am. J. Psychiatry*, **149**, 184–9.

Lennox, G., Lowe, J., Landon, M., Byrne, E.J., Mayer, R.J. & Godwin-Austen, R.B. (1989). Diffuse Lewy body disease: correlative neuropathology using anti-ubiquitin immunocytochemistry. *J. Neurol. Neurosurg. Psychiatry*, **53**, 1236–47.

Mayeux, R., Stern, Y. & Spanton, S. (1985). Heterogeneity in dementia of the Alzheimer type. Evidence of subgroups. *Neurology*, **35**, 453–61.

McKeith, I.G., Perry, R.H., Fairbairn, A.F., Jabeen, S. & Perry, E.K. (1992a). Operational criteria for senile dementia of Lewy body type (SDLT). *Psychol. Med.*, **22**, 911–22.

McKeith, I., Fairbairn, A., Perry, R., Thompson, P. & Perry, E. (1992b). Neuroleptic sensitivity in patients with senile dementia of Lewy body type. *BMJ*, **305**, 673–8.

McKeith, I.G., Fairbairn, A.F., Bothwell, R.A. et al. (1994). An evaluation of the predictive validity and inter-rater reliability of clinical diagnostic criteria for senile dementia of Lewy body type. *Neurology*, **44**, 872–7.

McKhann, G., Drachman, D., Folstein, M., Katzman, R., Price, D. & Stadlan, E.M. (1984). Clinical diagnosis of Alzheimer's disease: Report of the NINCDS-ADRDA work group. *Neurology*, **34**, 939–44.

McShane, R., Gedling, K., Reading, M., McDonald, B., Esiri, M.M. & Hope, T. (1995). Prospective study of relations between cortical Lewy bodies, poor eyesight and hallucinations in Alzheimer's disease. *J. Neurol. Neurosurg. Psychiatry*, **59**, 185–8.

Mortimer, J.A., Ebbitt, B., Jun, S. & Finch, M. (1992). Predictors of cognitive and functional progression in patients with probable Alzheimer's disease. *Neurology*, **42**, 1689–96.

Reisberg, B., Ferris, S.H., de Leon, M.J. & Crook, T. (1981). The global deterioration scale for assessment of primary degenerative dementia. *Am. J. Psychiatry*, **139**, 1136–9.

Richards, M., Stern, Y. & Mayeux, R. (1993). Subtle extrapyramidal signs can predict the development of dementia in elderly individuals. *Neurology*, **43**, 2184–8.

Rosen, J. & Zubenko, G.S. (1991). Emergence of psychosis and depression in the longitudinal evaluation of Alzheimer's disease. *Biol. Psychiatry*, **29**, 224–32.

Steele, C., Rovner, B.W., Chase, G.A. & Folstein, M. (1990). Psychiatric symptoms and nursing home placement of patients with Alzheimer's disease. *Am. J. Psychiatry*, **147**, 1049–51.

Stern, Y., Albert, M., Brandt, J. et al. (1994). Utility of extrapyramidal signs and psychosis as predictors of cognitive and functional decline, nursing home admission, and death in Alzheimer's disease: Prospective analyses from the Predictors Study. *Neurology*, **44**, 2300–7.

Wilcock, G.K., Hope, R.A., Brooks, D.N. et al. (1989). Recommended minimum data to be collected in research studies on Alzheimer's disease. *J. Neurol. Neurosurg. Psychiatry*, **52**, 693–700.

Williams, S., Byrne, E.J. & Stokes, P. (1993). The treatment of diffuse Lewy body disease: A pilot study. *Int. J. Geriatr. Psychiatry*, **8**, 731–9.

8

Neuropsychological aspects of Lewy body dementia

D. P. SALMON and D. GALASKO

Summary

Recent clinico-neuropathological studies have shown that approximately 25% of patients who manifest a syndrome similar to dementia of the Alzheimer type during life have diffuse Lewy body disease (DLBD), a condition characterized by neocortical and subcortical Lewy body pathology that occurs, in many cases, along with the typical cortical distribution of senile plaques and neurofibrillary tangles associated with Alzheimer's disease (AD). Studies of the neuropsychology of this disorder demonstrate that DLBD, without concomitant AD, can produce a global dementia characterized by particularly pronounced deficits in memory (i.e. retrieval), attention, visuospatial abilities and psychomotor speed. When both DLBD and AD pathology is present, patients exhibit severe deficits in memory, language, and executive functions, most likely due to the severe hippocampal and neocortical damage that occurs in AD, as well as particularly severe deficits in visuospatial abilities, attention, and psychomotor processes, which may reflect the additive effects of Lewy body pathology. This pattern of neuropsychological deficits has also been observed in recent prospective studies of patients with clinically diagnosed DLBD, and may prove to be an important addition to the diagnostic criteria for DLBD.

8.1 Introduction

Recent clinico-neuropathological studies have shown that approximately 25% of patients who manifest a syndrome similar to dementia of the Alzheimer type during life have Lewy bodies diffusely distributed throughout the neocortex (for review, see Hansen & Galasko, 1992).

99

This cortical Lewy body pathology occurs along with the typical subcortical changes of Parkinson's disease (i.e. Lewy bodies and cell loss) in the substantia nigra and other pigmented brainstem nuclei, and in many cases with the typical cortical distribution of senile plaques and neurofibrillary tangles associated with Alzheimer's disease (AD) (Hansen et al., 1990). Clinically, these patients present with insidious and progressive cognitive decline with no other significant neurologic abnormalities, inexorably progress to severe dementia, and are often diagnosed with probable or possible Alzheimer's disease during life (e.g. Hansen et al., 1990). A variety of designations have been given to this clinico-neuropathologic entity including diffuse Lewy body disease, the Lewy body variant of AD, Lewy body dementia, and senile dementia of the Lewy body type (Hansen & Galasko, 1992).

Despite the similarities in the clinical presentation of the two disorders, retrospective studies indicate that patients with diffuse Lewy body disease (DLBD), with or without concomitant AD, may be distinguishable from those with 'pure' AD on the basis of specific neurological and neuropsychiatric features. Hansen and colleagues (Hansen et al., 1990; Galasko et al., in press) for example, found that patients with Lewy body disease and concomitant AD pathology differed from patients with 'pure' AD in that a greater proportion had mild parkinsonian or extrapyramidal motor findings (e.g. bradykinesia, rigidity, masked facies, gait abnormalities; but no resting tremor). A retrospective study by McKeith et al. (1992) of patients with Lewy body disease without sufficient neurofibrillary tangles to reach criteria for concomitant AD revealed that these patients were significantly more likely than 'pure' AD patients to manifest fluctuating cognitive impairment, visual or auditory hallucinations, unexplained falls, and extrapyramidal features at some point during the course of the disease. Based upon these and similar retrospective studies, investigators have had some success in developing clinical criteria for the prospective diagnosis of dementia associated with Lewy body disease (McKeith et al., 1992; 1994; Galasko et al., in press).

Although knowledge of the neuropathological, neurological and psychiatric features of DLBD has grown over the past 5 years, little is known about the neuropsychological manifestation of the disorder. In this chapter we will first review the few studies in which detailed cognitive testing had been performed with patients who ultimately received a neuropathological diagnosis that indicated the presence of cortical Lewy body disease with or without concomitant AD pathology. We will then discuss a number of recent studies that prospectively compare the cognitive deficits associated with clinically diagnosed Lewy body disease and AD. Because of the importance of extrapyramidal features in distinguishing between AD and Lewy body disease in some retrospective studies (e.g. Hansen et al., 1990), we will also discuss several studies that have compared the cognitive deficits apparent in clinically diagnosed AD patients with and without extrapyramidal features.

8.2 Neuropsychological features of autopsy-proven Lewy body disease

While a number of studies have shown through retrospective review of records that patients with neuropathologically proven DLBD were demented, very few have provided evidence concerning the specific nature of the cognitive impairment engendered by this disease. In one study that addressed this issue, Gibb et al. (1985) reviewed the records of four patients with DLBD, two with significant concomitant AD pathology and two without, and found that all four evidenced memory impairment, three of the four had mild dysphasia or confrontation naming deficits, and one was impaired on the digit span, block design and object assembly subtests from the Wechsler Adult Intelligence Scale (WAIS). In a similar but larger study, Byrne et al. (1989) found that of 15 patients with confirmed DLBD (with or without concomitant AD) all had impaired memory, 10 had dyscalculia, nine had constructional and ideomotor dyspraxia, and eight had dysphasia.

To determine if DLBD produced a pattern of neuropsychological impairment distinguishable from that of 'pure' AD, Förstl et al. (1993) compared the cognitive deficits of eight patients having DLBD with that of eight age- and gender-matched patients with AD. The groups did not differ with regard to age at onset of symptoms, duration of illness, or initial severity of cognitive impairment as measured by the CAMCOG. Examination of the specific cognitive functions measured by CAMCOG subscores revealed no differences between the groups in level of impairment of language, praxis, or memory.

In a study by McKeith et al. (1992) the cognitive functioning of 21 patients with autopsy-verified DLBD (and some AD pathology) was compared with that of 37 patients having AD. Although the groups did not differ in age or gender distribution, the DLBD patients had a significantly shorter duration of illness at first presentation than the AD patients and performed significantly better on the standardized Mental Test Score of Blessed. Examination of the recall component of the Mental Test Score revealed that the memory of the DLBD patients was less severely impaired than that of the AD patients. The groups did not differ significantly on a test measuring temporal and parietal lobe function or on a behavior rating scale. McKeith et al. (1992) also reported that the case notes for the patients with Lewy body disease often referred to fluctuating disorders of language and visuospatial abilities.

In a quite detailed study, Hansen et al. (1990) compared the performances of patients with the Lewy body variant (LBV) of AD (DLBD with concomitant AD pathology) and 'pure' AD on a battery of neuropsychological tests designed to assess memory, attention, language, conceptualization and visuospatial abilities. Nine patients with LBV were matched one-to-one to nine patients with AD on the basis of age, education, overall level of global dementia as assessed by the Information–Memory–Concentration test of Blessed, and the interval between testing and death. The results indicated that despite equivalent levels of global dementia, the patients with LBV performed significantly worse than the patients with pure AD on a test of attention (the Digit Span subtest from the WAIS – revised), and on tests of visuospatial and constructional ability (the Block Design subtest from the Wechsler Intelligence Scale for Children – revised and the Copy-a-Cross test). In addition, the LBV and AD patients produced different patterns of impairment on tests of verbal fluency. The LBV group scored significantly lower than the pure AD group on the phonemically-based letter fluency task (generating words that begin with a particular letter), but the two groups performed similarly on the semantically based category fluency task (producing words that belong to a particular category). In contrast to these differences, the groups were equivalently impaired on tests of episodic memory, confrontation naming (e.g. the Boston naming test), and arithmetic.

Hansen and colleagues interpreted the pattern of cognitive deficits produced by the patients with LBV within a framework that distinguishes between so-called 'cortical' and 'subcortical' dementia syndromes (Cummings, 1990). Numerous studies have shown that AD, a prototypical 'cortical' dementia, is broadly characterized by prominent amnesia (due to ineffective consolidation and rapid forgetting) and additional deficits in language and semantic knowledge (aphasia), abstract reasoning, other 'executive' functions, and constructional and visuospatial abilities. In contrast, the dementia associated with Huntington's disease or Parkinson's disease, forms of 'subcortical' dementia, includes only a moderate memory disturbance (due primarily to a deficiency in retrieving stored information), bradykinesia and bradyphrenia, attentional dysfunction, problem solving deficits, visuoperceptual and construction deficits, and a deficiency in performing arithmetic. Subcortical dementia results in little or no aphasia, although patients may be dysarthric due to motor dysfunction.

When the results from the Hansen et al. (1990) study were viewed from the perspective of this framework, patients with LBV appeared to exhibit a superimposition of cortical and subcortical neuropsychological impairments. The two groups demonstrated equivalent deficits in cognitive abilities usually affected by AD (e.g. memory, confrontation naming), but the LBV patients displayed disproportionately severe deficits in cognitive abilities such as attention, verbal fluency and visuospatial processing that are prominently affected in subcortical dementia. This superimposition of the neuropsychological features of cortical and subcortical dementia in the LBV patients is consistent with the distribution of neuropathological changes in the brains of these patients. All of the patients in the Hansen et al. (1990) study had the typical neuropathological changes of AD in the hippocampus and association cortices, as well as the subcortical and diffusely distributed neocortical changes associated with diffuse Lewy body disease.

Although the Hansen et al. (1990) study suggests that the Lewy body pathology present in LBV contributes importantly to the dementia associated with the disease, the extent of this contribution, and the particular pattern of neuropsychological deficits that may be associated with the presence of cortical and subcortical Lewy bodies without concomitant AD, cannot be easily determined by studying these patients. This issue was addressed, however, in a recently completed study of five patients who clinically resembled patients with AD, or LBV, but who at autopsy were found to have DLBD with little or no AD pathology (Salmon et al., in press).

All five of the patients in the Salmon et al. (in press) study initially presented with cognitive decline that began insidiously and subsequently developed mild extrapyramidal motor dysfunction. By the time of their initial clinical evaluation, three of the five patients had developed visual, auditory or tactile hallucinations, and two had developed delusions. They were all clinically diagnosed with probable or possible AD or one of its variants (Lewy body variant of AD, mixed AD and vascular dementia). At autopsy, subcortical and diffusely distributed cortical Lewy bodies were observed in the brains of all five patients. Alzheimer disease pathology was absent in two of the cases and at a level comparable to that found in normal elderly individuals in the other three cases.

Despite only borderline to mild impairment on the Mini-Mental State Examination at the time of the neuropsychological evaluation (range = 22–26), all five DLBD patients demonstrated global cognitive decline on more rigorous testing, with deficits in memory, attention, language, executive functions, and visuospatial and visuoconstructional abilities. However, the pattern and severity of their neuropsychological deficits differed somewhat from that typically observed in patients with AD.

With regard to memory, for example, the DLBD patients scored 2 to 3 standard deviations below normal performance on key measures of the California Verbal Learning Test (CVLT), including learning on trials 1 through 5, recall on trial 5, short- and long-delay free recall, and recognition discriminability. These scores did not, however, reflect the very poor retention over delay intervals, increased propensity to produce intrusion errors in the cued recall condition, and very poor recognition discriminability typical of AD (Delis et al., 1991). Indeed, when the scores achieved by the DLBD patients on the CVLT were subjected to discriminant function equations that have been previously shown to effectively distinguish between patients with cortical (e.g. Alzheimer's disease) and subcortical (e.g. Huntington's disease) dementia syndromes, four of the five DLBD patients were classified as 'subcortical' and one as 'cortical'. Delis et al. (1991) have postulated that these distinct memory profiles arise from a consolidation deficit in patients with a cortical dementia syndrome, but a retrieval deficit in patients with a subcortical dementia syndrome.

The nature of the memory deficit associated with DLBD is consistent with the neuropathology of the disorder. Although some investigators have demonstrated that ubiquitin-immunoreactive dystrophic neurites are often present in the CA2/CA3 region of the hippocampus in DLBD (Dickson et al., 1991), the hippocampus and related structures (e.g. entorhinal cortex, parahippocampal gyrus) that are thought to underlie memory consolidation (storage) are generally less damaged than in AD. In contrast, DLBD patients have a particularly severe reduction in dopaminergic projection to the striatum (Perry et al., 1990), and striatal dysfunction has been linked to a retrieval deficit (Cummings, 1990).

To further examine the profile of neuropsychological deficits associated with DLBD and AD, Salmon and colleagues directly compared the performance of the DLBD patients with that of five patients having autopsy-proven 'pure' AD on a variety of cognitive tests. The DLBD and

AD patients were matched one-to-one on the basis of global level of dementia (as measured by the Dementia Rating Scale; DRS) at the time of testing.

Although the DLBD and AD patients were equally impaired on the WAIS-R Digit Span subtest, the Boston Naming Test, the letter and category versions of the Verbal Fluency test, and the WAIS-R Similarities subtest, significant differences between the groups were noted in a number of cognitive functions. For example, the DLBD and AD patients differed on two of the five subtests of the DRS. The DLBD patients were significantly worse than the AD patients on the Construction subtest, whereas the AD patients performed worse than the DLBD patients on the Memory subtest. When the subjects' subtest scores were subjected to discriminant function equations that distinguish between patients with cortical and subcortical dementia syndromes, all five DLBD patients exhibited a DRS subtest profile consistent with subcortical dementia while four of the five patients with Alzheimer's disease exhibited a profile consistent with cortical dementia.

One of the most striking differences between the DLBD and AD patients was evident on tests of visuospatial and visuoconstructive ability. Patients with DLBD performed significantly worse than the AD patients on the WISC-R Block Design subtest with four of the five DLBD patients performing at floor levels and the fifth severely impaired. A similarly severe deficit was evident on the Clock Drawing test with the DLBD patients performing significantly worse than the AD patients on the copy, but not the command, condition of this task. Qualitative analyses of the clocks revealed that the DLBD and AD groups performed similarly in terms of the proportion of subjects producing conceptual, stimulus bound and graphic errors in the command and copy conditions, but a significantly greater proportion of DLBD (five of five patients) than AD (one of five patients) patients produced errors related to the spatial layout of the clock in the copy condition. As Salmon et al. (in press) suggest, the DLBD patients' particularly severe deficit in visuospatial and visuoconstructive abilities may be the result of an additive effect of the two types of pathology producing worse impairment in the DLBD patients than in patients with only cortical (e.g. AD) or subcortical (e.g. Parkinson's disease) dysfunction.

A prominent difference between DLBD and AD patients was also observed on tests of psychomotor speed. All five DLBD patients were severely impaired on both parts A and B of the Trail-Making test, and were significantly slower than the AD patients in both conditions. It is unlikely that this severe deficit was due primarily to impaired executive functions since the patients were only mildly impaired, at worst, on other tests of executive functions such as the WAIS-R Similarities subtest and the Conceptualization subtest from the DRS.

The results of the study by Salmon et al. (in press) has important implications concerning the neuropsychological aspects of Lewy body disease and for the relationship between the clinical and neuropathological features of LBV. It is now clear that subcortical and diffusely distributed neocortical Lewy body pathology, without concomitant AD pathology, can produce global cognitive impairment with particularly severe deficits in visuospatial/visuoconstructive and psychomotor abilities. In LBV, this pathology is superimposed on the neuropathological changes that typically occur in AD, and the resulting neuropsychological impairment appears to reflect the effects of both. For example, patients with LBV, like patients with pure AD, have severe deficits in memory, language, and executive functions, most likely due to the severe hippocampal and neocortical damage that occurs in AD (Hansen et al., 1990). In addition, patients with LBV, like patients with DLBD, have particularly severe deficits in visuospatial abilities, attention, and psychomotor processes, which may reflect the effects of Lewy body pathology. Thus, both Lewy body pathology and AD pathology appear to contribute importantly to the clinical manifestation of LBV.

8.3 Neuropsychological deficits associated with clinically defined Lewy body disease

As mentioned previously, some investigators have established clinical criteria for the diagnosis of Lewy body dementia based on retrospective examination of the neurological and neuropsychiatric characteristics of autopsy verified cases (McKeith et al., 1992). The application of these criteria has allowed individuals with probable Lewy body disease to be identified and provided the opportunity for prospective studies of the neuropsychological features of the disorder. Although these criteria have been shown to provide relatively high diagnostic sensitivity and specificity when related to neuropathologic findings (e.g. McKeith et al., 1994), it should be kept in mind that the results of these prospective studies must remain tentative without autopsy confirmation of the disease.

A series of studies by Sahgal et al. (1992a,b) examined attention, learning, and memory in patients with probable senile dementia of the

Lewy body type (SDLT) using the Cambridge Neuropsychological Test Automated Battery, a microcomputer and touch-screen based test procedure. As demonstrated by McKeith et al. (1992), the clinical criteria for SDLT primarily identify individuals with DLBD and senile plaques, but without sufficient numbers of neurofibrillary tangles to support a diagnosis of concomitant AD. In an initial study in this series, Galloway and colleagues (Galloway et al., 1992) compared the performance of 10 patients with senile dementia of the Alzheimer type (SDAT), seven patients with SDLT, and 16 elderly normal control subjects on a recognition memory test and a conditional pattern-location paired-associated learning task. The SDAT and SDLT groups did not differ significantly in age or estimated premorbid verbal IQ and were equally demented as measured by the MMSE and the clinical dementia rating (CDR) scale. The recognition memory test involved the initial presentation of 12 abstract line pattern stimuli followed by a 12 trial two-choice recognition test in which one of the initial stimuli had to be discriminated from a paired distractor stimulus on each trial. The conditional pattern-location paired-associate learning task required subjects to identify the location of particular target stimuli which had been previously presented in one of six possible locations comprising a spatial array. The number of target stimuli to be paired with a particular location in the spatial array on each trial increased from one to eight (with the addition of two spatial locations) as the test progressed. Incorrect trials were repeated for a maximum of 10 trials at each stimulus level.

The results of this study indicated that both the SDAT and SDLT patients were impaired on the recognition test compared with control subjects, but did not differ from each other. In contrast, the SDLT patients performed significantly worse than the SDAT patients on the conditional pattern-location learning task in terms of the number of trials required to complete the task. Both patients groups were significantly worse than normal control subjects on this task.

A second study in this series compared the short-term recognition memory abilities of the same SDAT and SDLT subjects using simultaneous and delayed matching to sample tasks (Sahgal et al., 1992a). In this task, a sample stimulus was presented and the subject had to choose and respond to the same stimulus when it was presented in an array with three distractor stimuli. In the simultaneous condition, the sample remained visible until the subject made their response to one of the four choice stimuli. In the delay condition, the sample was extinguished after its presentation and the four choice stimuli were presented after a delay of

0, 4 or 12 s. The performances of the SDLT and SDAT patients in the simultaneous condition did not differ, but were both impaired relative to that of control subjects. Both patient groups also performed significantly worse than control subjects in the delayed condition; however, the SDLT patients performed worse than the SDAT patients in this condition at all delay intervals.

Sahgal and colleagues (Sahgal et al., 1992b) also examined the performance of these SDLT and SDAT patients on tests of visual attention. Focal attention was assessed with a visual search task in which a target stimulus (an abstract dot pattern) was presented in the center of a computer screen and, two seconds later, 1, 2, 4, or 8 choice stimuli appeared in eight surrounding locations. Subjects were required to touch the choice stimulus that was identical to the target stimulus as quickly as possible. To assess complex attentional processes, an attention set-shifting paradigm was used which included a simple two-choice discrimination problem with compound stimuli and shifts in the discrimination problem that were either intradimensional (i.e. the stimuli changed but the relevant dimension remained the same) or extradimensional (i.e. the stimuli and the relevant dimension changed).

The SDLT patients performed significantly worse than the SDAT patients and the normal control subjects on the visual search task, but the latter two groups did not differ significantly from each other. Thus, focal attention appears to be selectively impaired in SDLT patients. On the more complex set-shifting paradigm, both patient groups were impaired and did not differ significantly from each other in any of the conditions. The SDLT patients did, however, demonstrate a tendency to have more difficulty than the SDAT patients when an intradimensional shift was required. This tendency for a greater loss of attentional efficiency may be indicative of more severe frontal lobe dysfunction in SDLT patients than in SDAT patients.

The most recent study in this series compared the performance of SDLT and SDAT patients on a spatial working memory task which assessed both spatial memory and the ability to use an efficient search strategy (Sahgal et al., 1995). Subjects were required to search through a number of boxes (2, 3, 4, 6 or 8 per trial) presented on a computer screen in order to locate a hidden 'token'. Two types of errors were recorded in this task: within-search errors in which a subject re-examined an empty box before finding a token on the current trial, and between-search errors in which a subject searched a box where a token had already been found on the current trial (despite explicit instructions to the contrary).

Although both patient groups were equivalently impaired on a simple visual span task similar to the Corsi blocks test, they performed differently on the spatial working memory task. SDLT patients made more within-search errors and between-search errors than the SDAT patients, particularly on the larger set size trials (6 or 8 boxes). Both groups were impaired on this task relative to the control subjects at the larger set sizes. An examination of the search strategies used when performing the task showed no differences between the SDLT and SDAT patients. Because poor performance on the spatial working memory task has been linked to frontal lobe dysfunction, these results support Sahgal et al.'s (1995) suggestion that SDLT patients may have more severe frontal pathology than SDAT patients.

Taken together, the studies of Sahgal and colleagues reviewed above suggest that, despite equivalent levels of global dementia, SDLT patients perform significantly worse than patients with SDAT on tests of focal and complex attention, and on memory tests that have a conditional element (e.g. the conditional pattern-location paired-associate learning task) or that require efficient search strategies (e.g. the spatial working memory task). Tests of this nature have been shown previously to be sensitive to frontal lobe dysfunction and to disorders such as Parkinson's disease which are thought to interrupt the fronto-striatal circuits of the brain. Thus, the neuropsychological deficits that occur in patients with probable SDLT are similar in some respects to the pattern of cognitive deficits that have been observed in retrospective studies of patients with neuropathologically proven DLBD (particularly with concomitant AD), and may reflect the effects of neocortical and subcortical Lewy body pathology with a possible contribution from additional AD pathology.

Although extrapyramidal motor signs (EPS) are not used as one of the primary clinical diagnostic criteria for SDLT by McKeith and colleagues (1992), other investigators have emphasized the importance of this feature for differentiating between Lewy body disease and AD. Galasko, Hansen and colleagues (Hansen et al., 1990; Galasko et al., in press), for example, reported that mild EPS were present to a much greater degree in patients with autopsy-proven Lewy body disease than in those with pure AD, and suggested that this feature of the syndrome might play a key role in the development of clinical criteria for the disorder. Because of the close association between EPS in demented patients and the presence of Lewy body disease, studies that have compared the pattern of neuropsychological deficits in clinically diagnosed AD patients who do or do not exhibit EPS may provide information about cognitive aspects of Lewy body disease.

Studies that have compared the neuropsychological test performance of AD patients with and without EPS have generally found that those with EPS have the same degree of impairment as those without EPS in cognitive abilities that are prominently affected by AD, such as long-term memory and confrontation naming. However, AD patients with EPS often exhibit disproportionately severe cognitive deficits in cognitive abilities that are thought to be mediated, at least in part, by the fronto-striatal circuits that are disrupted in subcortical dementing disorders.

Richards et al. (1993) for example, found that AD patients with EPS performed significantly worse than those without EPS on measures of short-term verbal memory, orientation, naming, verbal fluency, and constructional ability. In contrast, the performance of the two AD groups did not differ on measures of long-term memory, abstract reasoning, phrase repetition, or verbal comprehension. These results, according to Richards et al. (1993) suggest that AD patients with EPS exhibit a pattern of cognitive deficits typical of AD along with disproportionately severe deficits in cognitive functions that are also affected in Parkinson's disease.

A similar finding was reported by Merello et al. (1994). These investigators found that AD patients with EPS performed worse than those without EPS on a number of tests sensitive to frontal lobe dysfunction (see also Girling and Berrios, 1990). AD patients with severe EPS (parkinsonism) performed significantly worse than the AD patients without EPS on the Wisconsin Card Sorting test, the Trail-Making test, a verbal fluency task, Raven's Progressive Matrices test, a backward digit span test, and the Block Design test. AD patients with milder and fewer EPS (isolated EPS) performed worse than those without EPS on the Wisconsin Card Sorting test, the Trail-Making test, Raven's Progressive Matrices test, a Block Design test, and Benton's Visual Retention test. It should be noted that despite these differences the three AD groups did not differ significantly on tests of long-term memory (the Buschke Selective Reminding test), verbal comprehension (the Token test), or confrontation naming (the Boston naming test).

Soininen et al. (1992) performed a longitudinal study of the cognitive decline that occurred in AD patients with and without EPS. In the initial evaluation there were no significant differences between the two AD patient groups on tests of a variety of cognitive functions (e.g. memory, language, praxis and visuospatial abilities). After one year, however, the AD patients without EPS had declined significantly only on a test of confrontation naming, while those with EPS had declined on tests of reasoning and abstraction, visuospatial abilities, praxis, verbal fluency, language processing, and confrontation naming. The AD patients with EPS also declined on the recall, but not the recognition, component of a verbal memory test.

The pattern of cognitive impairment exhibited by the AD patients with EPS in these studies is reminiscent of that of patients with autopsy-confirmed LBV or DLBD. In both cases patients display cognitive deficits indicative of fronto-striatal dysfunction superimposed upon deficits that are typically associated with the neuropathologic changes of AD. Thus, AD patients with EPS, like patients with LBV or DLBD, have deficits in memory and language which are equivalent to those of patients with 'pure' AD, as well as disproportionately severe deficits in cognitive functions that are mediated to some degree by fronto-striatal circuits, such as attention, retrieval, constructional abilities and psychomotor speed.

8.4 Conclusions

The available evidence now clearly supports the contention that DLBD, without concomitant AD pathology, can produce a global dementia characterized by particularly pronounced deficits in memory (retrieval), attention, visuospatial abilities and psychomotor speed, with additional impairment of language and executive functions. These neuropsychological deficits are consistent with the neocortical and subcortical brain damage that occurs in the disease. Neuropathological abnormalities in the neocortex of patients with DLBD may contribute to such cortical features of the dementia as impaired memory, language, executive functions, and visuospatial abilities, whereas neuropathological changes in the substantia nigra, and the corresponding depletion of dopaminergic input to the striatum, most likely contribute to the neuropsychological deficts that are usually associated with subcortical dysfunction, such as impaired learning, attention, visuoconstructive abilities and psychomotor speed (for review, see Cummings, 1990).

When the neuropathological changes of DLBD occur in conjunction with those of AD, as in the Lewy body variant of AD, the neuropsychological features of the disorder reflect the superimposition of the two types of pathology. Thus, LBV patients have severe deficits in memory, language, and executive functions, most likely due to the severe hippocampal and neocortical damage that occurs in AD, as well as particularly severe deficits in visuospatial abilities, attention, and psychomotor processes, which may reflect the additive effects of Lewy body pathology.

The pattern of neuropsychological deficits observed in retrospective studies of patients with autopsy-confirmed DLBD, with or without concomitant AD, have also been observed in recent prospective studies of patients with clinically diagnosed SDLT and in patients with clinically diagnosed AD who exhibit mild extrapyramidal motor dysfunction. Even at a relatively early stage of disease, demented patients with presumed Lewy body pathology often exhibit prominent deficits in attention, retrieval, visuospatial abilities, and other abilities affected by fronto-striatal dysfunction. Consideration of these neuropsychological features may improve the accuracy with which DLBD can be diagnosed during life.

Acknowledgement

Preparation of this chapter was supported in part by funds from NIA grants AG-05131 and AG-12963, and NIMH grant MH-48819.

References

Byrne, E.J., Lennox, G., Lowe, J. & Godwin-Austen, R.B. (1989). Diffuse Lewy body disease: Clinical features in 15 cases. *J. Neurol., Neurosurg. Psychiatry*, **52**, 709–17.

Cummings, J.L. (1990). *Subcortical Dementia*. New York: Oxford University Press.

Delis, D.C., Massman, P.J., Butters, N., Salmon, D.P., Cermak, L.S. & Kramer, J.H. (1991). Profiles of demented and amnesic patients on the California Verbal Learning Test: Implications for the assessment of memory disorders. *Psychol. Assess.*, **3**, 19–26.

Dickson, D.W., Ruan, D., Crystal, H. et al. (1991). Hippocampal degeneration differentiates diffuse Lewy body disease (DLBD) from Alzheimer's disease: Light and electron microscopic immunocytochemistry of CA2-3 neurites specific to DLBD. *Neurology*, **41**, 1402–9.

Förstl, H., Burns, A., Luthert, P., Cairns, N. & Levy, R. (1993). The Lewy-body variant of Alzheimer's disease: Clinical and pathological findings. *Bri. J. Psychiatry*, **162**, 385–92.

Galasko, D., Katzman, R., Salmon, D.P., Thal, L.J. & Hansen, L. (in press). Clinical and neuropathological findings in Lewy body dementias. *Brain and Cognition*.

Galloway, P.H., Sahgal, A., McKeith, I.G. et al. (1992). Visual pattern recognition memory and learning deficits in senile dementias of Alzheimer and Lewy body types. *Dementia*, **3**, 101–7.

Gibb, W.R.G., Esiri, M.M. & Lees, A.J. (1985). Clinical and pathological features of diffuse cortical Lewy body disease (Lewy body dementia). *Brain*, **110**, 1131–53.

Girling, D.M. & Berrios, G.E. (1990). Extrapyramidal signs, primitive reflexes and frontal lobe function in senile dementia of the Alzheimer type. *Br. J. Psychiatry*, **157**, 888–93.

Hansen, L.A. & Galasko, D. (1992). Lewy body disease. *Curr. Opin. Neurol. Neurosurg.*, **5**, 889–94.

Hansen, L., Salmon, D., Galasko, D. et al. (1990). The Lewy body variant of Alzheimer's disease: A clinical and pathologic entity. *Neurology*, **40**, 1–8.

McKeith, I.G., Perry, R.H., Fairbairn, A.F., Jabeen, S. & Perry, E.K. (1992). Operational criteria for senile dementia of Lewy body type (SDLT). *Psychol. Med.*, **22**, 911–22.

McKeith, I.G., Fairbairn, A.F., Bothwell, R.A. et al. (1994). An evaluation of the predictive validity and inter-rater reliability of clinical diagnostic criteria for senile dementia of Lewy body type. *Neurology*, **44**, 872–7.

Merello, M., Sabe, L., Teson, A. et al. (1994). Extrapyramidalism in Alzheimer's disease: Prevalence, psychiatric, and neuropsychological correlates. *J. Neurol., Neurosurg. Psychiatry*, **57**, 1503–9.

Perry, R.H., Irving, D., Blessed, G., Fairbairn, A. & Perry, E.K. (1990). Senile dementia of the Lewy body type: A clinically and neuropathologically distinct form of Lewy body dementia in the elderly. *J. Neurolog. Sci.*, **95**, 119–39.

Richards, M., Bell, K., Dooneief, G. et al. (1993). Patterns of neuropsychological performance in Alzheimer's disease patients with and without extrapyramidal signs. *Neurology*, **43**, 1708–11.

Sahgal, A., Galloway, P.H., McKeith, I.G. et al. (1992a). Matching-to-sample deficits in patients with senile dementias of the Alzheimer and Lewy body types. *Arch. Neurol.*, **49**, 1043–6.

Sahgal, A., Galloway, P.H., McKeith, I.G., Edwardson, J.A. & Lloyd, S. (1992b). A comparative study of attentional deficits in senile dementias of Alzheimer and Lewy body types. *Dementia*, **3**, 350–4.

Sahgal, A., McKeith, I.G., Galloway, P.H., Tasker, N. & Steckler, T. (1995). Do differences in visuospatial ability between senile dementias of the Alzheimer and Lewy body types reflect differences solely in mnemonic function? *J. Clin. Exp. Neuropsychol.*, **17**, 35–43.

Salmon, D.P., Galasko, D., Hansen, L.A. et al. (in press). Neuropsychological deficits associated with diffuse Lewy body disease. *Brain and Cognition*.

Soininen, H., Helkala, E.L., Laulumaa, V., Soikkeli, R., Hartikainen, P. & Riekkinen, P.J. (1992). Cognitive profile of Alzheimer patients with extrapyramidal signs: A longitudinal study. *J. Neural Transm.*, **4**, 241–54.

9

The neuroanatomical basis of cognitive deficits in Lewy body dementia

A. SAHGAL

Summary

Using computerized neuropsychological tests of nonverbal visual recognition memory and attention/planning (which require intact temporal and fronto-striatal circuitry respectively), we have obtained evidence to support the view that senile dementias of Alzheimer's (SDAT) and Lewy body (SDLT) type can be distinguished from each other. The main conclusions reviewed here are that while both SDAT and SDLT patients suffer severe mnemonic deficiencies, which reflect degeneration of temporal lobe structures, SDLT patients have, in addition, attentional impairments which could arise from damage to dopaminergic fronto-striatal mechanisms. In this latter respect, the cognitive aspects of the SDLT disorder resemble those seen in Parkinson's disease (PD) patients and others with frontal lobe dysfunctions.

9.1 Introduction

This review does not need to begin with a description of Lewy body dementia; the numerous reports in this book bear testimony to growing research interest in this disease. The aim is to provide a neuropsychological contribution to these efforts. But what can neuropsychology offer? By studying alterations in specific cognitive abilities under controlled conditions in a large group of subjects, we can obtain a precise idea of the nature of cognitive decline in the disorder and contrast it with related diseases such as senile dementia of the Alzheimer type. Moreover, experimental studies – usually on animal subjects – have, over many years, provided us with a great deal of evidence as to which neural pathways mediate what cognitive processes. Thus, neuropsychological studies can

114

help pinpoint the neuroanatomical focus of a given cognitive dysfunction. This is especially valuable, since cognitive ability can be studied in the early stages of a disease and we can therefore determine which circuits and/or neural structures start to degenerate first; this has obvious implications for therapy and care.

We shall discuss findings which we have reported with respect to senile dementias of Alzheimer's type (SDAT) and Lewy body type (SDLT), together with preliminary data on a cohort of patients with Parkinson's disease (PD), using the recently developed CANTAB (Cambridge Neuropsychological Test Automated Battery) (Galloway et al., 1992; Sahgal et al., 1991, 1992a,b,c, 1995; Owens et al., unpublished). Computerized methods have unique advantages, including: precise presentation of stimuli; automatic and accurate recording of response latencies; use of the same basic procedure to assess a range of different cognitive abilities; nonverbal response requirement; interesting tasks which help maintain a high level of motivation; built-in controls for any motor disability; use of titration procedures to automatically and continuously adjust the difficulty of a given task, depending on ongoing performance – this avoids 'ceiling' or 'floor' effects. Finally, and perhaps most importantly, the tasks included in CANTAB, which test visual memory, planning and attention, were carefully selected. Thus, there are tests of recognition memory sensitive to temporal lobe (cortical, hippocampal) damage. Other tasks require intact frontal or fronto-striatal structures and circuitry necessary to efficiently execute attentional, strategic planning and certain memory functions. These constitute some of the main deficiencies seen in dementia.

CANTAB has been used to test patients with mild to moderate SDAT or PD, and has provided clear insights into the differences that exist. The main conclusions to be drawn are that SDAT is characterized by impairments in mnemonic function, reflecting the involvement of temporal lobe structures and circuitry (Sahakian et al., 1988, 1990; Sahgal et al., 1991, 1992a,b and c, 1995; Galloway et al., 1992). In contrast, PD patients, and those with frontal lobe dysfunctions, show attentional/planning deficits, which point to fronto-striatal circuit damage (Sahakian et al., 1988; Downes et al., 1989; Owen et al., 1990, 1991, 1992, 1993; Chari et al., 1996; Owens et al., unpublished).

Neurochemical, neuropathological and clinical investigations of SDLT have confirmed that these patients share features with both SDAT and PD patients. For example, there is little, if any, nigro-striatal dopaminergic loss in SDAT, about 50% in SDLT and 80% in PD (Perry et al., 1990). Indeed, in some ways SDLT can be thought of as falling between the two extremes. It was thought of interest to apply the relevant CANTAB range of tests in order to further our understanding of the disease and to provide suggestions as to where its neuroanatomical foci may lie.

9.2 Preliminary procedures

9.2.1 Subjects

All subjects were matched for age (mean of around 75 years). SDAT patients were diagnosed as having probable SDAT using the NINCDS–ADRDA criteria (McKhann et al., 1984), and SDLT was established according to clinical criteria for this disease (McKeith et al., 1992, 1994). Data for 16 healthy controls and for the two spatial tests (SS and SWM) 9 SDAT and 10 SDLT patients are reviewed; in the four nonspatial tests, 10 SDAT and 7 SDLT patients participated. In the PD study, there were 10 controls and 9 PD patients.

Preliminary tests were carried out to ensure that the SDAT and SDLT groups were evenly matched for pre-morbid ability, screen the elderly control subjects for possible dementia, and ensure that all subjects possessed adequate sensorimotor capabilities. A number of standard psychometric (for example, the Mini-Mental State Examination (MMSE) and the National Adult Reading Test (NART)) and motor tests were used. In brief, both the dementing groups were evenly matched for global cognitive ability and were in the milder stages of dementia. However, the tests indicated that both were impaired relative to control (as we might expect). None of the control subjects were found to be in the dementing range. Motor screening tests suggested that the SDAT group was not significantly different from control, but that the SDLT group was slower than both control and SDAT groups. Details of these tests may be found elsewhere (Galloway et al., 1992; Sahgal et al., 1995).

Care was taken to ensure that SDLT patients were not tested during a period of marked confusion. None of the patients was taking any drugs which might have affected performance. The studies were approved by the local ethics committee, and informed consent was also obtained from all participants and/or carers.

9.3 CANTAB procedures and results

Stimuli were generated by microcomputer (British Broadcasting Corporation Master 128, manufactured by Acorn Computers Ltd, Cambridge, UK) and presented on a 14-inch (36-cm) colour monitor fitted with a touch-screen (Microvitec plc, Bradford, UK; models 1451 and 501 respectively). For some tests, a nonlatching, hand-operated, switch fitted with a light spring for comfortable hand operation was connected to the computer. Subjects sat in a comfortable position about 0.5 m from the touch-screen. The computer, which was handled only by the experimenter, was placed a short distance away. Thus, subjects responded only via the touch-screen.

The experimenter first explained the nature of each task to the subject, and all procedures and response requirements were demonstrated in a number of practice trials. Audio-visual feedback (tones and ticks or crosses) was provided in most cases. The tests reported here took about 3 hours to complete, and were not necessarily completed in a single session.

Data concerning performances measured as percentage correct, trials completed (or to criterion) errors, stimulus/response choice and latencies were automatically recorded as appropriate. Statistical analysis employed both parametric analysis of variance (ANOVA) as well as nonparametric methods if the data required it. Means were compared using appropriate tests such as the Newman-Keuls.

9.3.1 Pattern recognition (PR)

This memory task is sensitive to temporal, but not frontal, lobe damage.

Twelve abstract line patterns, enclosed by a 4 × 4 cm square outline, were sequentially presented for 3 seconds each on the centre of the screen and had to be memorized. When the entire list had been presented, and 5 seconds after the last stimulus, 12 pairs of stimuli were sequentially presented side by side. One stimulus in each pair was novel, the other had occurred in the original list; the subject had to point to the familiar one. A second list of 12 new stimuli was presented soon after testing on the first list had finished. Examples of the stimuli are given elsewhere (Owen et al., 1993).

With respect to percentage correct (accuracy), there was a main effect of group ($p < 0.001$), which further analysis showed was due to differences between the SDAT and SDLT groups compared with control; the two patient groups were not different from each other (Fig. 9.1). In the PD study, no group difference was found.

In terms of latency of responding the SDAT and SDLT groups did not differ from each other significantly, but both groups, as well as PD patients, responded slower than their respective controls ($p < 0.01$). The means, in seconds were: (SDAT/SDLT study) control 2.87 ± 0.24; SDAT 4.99 ± 0.46 and SDLT 8.93 ± 2.74.

9.3.2 Matching to sample (MTS)

This recognition memory task is sensitive to temporal lobe damage.

MTS involved the opening of a 4 × 4 cm red box, located at the top centre of the screen, to reveal a sample stimulus which was one of a number of abstract dot patterns involving different arrangements of two components: four types of shape and four colours, measuring 2 cm long × 1 cm high. This was followed by the opening of four boxes which revealed four different choice stimuli in a row along the screen. One stimulus was always identical in shapes and colours to the sample stimulus, a second differed in shapes but had the same colour components, the

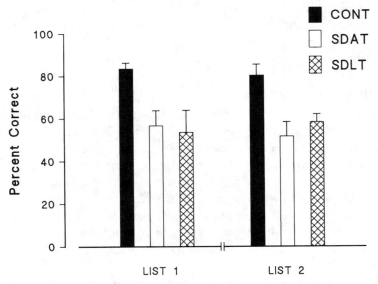

Fig. 9.1 PR percent correct (± SEM; CONT = control group); both SDAT and SDLT patients were equivalently impaired. From Galloway et al., 1992, reproduced with permission from Karger, Basel.

third in colours but not shapes, and the fourth (a distractor) was different in both shapes and colours (see Owen et al., 1993).

In simultaneous matching to sample (SMTS), a 'control' condition which helps to rule out the influence of nonspecific factors such as comprehension and sensory disabilities, the sample stimulus remained on when the choice stimuli appeared. In delayed matching to sample (DMTS) the sample was presented for 4.5 seconds, then disappeared, and choice stimuli were presented 0, 4 or 12 seconds later. When the choice stimuli appeared (and they remained on indefinitely until a response was made), subjects had to point to the one on the lower row which resembled the sample. The trial continued until a correct response was made. Different delays (including the simultaneous condition) were programmed in a pseudo-random order, with 10 trials at each value; however, the test always began with practice trials on the simultaneous condition, followed by 0 and 12 second delay conditions. Thus, the DMTS task systematically varies the load on memory by imposing different delays and enables forgetting curves (performance versus delay) to be calculated and compared between groups. Since memory is the retention of information over time, poor performance should manifest itself in terms of a steeper (relative to control) forgetting curve.

The SDAT and SDLT groups' simultaneous matching (SMTS) accuracy was impaired relative to control ($p < 0.01$), but the two groups did not differ from each other. In delayed matching (DMTS) both patient groups performed worse than control ($p < 0.01$), but the SDLT group was more impaired than SDAT. The percent correct scores for the groups and delay conditions are shown in Fig. 9.2.

The corresponding latency analyses indicated that both SDAT and SDLT groups responded slower than control ($p < 0.01$), but were not different from each other. The SMTS and DMTS means were: control 3.85 ± 0.34 and 4.45 ± 0.23; SDAT 11.35 ± 2.63 and 10.07 ± 1.30; SDLT 16.56 ± 3.70 and 9.81 ± 1.71 seconds respectively.

9.3.3 Spatial span (SS)

This computerized version of the Corsi block-tapping task (Milner, 1971) was originally developed to investigate nonverbal memory span deficits in patients with right hippocampal damage.

An array of nine boxes (3 cm square) was displayed at pseudo-random locations on the screen (see Owen et al., 1992). The test began with a box changing colour for 3 seconds before reverting back to its former state.

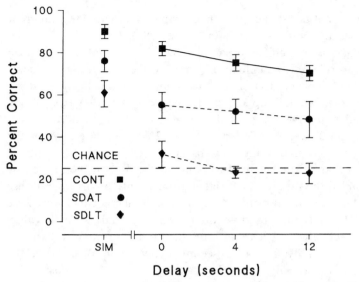

Fig. 9.2 MTS percent correct (± SEM; SIM = simultaneous condition; CONT = control group). In general, SDLT performance was worse than both control and SDAT. From Sahgal et al., 1992b, reproduced with permission from the publishers (Copyright 1992, American Medical Association).

One or more other boxes then changed colour sequentially, an audible tone signifying the end of the sequence. The subject's task was to point to the boxes in the order in which they had changed colour. At first only two boxes were involved, but this increased progressively to a maximum of nine boxes. There were three lists at each level, and the test terminated when an individual subject failed on all three lists at a particular level. The subject's spatial span was equal to the longest correctly reproduced sequence.

The group effect was significant ($p < 0.001$). However, the control group performed significantly ($p < 0.01$) better than both SDAT and SDLT groups, but the two demented groups were no different from each other. Mean sequence (span) lengths were: control 4.81 ± 0.13; SDAT 3.11 ± 0.37; and SDLT 3.00 ± 0.32. PD patients were not impaired relative to their controls, but the data tended towards significance ($p < 0.08$).

9.3.4 Conditional learning: pattern-location paired associates (CLPA)

The CLPA test is sensitive to right-sided hippocampal, but especially frontal lobe damage.

In this task, 6 white boxes measuring 4 ×4 cm appeared in a circular arrangement on the screen. These opened for 3 seconds, in a random order, to reveal one of a number of abstract colour stimuli (see Owen et al., 1993); the boxes could also be empty. A stimulus appeared at the centre after all boxes had been opened, and the subject was required to point to the box where it had originally appeared. At first, only one stimulus was hidden in one of the six locations. If a correct response was made, a further replication of the test, using a novel stimulus, was presented. An incorrect response resulted in the whole cycle of stimulus presentation being repeated for a maximum of 10 cycles in all. At this point, the test would terminate. Otherwise, the stimulus set size was increased from 1 to 2, 3, 6 and finally 8 different stimuli (two extra boxes being added to the display on the latter occasion). A replication at set sizes 1, 2 and 3 was included, and any errors again resulted in a repeat of the cycle for up to 10 cycles. Performance can be measured in terms of maximum set size (1, 2, 3, 6 or 8) achieved. A more precise measure is the total number of trials taken to complete the test, cumulated over all sets and replications. The maximum score of 10 was inserted for each stage not attempted.

All control subjects reached the maximum set size of 8, but none of the SDAT or SDLT subjects did. Two out of 10 SDAT subjects attempted set size 6; however, the best performance in the SDLT group was one patient who attempted set size 3. These data are shown in Fig. 9.3. In terms of total trials to completion, the control group scored on average 16.6 ± 1.2, the SDAT group 50.1 ± 3.6 and the SDLT group 65.4 ± 2.0 trials. There was an overall group effect ($p < 0.001$), which analysis showed was due to both patient groups being worse than control, as well as being different from each other. PD patients also performed worse than their controls ($p < 0.01$).

9.3.5 Spatial working memory (SWM)

Performance in this test is affected by temporal and especially frontal lobe damage.

This task determines the subject's ability to find tokens hidden behind a (variable) number of boxes. It began with a demonstration where two coloured boxes (2.5 cm square) were shown on the main part of the screen. The far right-hand side of the screen displayed a rectangular column where subjects could 'store' the tokens discovered, and this was just large enough to accommodate all the tokens available. The

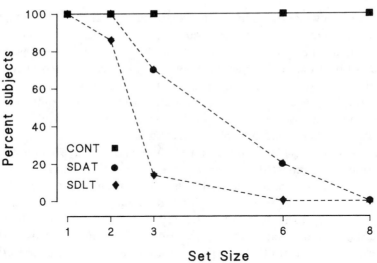

Fig. 9.3 CLPA percent subjects reaching a given set size (CONT = control). Analysis showed that SDLT performance was worse than SDAT, which in turn was worse than control. From Galloway et al., 1992, reproduced with permission from Karger, Basel.

experimenter touched one of the boxes which opened to reveal a blue token, which was 'moved' to the token store by pointing to that part of the screen. The second box was then touched and this also revealed a token, which was similarly transferred. In the next (practice) trial the subject was presented with two boxes in different locations. The first box to be touched was always empty. The subjects were then encouraged to try the other box. This contained a token which they transferred to the store. On returning to the first box they found a token which was moved as before. The test proper then commenced: four blocks of trials were given using 2, followed by four blocks at 3, then 4, 6 and finally 8 boxes (see Owen et al., 1992 for an illustration). Performance was measured by analysing the errors made and the time taken to complete the whole task. Three different types of error were possible: (a) 'between' errors, which occurred when subjects, on any particular search, revisited a box from which a token had already been removed on that block; (b) 'within' errors, which were committed when the subject returned to an empty box before finding the next token in that search sequence; and (c) 'double' errors, which were a combination of between and within errors. These occurred when the subject repeated a between error before finding the next token, again in that particular search sequence.

Although subjects may adopt various search strategies to sample the boxes (Sahgal et al., 1995), an efficient and frequently observed strategy is to follow a predetermined search sequence, starting with a particular box and returning to it to start a new sequence as soon as a token has been found – providing, of course, that it did not itself contain a token (Owen et al., 1990; Joyce and Robbins, 1991; Sahgal et al., 1992c, 1995). A numerical index for this strategy can be estimated by counting the number of times unique boxes were used to start each of the four search sequences at 6 and 8 box problem levels. For technical reasons, the lowest (most efficient) possible score is 20 and the highest, 56. By subtracting 19 from each score a linear scale in the range of 1 to 37 is achieved.

(a) Errors

As expected, the number of (any type of) errors made increased with the number of boxes to be searched (all ps <0.01). All groups made many more 'between' errors than 'within' or 'double' errors: they tended to return to boxes from which the token had already been removed. However, there were group differences. In general, the SDLT group made more errors than SDAT (who in turn were worse than control), especially as set size increased. Likewise, the PD study showed that those patients made significantly more ($p < 0.01$) 'between' – but not 'within' or 'double' errors.

(b) Strategy analysis

None of the groups differed in the extent to which they used a search strategy. The mean values for the strategy index were: control 18.13 ± 0.74; SDAT 17.25 ± 1.10; SDLT 18.88 ± 1.22. In contrast, PD patients were much worse (mean score 21.1; control 15.3; $p < 0.01$).

9.3.6 Visual search matching to sample (VSMTS)

This tests focal attentional ability, and evidence suggests that intact fronto-striatal circuits are necessary for efficient performance in this task. Prior to testing, subjects were trained on the use of the hand switch.

The stimuli presented consisted of abstract rectangular (2 cm long × 1 cm high) dot patterns involving different arrangements of four types of shape and four colours. The stimuli used were similar to the type described for matching to sample (see Downes et al., 1989 for a diagram of the stimuli used). Depression of the switch opened a central red box to reveal the (sample) stimulus and, 2 seconds later, choice stimuli (1, 2, 4 or 8) appeared in eight surrounding boxes: one choice stimulus was identical to the sample. Initially, subjects were shown the array of filled boxes and instructed to find the correct choice stimulus as quickly as possible. Three practice trials were given before the 48 test trials (12 at each of the 4 set sizes, presented in a random manner).

The main group ANOVA demonstrated no difference between control and SDAT performance, but the SDLT group performed significantly worse than both other groups ($p < 0.001$). All three groups' VSMTS performance depended on set size ($p < 0.001$). Further analysis indicated that set sizes 1 and 2 gave similar performance, which then declined as the number of stimuli increased. These data are illustrated in Fig. 9.4. Interestingly, patients in our preliminary PD study were not impaired.

9.3.7 Intra- and extradimensional set-shifting (IDED)

This paradigm assesses complex aspects of attentional processing, including selective perception, and it is indirectly related to the familiar Wisconsin card sorting test. Performance is affected by frontal lobe damage.

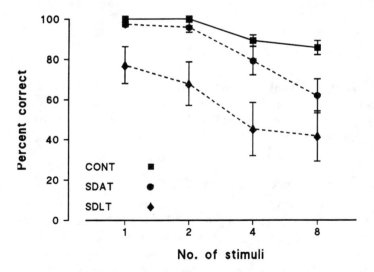

Fig. 9.4 VSMTS percent correct ($\pm$ SEM; CONT = control). SDLT performance was worse than SDAT or control; the latter two groups did not differ. From Sahgal et al., 1992a, reproduced with permission from Karger, Basel.

Theoretical and practical details for this task have been described elsewhere (Downes et al., 1989; Sahakian et al., 1990). All subjects were first trained on a simple discrimination task, in which they were asked to point repeatedly to the smaller of two discs and then to switch to the larger. The subsequent protocol required the subject to learn, in a sequential manner, a set of visual discrimination tasks in which one of two stimuli was correct, feedback being provided by the machine. The screen was cleared 1.5 seconds after a response, and the next trial began 1 second later. Response latency data were also recorded. The procedure gives a measure of the ability to make attentional shifts to exemplars (white, abstract line drawings or simple purple-coloured shapes) either (a) within the stimulus dimension presently being attended to (an intradimensional shift, IDS: for example, switching from one line drawing to the other), or (b) shifts to the previously irrelevant dimension (an extradimensional shift, EDS: for example, switching from lines to shapes).

The task involved nine successive stages, the subject proceeding to the next stage when a criterion of eight successive correct responses was reached; however, the whole test terminated if criterion was not reached within 50 trials at any level. The different stages were as follows:

1. Simple discrimination (SD). Four boxes appeared on the screen, any two of which, from trial to trial, contained (different) line stimuli. The subject had to discover which of the two stimuli was correct.
2. The next stage involved a reversal (SDR), where the previously incorrect stimulus became the correct one, and vice-versa.
3. A second dimension (shape) was introduced, with one exemplar of each dimension paired to give a compound stimulus (C_D) in any two of the four boxes; in this stage, the dimensions were spatially separate and subjects had to respond to the exemplar from the previous stage. From now on, exemplars were paired in a pseudorandom manner.
4. This stage (CD) was similar to the previous one, but the exemplars were superimposed, the line always in the foreground.
5. This was a reversal of the above (CDR).
6. Novel exemplars for both dimensions were introduced, but the relevant dimension remained the same; an intradimensional shift (IDS).
7. A reversal occurred at this stage (IDR).

8. New exemplars were again introduced, and subjects had to make an extradimensional shift (EDS) to the exemplars of the formerly irrelevant dimension.

9. At this final stage, contingencies were reversed (EDR) to the previously incorrect exemplar of the new dimension.

Group analysis of the learning stage reached indicated that the groups differed ($p < 0.001$). Subsequent analysis showed that both dementing groups were significantly different from control, but not from each other. These data are illustrated in Fig. 9.5.

Inspection of the data demonstrated that although both dementing groups were severely impaired, none of the SDLT patients solved the IDS stage. A comparison at this level suggested that SDLT performance was worse than SDAT ($p = 0.057$); data from the PD study are at present incomplete.

9.4 Discussion

Standard psychometric tests such as the MMSE indicated that both the SDAT and SDLT groups had very similar overall levels of cognitive

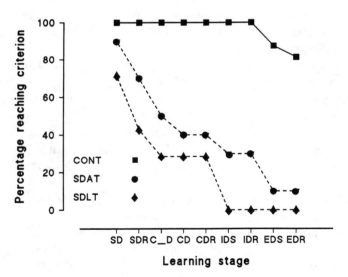

Fig. 9.5 IDED percent subjects reaching a given learning stage (see text for abbreviations; CONT = control). Both SDLT and SDAT groups were impaired, and further analysis indicated that SDLT performance tended to be worse than SDAT. From Sahgal et al., 1992a, reproduced with permission from Karger, Basel.

impairment. However, our previous studies (Galloway et al., 1992; Sahgal et al., 1992b, 1995) indicated that these tests generally failed to discriminate between the two groups, reinforcing the need to use more sensitive neuropsychological tests, such as the ones present in CANTAB.

Both SDAT and SDLT groups of dementing subjects performed at, or near, chance (50%) on the pattern recognition (PR) test (Galloway et al., 1992). This 'floor' effect might explain the lack of dissociation between SDAT and SDLT, but it also suggests that this task, unlike CLPA discussed below, is particularly sensitive to disruption in dementia.

All groups were able to do simultaneous matching (SMTS), even though both patient groups were impaired relative to control (Fig. 9.2). This finding suggests that the mild to moderately impaired patients tested in this study had understood, and were perceptually capable – in terms of visual acuity – of performing the task at its simplest level: in other words, procedural memory was not severely impaired. On the other hand, delayed matching (DMTS) data distinguished between groups: although SDAT performance was impaired relative to control, it was better than chance (25%), and superior to the SDLT group (Sahgal et al., 1992b). The latency analysis indicated that both SDAT and SDLT subjects were slow to respond, but their latencies did not differ from each other. This demonstrates that differences in general responsiveness cannot account for the substantial group difference in performance accuracy (percent correct).

Evidence from animal and human studies indicates that PR and DMTS accuracy is disrupted by posterior temporal cortical lesions, including hippocampal damage. In particular, posterior inferotemporal lesions disrupt visual discrimination and the encoding of information, while more anterior ones disrupt retrieval processes (Iversen, 1973; Sahgal & Iversen, 1978a,b). In other words, we may surmise that these structures are severely affected in both SDAT and SDLT. It is tempting to speculate that the exceptionally marked impairment demonstrated by the SDLT group, who were unable to tolerate even short delays (Fig. 9.2), reflects relatively severe degeneration of these temporal lobe structures in the early stages of the disease.

The spatial span (SS) test showed that SDAT and SDLT patients were impaired in their ability to execute a plan of action which involved pointing to a number of spatial locations sequentially. Thus, we can conclude that hippocampal structures are affected (cf. Milner, 1971) during early SDAT and SDLT.

   Group differences were found in the conditional learning paired associated (CLPA) task. In this test the SDLT group were more severely
impaired than SDAT patients, who in turn performed worse than control
subjects. PD patients also performed worse than their controls. All subjects responded with good accuracy at the smallest set sizes, indicating
that they had understood the basic nature of the task. The CLPA test is
similar to the test of object place memory used by Smith and Milner
(1981), and is sensitive to right-sided hippocampal damage. The learning
aspect of the test also has a conditional element, analogous to tasks used
by Petrides (1985) to demonstrate frontal lobe dysfunctions, although
there are procedural differences which may make them differentially susceptible to temporal/frontal lobe damage. For example, the Petrides
learning test is 'self-ordered' in that the subjects have to find out from
their own responses which stimuli are associated with one another,
whereas in the test used here this is made explicit to the subject from
the outset. Thus, the marked impairment demonstrated by the SDLT
(and PD) group might reflect *relatively* severe degeneration of medial
temporal, and perhaps frontal, lobe structures.
   Evidence from the spatial working memory (SWM) task, which represents a development of the radial maze techniques used to assess memory
in rodents (Olton et al., 1977), leads to a similar conclusion. Inspection of
the errors and search patterns showed that the SDLT (and PD) patients
made more errors, but both SDAT and SDLT subjects were capable of
formulating a search strategy. A tendency to re-sample previous boxes
which have *not* contained a token is a useful strategy for reducing the
spatial working memory load and is generally significantly correlated
with superior performance in normal control subjects. By contrast, deficiencies in the use of this strategy have been found in patients with frontal
lobe damage (Owen et al., 1990) and Korsakoff's syndrome (Joyce &
Robbins, 1991), which presumably contribute to their spatial working
memory deficit.
   Two tasks sensitive to attentional dysfunction have also been
described. These were the visual search matching to sample (VSMTS),
which provides a measure of 'focal' attention, and the attentional set
shifting (IDED) paradigm, which assesses complex aspects of attentional
processing, including selective perception, and which is indirectly related
to the Wisconsin card sorting test. These tasks, it was hoped, would
qualitatively distinguish SDLT from SDAT, since nigro-striatal deficiencies have been reported in SDLT but not SDAT (Perry et al., 1990).
Attentional abilities depend on intact frontal lobe and basal ganglia

structures (Passingham, 1972; Downes et al., 1989). Neurodegeneration involving the substantia nigra might therefore produce specific attentional deficits, and this has been confirmed in PD (Downes et al., 1989; Owen et al., 1992) and in patients with frontal lobe excisions (Owen et al., 1991). Data from the visual search task (VSMTS) indicated that only the SDLT patients were impaired (Sahgal et al., 1992a), and that the SDAT patients performed at or about control levels (Sahgal et al., 1991, 1992a). In other words, there was a qualitative difference between the two groups, and it provides strong evidence to suggest that 'focal' attentional ability is selectively impaired in SDLT. On the other hand, data from the attentional set shifting (IDED) paradigm are more difficult to interpret, since both SDLT and SDAT groups were impaired (Sahgal et al., 1992a). However, the indication was that, unlike SDAT subjects, none of the SDLT patients were able to make intradimensional shifts (IDS) (Fig. 9.5). This is the stage where efficient attentional capacity, mediated by frontal lobe structures, is particularly necessary (Downes et al., 1989). In this respect, the present IDED data support findings from the VSMTS task described above. However, this aspect of attentional ability requires more detailed study, involving much larger group sizes than those used here.

In conclusion, our studies have demonstrated qualitative differences between SDAT and SDLT even when global estimates of cognitive abilities indicate that the degree of cognitive decline in the two dementing groups is similar. The CANTAB tests chosen focus on fronto-striatal and temporal lobe processes (attention/planning and memory respectively), that is, precisely those processes which could be impaired in the SDAT/SDLT/PD spectrum of diseases. Unfortunately, there is as yet no strong evidence for a 'double dissociation' between SDAT and SDLT (where one disorder affects Task A but not Task B, and vice versa). This can, however, be expected if we argue that SDLT involves extra (for example dopaminergic fronto-striatal) degeneration in addition to the marked temporal lobe damage occurring in (early) SDAT/SDLT. Thus, these studies suggest that the neuroanatomical foci of the two diseases reflect more or less equivalent temporal lobe and hippocampal involvement, but the generally poorer (attentional) performance of the SDLT patients reflects greater damage to fronto-striatal structures and circuits, similar to, but less than, that seen in PD. Thus, our neuropsychological data support neurochemical and neuropathological findings reviewed elsewhere in this volume. Studies, using other tests available in the CANTAB package (e.g. the 'Tower of London' planning test, and a light-tracking attentional task), as well as new, computerized, and hopefully more sensitive attentional/planning tasks are currently underway, which should help characterize cognitive dysfunctions in SDLT more clearly.

Acknowledgements

I thank Mr A.E. Oakley for photography. The data reviewed in this article have been published elsewhere (see citations in text and figure legends). CANTAB (including IBM compatible equipment) can be purchased from Paul Fray Ltd, Flint Bridge, Ely Road, Waterbeach, Cambridge CB5 9PG (UK).

References

Chari, G., Shaw, P.J. & Sahgal, A. (1996). Nonverbal visual attention, but not recognition memory or learning, processes are impaired in motor neurone disease. *Neuropsychologia*, **34**, 377–85.

Downes, J.J., Roberts, A.C., Sahakian, B.J., Evenden, J.L., Morris, R.G. & Robbins, T.W. (1989). Impaired extra-dimensional shift performance in medicated and unmedicated Parkinson's disease: evidence for a specific attentional dysfunction. *Neuropsychologia*, **27**, 1329–43.

Galloway, P.H., Sahgal, A., McKeith, I.G. et al. (1992). Visual pattern recognition memory and learning deficits in senile dementias of Alzheimer and Lewy body types. *Dementia*, **3**, 101–7.

Iversen, S.D. (1973). Visual discrimination deficits associated with posterior inferotemporal lesions in the monkey. *Brain Res.*, **62**, 89–101.

Joyce, E.M. & Robbins, T.W. (1991). Frontal lobe function in Korsakoff and non-Korsakoff alcoholics: planning and spatial working memory. *Neuropsychologia*, **29**, 709–23.

McKeith, I.G., Perry, R.H., Fairbairn, A.F., Jabeen, S. & Perry, E.K. (1992). Operational criteria for senile dementia of Lewy body type. *Psychol. Med.*, **22**, 911–22.

McKeith, I.G., Fairbairn, A.F., Bothwell, R.A. et al. (1994). An evaluation of predictive validity and inter-rater reliability of clinical diagnostic criteria for senile dementia of Lewy body type (SDLT). *Neurology*, **44**, 872–7.

McKhann, G., Drachman, D., Folstein, M., Katzman, R., Price, D. & Stadlan, E.M. (1984). Clinical diagnosis of Alzheimer's disease: report of the NINCDS–ADRDA work group under the auspices of Department of Health and Human Services Task Force on Alzheimer's disease. *Neurology*, **34**, 939–44.

Milner, B. (1971). Interhemispheric differences in the localization of psychological processes in man. *Br. Med. Bull.*, **27**, 272–7.

Olton, D.S., Collison, C. & Werz, M.A. (1977). Spatial memory and radial arm maze performance of rats. *Learn. Motiv.*, **8**, 289–314.

Owen, A.M., Downes, J.J., Sahakian, B.J., Polkey, C.E. & Robbins, T.W. (1990). Planning and spatial working memory following frontal lobe lesions in man. *Neuropsychologia*, **28**, 1021–34.

Owen, A.M., Roberts, A.C., Polkey, C.E., Sahakian, B.J. & Robbins, T.W. (1991). Extra-dimensional versus intra-dimensional set shifting performance following frontal lobe excisions, temporal lobe excisions or amygdalo-hippocampectomy in man. *Neuropsychologia*, **29**, 993–1006.

Owen, A.M., James, M., Leigh, P.N. et al. (1992). Fronto-striatal cognitive deficits at different stages of Parkinson's disease. *Brain*, **115**, 1727–51.

Owen, A.M., Beksinska, M., James, M. et al. (1993). Visuospatial memory deficits at different stages of Parkinson's disease. *Neuropsychologia*, **31**, 627–44.

Passingham, R. (1972). Non-reversal shifts after selective pre-frontal ablation in monkeys (*Macaca mulatta*). *Neuropsychologia*, **10**, 41–6.

Perry, E.K., Marshall, E., Perry, R.H. et al. (1990). Cholinergic and dopaminergic activities in senile dementia of Lewy body type. *Alzheimer Dis. Assoc. Disord.*, **4**, 87–95.

Petrides, M. (1985). Deficits on conditional associative learning tasks after frontal- and temporal-lobe lesions in man. *Neuropsychologia*, **23**, 601–14.

Sahakian, B.J., Morris, R.G., Evenden, J.L. et al. (1988). A comparative study of visuospatial memory and learning in Alzheimer-type dementia and Parkinson's disease. *Brain*, **111**, 695–718.

Sahakian, B.J., Downes, J.J., Eagger, S. et al. (1990). Sparing of attentional relative to mnemonic function in a subgroup of patients with dementia of the Alzheimer type. *Neuropsychologia*, **28**, 1197–213.

Sahgal, A. & Iversen, S.D. (1978a). Categorization and retrieval after selective inferotemporal lesions in monkeys. *Brain Res.*, **146**, 341–50.

Sahgal, A. & Iversen, S.D. (1978b). The effects of foveal prestrate and inferotemporal lesions on matching to sample behaviour in monkeys. *Neuropsychologia*, **16**, 391–406.

Sahgal, A., Sahakian, B.J., Robbins, T.W. et al. (1991). Detection of visual memory and learning deficits in Alzheimer's disease using the Cambridge Neuropsychological Test Automated Battery. *Dementia*, **2**, 150–8.

Sahgal, A., Galloway, P.H., McKeith, I.G., Edwardson, J.A. & Lloyd, S. (1992a). A comparative study of attentional deficits in senile dementias of Alzheimer and Lewy body types. *Dementia*, **3**, 350–4.

Sahgal, A., Galloway, P.H., McKeith, I.G. et al. (1992b). Matching-to-sample deficits in patients with senile dementia of the Alzheimer and Lewy body types. *Arch. Neurol.*, **49**, 1043–6.

Sahgal, A., Lloyd, S., Wray, C.J. et al. (1992c). Does visuospatial memory in senile dementia of the Alzheimer type depend on the severity of the disorder? *Int. J. Geriatr. Psychiatry.*, **7**, 427–36.

Sahgal, A., McKeith, I.G., Galloway, P.H., Tasker, N. & Steckler, T. (1995). Do differences in visuospatial ability between senile dementias of the Alzheimer and Lewy body types reflect differences solely in mnemonic function? *J. Clin. Exp. Neuropsychol.*, **17**, 35–43.

Smith, M.L. & Milner, B. (1981). The role of the right hippocampus in the recall of spatial location. *Neuropsychologia*, **19**, 781–93.

10

The clinical and functional imaging characteristics of parkinsonian dementia

B.L. MILLER, L.E. URRUTIA,
M. CORNFORD and I. MENA

Summary

We describe the clinical and single photon emission computerized tomography (SPECT) characteristics of nine patients with parkinsonian-dementia (PD) and contrast their clinical and SPECT characteristics with nine MMSE matched Alzheimer's disease (AD) patients. In six of the PD patients there was pathological confirmation of the diagnosis while in three others the diagnosis was based upon the clinical presentation. The PD patients significantly differed from the AD patients due to the high frequency of visual hallucinations, delusions, and atypical (SPECT) patterns. The clinical and SPECT patterns in PD differ from AD.

10.1 Introduction

There is an emerging literature on the neurologic (Perry et al., 1989; Crystal et al., 1990), neuropsychiatric (Perry et al., 1990a and 1990b), neuropsychological (Sakahian et al., 1988; Sahgal et al., 1992), neurochemical (Perry et al., 1990b,c; Dickson et al., 1991) and neuropathologic (Hansen et al., 1990; Dickson et al., 1991; Kosaka, 1993) features of patients who present with a mixture of parkinsonism and dementia (PD). There are three differing hypotheses regarding the classification of these PD patients. One theory emphasizes that senile plaques are commonly found with PD and suggests that PD patients are part of the spectrum of Alzheimer's disease (AD) (Hansen et al., 1990). In contrast, Perry et al. (1989) have hypothesized that the cortical Lewy bodies found at pathology in PD represent a unique disorder for which they coined the term senile dementia of the Lewy body type (SDLT). These researchers have noted that SDLT patients do not show sufficient neurofibrillary tangles to meet AD research criteria and emphasize that the neurochemical features of these patients distinguish them from AD. Others (Gibb et al., 1987) note that cortical Lewy bodies are present in patients with idiopathic Parkinson's disease. Similarly, Kazee and Han (1995) have found that cortical Lewy bodies are commonly found in AD so that the specificity of these lesions for SDLT is debated.

Because the PD syndrome is just beginning to attract active study, there have been few efforts to compare the clinical and imaging features of patients with PD. This is unfortunate as a clearer definition of the neuroimaging characteristics of PD patients could help to delineate the clinical features of this condition, and might offer indirect clues as to the category of disease that these patients represent. The two main functional imaging techniques that have been used to evaluate dementia are single photon emission computerized tomography (SPECT) and positron emission tomography (PET) (Miller et al., 1995). Most of the SPECT studies in dementia have measured regional cerebral blood flow (rCBF) while the PET studies have evaluated glucose metabolism (uptake).

In the setting of primary degenerative dementia the findings with SPECT and PET are similar. Therefore, areas with decreased rCBF with SPECT tend to show diminished glucose uptake with PET. AD patients show symmetrical posterior temporal-parietal hypoperfusion with SPECT (Johnson et al., 1987) or hypometabolism with PET (Mazziotta et al., 1992). In contrast, the fronto-temporal dementias (FTD) show frontal and anterior temporal abnormalities with SPECT (Neary et al., 1987; Miller et al., 1991; Risberg et al., 1993) and PET (Friedland et al., 1993). In most instances the SPECT or PET patterns seen with AD and FTD reliably predict pathology (Read et al., 1995) and although the functional imaging features of AD and FTD have been well-characterized, there are few studies which have determined the SPECT or PET patterns in patients with pathologically confirmed PD.

We report upon the clinical, neuropsychiatric and SPECT characteristics of nine patients with PD compared with nine Mini-Mental State Examination (MMSE) matched AD patients. In six PD patients there was pathological confirmation of the diagnosis; in three others the diagnosis was based upon the clinical presentation. The similarities and differences in the clinical symptoms and SPECT pattern in PD versus typical AD are discussed.

10.2 Methods

Patients with PD and AD are actively recruited and studied through the University of California at Los Angeles, Alzheimer Disease Center (UCLA ADC). Through the ADC all patients receive extensive neurobehavioral, neuropsychological and neuroimaging examinations. The MMSE (Folstein, 1975) and bedside cognitive testing are administered to all patients. Additionally, most are imaged with SPECT.

For this study nine patients with PD were compared with nine who met a National Institutes of Neurological and Communicative Disorders and Alzheimer's Disease and Related Disorders Association (NINCDS–ADRDA) research diagnosis for probable AD (McKhann et al., 1984). The AD patients were randomly chosen based upon the MMSE from a larger cohort of patients within the UCLA ADC. Six of the nine PD patients had a pathologic study which demonstrated either substantia nigra degeneration or cortical Lewy bodies. Three PD patients are still living with clinical symptoms which include both parkinsonism and dementia. The clinical features, neuropsychiatric symptoms, SPECT findings and pathology of the PD and AD patients were retrospectively reviewed and the following were determined.

1. *Clinical features*: The clinical features including age, sex, first symptom and MMSE examination score at the time of first evaluation were documented.
2. *Neuropsychiatric symptoms*: The neuropsychiatric symptoms present in each patient were noted. We documented the presence of visual and auditory hallucinations, delusions and depression.
3. *SPECT*: SPECT was performed with ^{133}xenon and $[^{99m}$Tc]Hexamethy-propyleneamine-oxime (HMPAO). ^{133}xenon was used to obtain an absolute measure of rCBF (Kanno & Lassen, 1979) while HMPAO gave a high resolution qualitative image of cerebral perfusion. Patients were studied awake with eyes open in the supine position with low ambient light and noise. Following inhalation of 30 mCi (100 MBq) of ^{133}xenon gas rCBF was measured using high sensitivity collimation with a brain-dedicated unit (Headtome II, Shimadzu, Kyoto Japan) (Kanno et al., 1981). Three brain slices were acquired simultaneously. Next, each patient received 20 mCi (740 MBq) of HMPAO (Ceretec, Amersham, Arlington Heights, IL) injected intravenously. Scanning started 2 hours after injection so that soft tissue background activity could clear. For HMPAO imaging, the first acquisitions were com-

pleted in 10 minutes followed by two body shifts of 16 mm each that imaged the 32 mm of blind interslice space. Nine transaxial cuts of the brain were acquired in 30 minutes converting an extension of 14.4 cm, without blind regions. Transaxial scans were parallel and started at the orbito-meatal line. One patient could not tolerate the [133]xenon inhalation. Two others could not be studied in the high resolution scanner for HMPAO scanning for technical reasons and these patients had HMPAO imaging in a single headed SOPHY scanner.

Two raters (B.L.M., L.E.U.) obtained a consensus rating on the SPECT pattern for both the [133]xenon and HMPAO scans. Scans were rated as showing one of four general patterns, 'temporal-parietal', 'fronto-anterior temporal', 'normal' or 'other'. The abnormalities for patients with 'other' were subjectively described. With this system a 93% intra-rater and 91% inter-rater reliability was obtained (Masterman & Cummings, 1995).

4. *Pathology*: The six patients with pathology were rated by a board-certified neuropathologist (M.C.) with regards to the cortical concentration of amyloid plaques, neurofibrillary tangles and Lewy bodies and for the severity of substantia nigra cell loss and Lewy body concentration. M.C. determined whether patients met the Khachaturian Research Criteria for Alzheimer's disease.

10.3 Results

10.3.1 Clinical

No PD patients had a presenile onset of disease and their mean age was 72.7 years. This contrasted with the randomly-matched AD patients whose mean age was 64.8 years. Seven of the nine PD patients were male while four AD patients were male. The first symptom for five of the PD patients was memory disturbance or word-finding difficulty. In three PD patients the first symptom was either delusion, hallucinations or delirium while in one a depression seemed to herald the onset of the disease. In contrast, all of the AD patients had cognitive symptoms as the first manifestation of the disease. Six PD patients had parkinsonism while three did not (the three without parkinsonian features all had pathologic findings of PD). In the PD patients the extrapyramidal findings were variable although no PD patient had the classical triad of cogwheel rigidity, bradykinesia and tremor. No AD patient had parkinsonism. See Table 10.1 for clinical features of the PD patients.

Table 10.1. *PD clinical features*

Patient	Age	Sex	First symptom	MMSE*	Parkinson features
AA	73	F	Memory/word-finding	16	Bradykinesia/cogwheeling
BB	76	M	Memory	17	Tremor/shuffling gait
CC	73	F	Insomnia/delusions	23	Cogwheeling
DD	70	M	Hallucinations/cognition	20	Tremor/cogwheeling
FF	71	M	Memory	25	None
GG	69	M	Depression	20	Bradykinesia/cogwheeling
HH	76	M	Memory/word-finding	20	None
EE	74	M	Delirium	8	None
II	72	M	Memory/word finding	17	Bradykinesia/jaw tremor

* Mini-Mental Status Exam

10.3.2 Neuropsychiatric symptoms

The psychiatric symptoms in PD were distinct from AD. Eight of nine patients had visual hallucinations which were florid and complex, often characterized by colored scenes of people, animals, imaginary creatures (like dwarfs) or cartoon characters. The hallucinations tended to be highly idiosyncratic and none of the eight patients described similar visual distortions. The PD group endorsed the hallucinations as real. Although dopamine replacement can precipitate visual hallucinations, in most of the patients the hallucinations occurred off dopamine compounds. Auditory hallucinations were present in only one patient who stated that some of the people within his visual hallucination mumbled. Also common in PD were paranoid delusions which were present in seven of nine subjects. The delusions tended to be stereotyped with complaints of imaginary intruders, theft, or Capgras syndrome accounting for the delusions in all seven patients. Depression heralded the dementia in one patient but was found in only two of nine subjects (Table 10.2).

In contrast, no AD had hallucinations and only one had delusions at the time of presentation. Four AD patients had mild depressive symptoms although none suffered from sustained depression. With Fisher's Exact Test the differences between the two groups were highly significant with regards to visual hallucinations ($p < 0.0004$) and delusions ($p < 0.02$).

Table 10.2. *PD neuropsychiatry*

Patients	Visual hallucinations	Auditory hallucinations	Delusions	Depression
AA	Friendly cartoon characters	Mumbling voices	Paranoid; Theft of personal items	None
BB	Sees and talks with his dead brother	None	Theft	None
CC	Tall, short and dark haired people	None	Capgras syndrome	Mild
DD	Groups of hippies, armed men and church related men	None	Paranoid; neighbor shrinks people	None
FF	Chocolate colored dwarves and faces	None	None	None
GG	Small black crows and children	None	Capgras syndrome[*]	Yes
HH	Cats under his bed	None	People living in his house	None
EE	None	None	None	Yes
II	People dressed in black, young guitar players	None	Capgras syndrome	None

[*] Reduplicative paramnesia also present

10.3.3 SPECT

Nearly all PD and AD patients showed focal areas of hypoperfusion and in the regions with diminished rCBF, perfusion was measured in the 15–25 ml/100 gm tissue/min range. Only one of the eight PD patients showed a simple temporal-parietal hypoperfusion pattern as is seen with AD with ^{133}xenon and HMPAO. Although all of the PD patients had temporal-parietal hypoperfusion, eight of the nine also showed additional cortical areas with severe rCBF abnormalities (Table 10.3). In addition to the temporal-parietal hypoperfusion, there was lower rCBF in the frontal and occipital areas. The frontal hypoperfusion was nearly as severe as the temporal-parietal hypoperfusion. In contrast, 7/9 AD patients had an AD pattern with ^{133}xenon and 6/8 demonstrated an AD pattern with HMPAO. One of two AD patients with an atypical SPECT showed excessive frontal involvement with both while the other

Table 10.3. *PD brain imaging*

Patient	^{133}Xenon AD pattern (temporal parietal)	^{133}Xenon Other (describe)	Cerebral blood flow (mg/min/100g)	HMPAO AD pattern (temporal parietal)	HMPAO Other (describe)
AA	Yes Symmetrical	Occipital and bifrontal hypoperfusion	17	Yes Asymmetrical	No
BB	No	Bilateral frontal Bilateral parietal Bilateral temporal	20 15–25 15–25	No	Bilateral basal frontal Right parietal Bilateral temporal
CC		Not performed		No	Front parietal Right parietal > Left
DD	No	Right frontal Right parietal Bilateral temporal	25 17 <17	No	Bilateral frontal Biparietal and deep
EE	No	Frontal Parietal Bilateral temporal	22 22 20	No	Fronto-parietal Left > Right Temporal
FF	No	Bilateral frontal Bilateral parietal Bilateral temporal	20–22 20	No	Bilateral frontal Bilateral parietal Occipital
GG	No	Bilateral occipital Bilateral parietal	14–28	No	Bilateral parietal Bilateral occipital
HH	No	Left dorsal frontal Bilateral parietal	23–33 23	No	Bilateral frontal Temporal/parietal and deep
II	No	Bilateral temporal Bilateral frontal Temporal/parietal	23 20–44 14–28	No	Bilateral frontal Temporal and parietal

had a normal SPECT. With Fisher's Exact Test the differences between the PD and AD SPECT patterns were highly significant ($p < 0.02$).

10.3.4 Neuropathology

The neuropathology differed in each patient. (See Table 10.4 for the neuropathologic features of the six PD patients.) Two had few cortical plaques or tangles, abundant cortical and substantia nigra Lewy bodies and severe neuronal loss in the substantia nigra. Two others showed an insufficient number of plaques or tangles to meet a research diagnosis of AD but had moderate numbers of cortical Lewy bodies and mild to moderate substantia nigra degeneration. Two others met a research diagnosis for AD and both showed moderate numbers of cortical Lewy

Table 10.4. *PD pathology*

Patient	Plaques	Neurofibrillary tangles	Cortical Lewy bodies	Substantia nigra
BB	Insufficient no. for AD	Neocortical Sufficient no. for AD	Cingulum, insula, temporal moderate concentration	Severe cell loss LB present
CC	Hippocampal and neocortical abundant	Hippocampal and neocortical abundant	Frontal and temporal Abundant concentration	Severe cell loss LB present
DD	None	None	Rare	Severe cell loss LB present
FF	Rare	Rare	Cingulum, temporal Abundant concentration	Severe cell loss Abundant Lewy bodies
HH	Sufficient for AD	Parahippocampus and superior temporal lobe Insufficient no. for AD	Neocortex, cingulum, superior temporal Abundant concentration	Moderate cell loss Abundant Lewy bodies
EE	Frontal and occipital Insufficient no. for AD	Neocortical and subcortical insufficient no. for AD	Frontal moderate concentration	Mild cell loss Abundant Lewy bodies

LB = Lewy bodies

bodies. One showed severe substantia nigra degeneration while the other showed mild substantia nigra degeneration.

10.4 Discussion

In this study the clinical, neuropsychiatric and SPECT findings in the PD patients were strikingly different from those with AD. As a group the PD patients were older than the AD patients and there was a predominance of men. The older age at onset for the SDLT population is supported by other studies, and PD with dementia appears to be less common in patients under the age of 65 (Hansen et al., 1990; Perry et al., 1990a). At the time of initial evaluation, parkinsonian features were detected in six of nine subjects with PD, but none with AD. In the three PD patients in whom parkinsonian features were not detected, Lewy bodies were present in the substantia nigra and cell loss in the three patients was respectively mild, moderate and severe. In the patients in whom substantia nigra cell loss was found to be moderate and severe at pathology, parkinsonian features eventually developed.

The PD patients also had more psychiatric symptoms. As was originally reported by Perry et al. (1990a) PD patients exhibit visual hallucinations, often characterized by formed complex scenes with animals, cartoon characters or small people. Our study confirms this important observation and formed complex scenes occurred in eight of nine patients. In our PD patients, the visual hallucinations were extremely variable and none of the eight with hallucinations had similar visual phenomenology. Previously, the visual hallucinations found in PD have been attributed to the dopamine agonists used to treat these patients (Cummings & Miller, 1987). However, most of eight PD patients in this study developed spontaneous visual hallucinations off dopamine agonists, suggesting a special vulnerability to hallucinations in PD. The balance between monoaminergic and cholinergic systems has been hypothesized as producing this special vulnerability (Perry et al., 1990c).

Almost as common as visual hallucinations were delusions which were present in seven of nine patients. In contrast to the rich and complex phenomenology found in the PD patients, the delusions present in AD were more stereotyped; nearly all of the patients had either delusions of theft, infidelity or Capgras syndrome. In another study, Cummings et al. (1987) described similar 'simple' delusions associated with AD. The differences in depression between the two populations was not clinically significant. The almost invariable presence of visual hallucinations or delusions in our PD population strongly supports the concepts regarding PD that were developed by Perry et al. (1990a). Whether or not this PD is determined to be a variant of AD or a separate disease entity, the clinical phenomenology is so striking that separation of these patients seems warranted.

Previous imaging studies of patients with Parkinson's disease have shown variable results. The first studies of patients with Parkinson's disease looked at non-demented patients and showed subtle or no defects in brain rCBF or metabolism. In 1979 Lavy et al. showed global rCBF decreases (Lavy et al., 1979) and frontal hypoperfusion (Bes et al., 1983) in Parkinson's disease. With PET in four non-demented parkinsonian patients, Rougemont et al. (1984) showed normal brain metabolism prior to and after dopamine therapy. Subsequently, Costa et al. (1988) showed normal cortical rCBF in Parkinson's disease, but decreased caudate and increased thalamic rCBF during the 'off' phase.

Most studies of PD have reported widespread abnormalities in rCBF or glucose metabolism (Wolfson et al., 1985). Sawada et al. (1992) compared 13 parkinsonian patients without dementia, 13 with dementia (PD) and 10 age-matched controls. The nondemented subjects showed no significant differences from the controls, while there was significantly lower rCBF in the frontal, parietal and left temporal regions in the PD group. The authors did not describe an AD pattern in these subjects and emphasized the consistency of frontal abnormalities in PD. Peppard et al. (1992) studied 14 parkinsonian patients with variable changes in cognition. Those without dementia showed widespread cortical glucose hypometabolism while the demented patients showed both widespread and temporal-parietal hypoperfusion which resembled AD. Similarly, Kuhl et al. (1985) found temporal-parietal hypometabolism in patients with PD. Hence, most of the previous studies suggest marked cortical abnormalities in cerebral metabolism and rCBF in patients with PD with more subtle changes in parkinsonian patients without dementia. However, in none of the previous studies could we find a direct visual comparison between PD and AD.

In our study, most PD patients showed SPECT changes that were qualitatively distinct from the AD patients. The main difference between the two groups was that the PD patients showed more extensive frontal hypoperfusion than did the AD group. This parallels the findings of Sawada et al. (1992). Surprisingly, two PD patients also showed extensive occipital hypoperfusion. Hence, MMSE-matched AD patients showed temporal-parietal hypoperfusion while the PD group showed both temporal-parietal hypoperfusion with additional abnormalities in the frontal and sometimes occipital regions.

Because there was substantial overlap between the SPECT patterns seen with PD and AD it seems unlikely that functional imaging will reliably differentiate these patient groups with high sensitivity or specificity. Similarly, the mechanism for the SPECT differences between PD and AD is still undetermined. It is possible that the dopamine deficiency associated with PD accounts for the frontal hypoperfusion in PD as there are extensive basal-ganglia-frontal circuits. Another possible mechanism is that the cortical Lewy bodies, by themselves, alter cerebral perfusion. Unfortunately, the rCBF changes with functional imaging do not answer the fundamental question as to whether PD is a variant of AD or represents a separate biological disorder. As the clinical and neuropsychiatric features of these patients differ, it is possible that the combination of functional imaging and imaging of dopamine concentration (Martin et al., 1989) could reliably differentiate patients with AD from those with PD. Only careful clinical, imaging and pathologic correlations will definitively help to answer these important questions.

References

Bes, A., Guell, A., Fabre, N. et al. (1983). Cerebral blood flow studied with xenon-133 inhalation technique in Parkinsonism loss of hyperfrontal pattern. *J. Cereb. Blood Flow Metab.*, **3**, 33–7.

Costa, D.C., Ell, P.J., Burns, A., Philpot, M. & Levy, R. (1988). CBF tomograms with [^{99m}Tc]-HMPAO in patients with dementia (Alzheimer Type and HIV) and Parkinson's disease – initial results. *J. Cereb. Blood Flow Metab.*, **8** S109–15.

Crystal, H.A., Dickson, D.W., Lizardi, J.E., Davies, P. & Wolfson, L.I. (1990). Antemortem diagnosis of diffuse Lewy body disease. *Neurology*, **40**, 1523–8.

Cummings, J.L. & Miller, B.L. (1987). Visual hallucinations: an overview. *West. J. Med.*, **146**, 46–51.

Cummings, J.L., Miller, B.L., Hill, M.A. & Neshkes, R. (1987). Neuropsychiatric aspects of multi-infarct dementia and dementia of the Alzheimer type. *Arch. Neurol.*, **44**, 389–93.

Dickson, D.W., Ruan, D., Crystal, H. et al. (1991). Hippocampal degeneration differentiates diffuse Lewy body disease (DLBD) from Alzheimer's disease: light and electron microscopic immunocytochemistry of CA2-3 neurites specific to DLBD. *Neurology*, **41**, 1402–9.

Folstein, M.F., Folstein, S.E. & McHugh, P.R. (1975). 'Mini-Mental State': A practical method for grading the cognitive state of patients for the clinician. *J. Psychiat. Res.*, **12**, 185–98.

Friedland, R.P., Koss, E., Lerner, A. et al. (1993). Functional imaging of the frontal lobes, and dementia. *Dementia*, **4**, 192–203.

Gibb, W.R.G., Esiri, M.M. & Lees, L.J. (1987). Clinical and pathological features of diffuse cortical Lewy body disease (Lewy body dementia). *Brain*, **110**, 1131–53.

Hansen, L., Salmon, D., Galasko, D. et al. (1990). The Lewy body variant of Alzheimer's disease: a clinical and pathologic entity. *Neurology*, **40**, 1–8.

Johnson, K., Davis, D.R., Buonanno, F.S. et al. (1987). Comparison of magnetic resonance imaging and roentgen ray computerized tomography in dementia. *Arch. Neurol.*, **44**, 1075–80.

Kanno, I. & Lassen, N.A. (1979). Two methods for calculating regional cerebral blood flow from emission computed tomography of inert gas concentrations. *J. Comp. Assist. Tomogr.*, **3**, 71–6.

Kanno, I., Uemura, K., Miura, S. & Miura, Y. (1981). Headtome: a hybrid emission single-photon and positron emission tomograph for imaging of the brain. *J. Comp. Assist. Tomogr.*, **5**, 216–24.

Kazee, A.M. & Han, L.Y. (1995). Cortical Lewy bodies in Alzheimer's disease. *Arch. Pathol. Lab. Med.*, **119**, 448–53.

Kosaka, K. (1993). Dementia and neuropathology in Lewy body disease. *Adv. Neurol.*, **60**, 456–64.

Kuhl, D.E., Metter, E.J. & Riege, W.H. (1985). Similarities of cerebral glucose utilization demented in Alzheimer's disease and Parkinsonian dementia. *J. Cereb. Blood Flow Metab.*, **5**(suppl 1), S169–70.

Lavy, S., Melamed, E., Cooper, G. & Bentin, S. (1979). Regional cerebral blood flow in patients with Parkinson's disease. *Arch. Neurol.*, **36**, 344–8.

Martin, W.R.W., Palmer, M.R., Patlka, C.S. & Calne, D.B. (1989). Nigrostriatal function in humans studied with positron emission tomography. *Ann. Neurol.*, **26**, 535–42.

Masterman, D. & Cummings, J.L. (1995). Sensitivity and specificity of Tc-99-HMPAO SPECT in discriminating Alzheimer's disease patients from other patients with memory complaints. *Neurology*, **45**(Suppl 4), A405.

Mazziotta, J., Frackowiak, R.S.J. & Phelps, M.E. (1992). The use of positron emission tomography in the clinical assessment of dementia. *Semin. Nucl. Med.*, **12**(4), S123–6.

McKhann, G., Drachman, D., Folstein, M. et al. (1984). Diagnosis of AD disease: a report of the NINCDS–ADRDA work group under the auspices of the Dept. of Health and Human Services Task Force on Alzheimer's disease. *Neurology*, **34**, 939–44.

Miller, B.L., Cummings, J.L., Villanueva-Meyer, J. et al. (1991). Frontal lobe degeneration: clinical neuropsychological and SPECT characteristics. *Neurology*, **41**, 1374–82.

Miller, B.L., Mena, I., Cummings, J.L. & Darcourt, J. (1995). Neuroimaging in Clinical Practice. In: *Comprehensive Textbook of Psychiatry*, 6th edn, ed. H.I. Kaplan & B.J. Sadock, pp. 257–6. Baltimore, MD: Williams and Wilkins.

Neary, D., Snowden, J.S. & Shields, R.A. (1987). Single photon emission tomography using [99]mTc-HMPAO in the investigation of dementia. *J. Neurol. Neurosurg. Psychiatry*, **50**, 1101–9.

Peppard, R.F., Martin, W.R.W., Clark, G.D. et al. (1992). Cortical glucose metabolism in Parkinson's and Alzheimer's disease. *J. Neurol. Sci.*, **27**, 561–8.

Perry, R.H., Irving, D., Blessed, G., Perry, E.K. & Fairbairn, A.F. (1989). Clinically and neuropathologically distinct form of dementia in the elderly. *Lancet*, **i**, 166.

Perry, R.H., Irving, D., Blessed, G., Fairbairn, A. & Perry, E.K. (1990a). Senile dementia of the Lewy body type: a clinically and neuropathologically distinct form of Lewy body dementia in the elderly. *J. Neurol. Sci.*, **95**, 119–39.

Perry, E.K., Kerwin, J., Perry, R.H. et al. (1990b). Cerebral cholinergic activity is related to the incidence of visual hallucinations in senile dementia of Lewy body type. *Dementia*, **1**, 2–4.

Perry, E.K., Marshall, E., Kerwin, J. et al. (1990c). Evidence of monoaminergic-cholinergic imbalance related to visual hallucinations in Lewy body dementia. *J. Neurochem.*, **55**, 1454–6.

Read, S., Miller, B.L., Mena, I., Kim, R. & Darby, A. (1995). SPECT/ pathology corelations in dementia. *J. Am. Geriatr. Soc.*, **43**, 243–7.

Risberg, J., Passant, U., Warkentin, S. & Gustafson, L. (1993). Regional cerebral blood flow in frontal lobe dementia of non-Alzheimer's type. *Dementia*, **4**(3–4), 186–7.

Rougemont, D., Baron, J.C., Collard, P. et al. (1984). Local cerebral glucose utilization in treated and untreated patients with Parkinson's disease. *J. Neurol. Neurosurg. Psychiatry*, **47**, 824–30.

Sahgal, A., Galloway, P.H., McKeith, I.G. et al. (1992). Matching to sample deficits in patients with senile dementias of the Alzheimer and Lewy body types. *Arch. Neurol.*, **49**(10), 1043–6.

Sakahian, B.J., Morris, R.G., Evenden, J.D. et al. (1988). A comparative study of visuospatial memory and learning in Alzheimer-type dementia and Parkinson's disease. *Brain*, **111**, 695–718.

Sawada, H., Udaka, F., Kameyama, M. et al. (1992). SPECT findings in Parkinson's disease associated with dementia. *J. Neurol. Neurosurg. Psychiatry*, **55**(10), 960–3.

Wolfson, L.I., Leenders, K.L., Brown, L.L. & Jones, T. (1985). Alterations of cerebral blood flow and oxygen metabolism in Parkinson's disease. *Neurology*, **35**, 1399–405.

11

Positron emission tomography findings in Parkinson's disease and Lewy body dementia

N . T U R J A N S K I and D . J . B R O O K S

Summary

The pathological correlate of parkinsonism and dementia (PD-dementia) may be diffuse Lewy body disease (DLBD), Alzheimer's disease (AD) or a combination of both pathologies. Positron emission tomography (PET) studies show a resting pattern of fronto-temporo-parietal hypometabolism in both AD and in PD-dementia patients. Diagnostic criteria have been recently devised to try and distinguish between AD and dementia of the Lewy body type. We have studied three PD-dementia patients fulfilling the clinical criteria for DLBD with ^{18}F-fluorodeoxyglucose (FDG) PET. The results showed an AD pattern of fronto-temporo-parietal hypometabolism, although these patients had only mild cognitive dysfunction. These preliminary results suggest that metabolic PET studies are unable to distinguish the cortical deficit of PD-dementia from AD, though the PD-dementia patients may have relatively greater frontal hypometabolism. Further studies with postmortem confirmation will be required to establish whether DLBD is associated with a distinctive pattern of resting hypometabolism.

11.1 Introduction

Patients with postmortem evidence of diffuse Lewy body disease (DLBD) present clinically with either isolated parkinsonism, dementia or a combination of both (PD-dementia). PD-dementia may also be a manifestation of patients who show isolated Alzheimer's (AD) type changes at postmortem, or a mixture of both Alzheimer and Lewy body pathologies.

Initially, Lewy body disease was categorized according to its distribution in the central nervous system, diffuse (DLBD), transitional and isolated brainstem subtypes being recognized (Kosaka et al., 1984). Anti-ubiquitin staining however, has shown that cortical Lewy bodies are present in nearly all patients with clinically typical Parkinson's disease (PD) (Perry et al., 1991; Schmidt et al., 1991; Hughes et al., 1993). These findings suggest that patients with brainstem but few cortical Lewy bodies present with parkinsonism while those with profuse cortical Lewy bodies present with either parkinsonism or dementia, or more usually, a combination of both. Severity of dementia has been reported to correlate with density of cortical Lewy bodies (Lennox et al., 1989).

Currently, postmortem clinical diagnostic criteria for DLBD only apply to dementia cases. Dementia is thought to occur in 10–20% of patients with PD (Brown & Marsden, 1984; Tison et al., 1995) while extrapyramidal signs are found in 30–90% of patients with AD (Molsa et al., 1984; Tyrrell et al., 1990). Is it possible to clinically distinguish PD-dementia of Lewy body type from that of the AD type? It has been suggested that the dementia of the Lewy body type may differ from AD in that it shows fluctuating severity (Byrne et al., 1989; McKeith et al., 1992) and greater impairment of frontal function (Hansen et al., 1990). Additionally, DLBD patients may be more prone to develop hallucinations and be more sensitive to neuroleptics (McKeith et al., 1992). Based on these distinctions a criteria to diagnose PD-dementia of Lewy body type has been recently devised (McKeith et al., 1992). It has been also suggested that the parkinsonian syndrome in DLBD may have atypical features such as early gait involvement, poor levodopa response, or supranuclear gaze palsy (Crystal et al., 1990). However, no current criteria are available to detect DLBD patients if they have normal cognition.

Positron emission tomography (PET) and single photon emission tomography (SPECT) provide a mean of examining brain function in vivo, in patients. To date, they have been extensively used to explore the neuropharmacological, metabolic and blood flow changes associated with isolated dementia and parkinsonism. In this study we have used PET to examine cerebral metabolism in cases of possible DLBD.

11.2 PET and SPECT studies in Alzheimer's disease

PET studies either with $^{15}O_2$ and ^{19}F-fluorodeoxyglucose (FDG) in patients with established AD have shown global reductions of cerebral metabolism. The localization of focal deficits and their magnitude generally correlates with the clinical severity and type of cognitive impairment (Frackowiak et al., 1981; Friedland et al., 1983; Kennedy et al., 1995). Patients with mild cognitive deficits have most pronounced metabolic reduction in temporo-parietal cortices while those with advance disease or dysphasia show additional prefrontal hypometabolism (Frackowiak et al., 1981; Friedland et al., 1983; Chase et al., 1984; Alavi et al., 1986; Kennedy et al., 1995). SPECT studies with [^{99m}Tc]-HMPAO have shown similar patterns of cerebral hypofunction to PET, which also correlate with the type and severity of cognitive deficit (Costa et al., 1988; Smith et al., 1988).

More than 10 years ago, Garnett et al. (1984) demonstrated bilateral reductions in putamen ^{18}F-dopa uptake in Parkinson's disease (PD). These results have been reproduced in a number of PET studies which consistently have found a greater involvement of nigro-putaminal than nigro caudate projections and an inverse correlation between putaminal ^{18}F-dopa uptake and degree of motor impairment in parkinsonian subjects (Piccini et al., 1995).

Patients with AD and associated extrapyramidal rigidity studied with ^{18}F-dopa PET have shown a mean striatal uptake that is within the normal range. Although some AD individuals have mildly reduced levels of putamen tracer uptake, they never fall to the levels seen in idiopathic PD (Tyrrell et al., 1990).

11.3 PET and SPECT studies in Parkinson's disease and dementia

Metabolic PET studies in PD patients with early asymmetric disease generally show increased metabolism in the contralateral lenticular nucleus (Miletich et al., 1988). As the disease generalizes this raised lentiform glucose metabolism tends to normalize (Eidelberg et al., 1990).

Cortical metabolism in nondemented PD patients, is either normal (Otsuka et al., 1991; Karbe et al., 1992; Goto et al., 1993), or mildly reduced to levels lying in between the means observed for controls and demented PD groups (Kuhl et al., 1984b; Okada et al., 1989). Covariance analysis has shown an abnormal inverse relationship between resting striatal and frontal glucose metabolism (Eidelberg et al., 1994). Kuhl et al. (1984a) studied a mixed group of demented and nondemented parkinsonian patients and found a global reduction in ^{18}FDG uptake that correlated inversely with both the severity of bradykinesia and dementia. Severe cognitive impairment was associated with a metabolic reduction in parietal cortex similar to that observed in patients with AD (Kuhl et al., 1984a; Peppard et al., 1988). One PD-dementia patient who showed reduced fronto-temporo-parietal glucose metabolism has come to post-mortem. He showed isolated brainstem Lewy body disease without cortical involvement confirming that this pattern of metabolic deficit is not specific for AD (Schapiro et al., 1990). SPECT has shown normal cerebral blood flow in nondemented PD patients, while in demented patients either an isolated reduction of frontal flow or a fronto-temporo-parietal pattern of hypoperfusion has been seen (Sawada et al., 1992).

We have recently performed a metabolic study with [18]FDG and PET in three cases with cognitive dysfunction and parkinsonism that fulfilled the clinical criteria for PD-dementia of Lewy body type (McKeith et al., 1992).

Case 1

A 71-year-old right-handed man first noticed progressive memory loss five years earlier followed by impaired verbal fluency and confabulation. More recently, he developed tremor of the right arm. On examination at the time of his PET scan he showed resting and postural tremor of the right limbs associated with increased rigidity, bradykinesia and decreased armswing of the right hand. His minimental scale (MMSE) score was 27/30. He had formal psychometric testing performed twice over three years; the second testing, a few months before PET, revealed progressive impairment of frontal function but improvement in his performance IQ. His brain CT showed involutional changes without focal abnormalities. At the time of the PET study he was not receiving any medication.

Case 2

A 72-year-old right-handed woman presented with a two year history of a shuffling gait. Diagnosed as having Parkinson's disease, she was started on levodopa/carbidopa preparation with immediate improvement of her symptoms. After a few months she developed end-dose akinesia and peak-dose dyskinesias in response to levodopa. Two years later she noticed a deterioration of her memory. At the time of the PET study she was experiencing depression, geographical and temporal disorientation, confusion in the mornings and visual hallucinations (mainly in the evenings). On examination while off medication, she had hypophonia, a bilateral resting tremor, mild rigidity of the right side and decreased armswing bilaterally. She had a shuffling gait and impaired postural

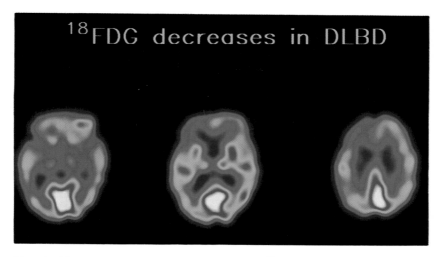

Plate 1 Three representative planes of integrated[18]FDG activity collected during the last 25 minutes of a 60-minute study.

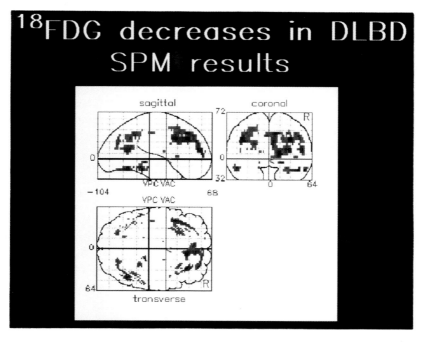

Plate 2 SPM transverse projections from the same normalized CMRGlc study. The black areas represent those regions in which the regional deficit was greater than 3 Z scores from the normal mean.

reflexes. Her MMSE was 22/30 and on bedside testing there was a deficit of recent recall, attention and praxis. Her brain CT showed basal ganglia calcification. At the time of the PET study she was receiving 400 mg of controlled release levodopa/carbidopa, fluoxetine 20 mg and diazepam 5 mg daily.

Case 3

A 73-year-old right-handed man had a thirteen year history of action tremor and a two year history of occasional geographical disorientation, gradual loss of memory, and an episode of visual hallucinations. At the time of PET he was complaining of fluctuating memory disturbance and depression. On examination he had hypophonia, mild bilateral resting and action tremor, absent armswing and bradykinesia most noticeable in the right hand. He had a stooped posture, a shuffling gait and impaired postural reflexes. The MMSE was 26/30 and he exhibited attentional deficit and apraxia. His brain CT showed mild involutional changes without focal abnormalities. At the time of the PET study he was receiving selegiline 10 mg/day.

Results were individually compared with those obtained for a group of 15 age-matched normal controls using statistical parametric mapping (SPM) to demonstrate focal reductions in resting glucose metabolism. Differences in global glucose metabolism (CMRglc) between subjects were normalized using an analysis of covariance (ANCOVA) with global metabolism as the confounding variable. Focal glucose metabolism for each individual was then compared on a pixel by pixel basis with that of a group of normals applying Z scores to each pixel. Due to the preliminary character of this study the results are expressed for those voxels in which the individual reduction of glucose metabolism from the control mean had a Z score greater than three.

Patient 1: Decreases in rCMRglc were most pronounced in bilateral mesial and lateral prefrontal cortex (areas 8 and 9), inferior temporal cortex, hippocampal gyrus, and right parietal area 40 – see Plates 1 and 2.

Patient 2: Decreases in rCMRglc were found in bilateral dorsal prefrontal area 9, anterior supplementary motor area and anterior cingulate, inferior temporal cortex, hippocampal gyrus, and bilateral parietal area 40.

Patient 3: Decrease in rCMRglc were seen in left mesial and lateral prefrontal cortex (areas 8 and 9), anterior supplementary motor area,

Broca's area 44, posterior cingulate/retrosplenial cortex (23) and bilateral inferior temporal cortex.

These preliminary results in our three patients showed a reduction in rCMRglc in fronto-temporo-parietal cortices, similar to that previously described in patients with AD and PD-dementia. Although these three patients only had mild cognitive failure they all showed a frontal metabolic deficit, while in AD patients with mild dementia the metabolic deficit is reported to be restricted to temporo-parietal areas (Frackowiak et al., 1981; Foster et al., 1983; Friedland et al., 1983; Kennedy et al., 1995). The only reported patient with pathological confirmed PD and mild dementia also showed glucose hypometabolism in fronto-temporo-parietal areas (Schapiro et al., 1990).

In summary, parkinsonism-dementia may be a clinical expression of either isolated brainstem or diffuse Lewy body disease or a combination of Lewy body and AD pathologies, although recent findings suggest that isolated brainstem pathology is extremely rare. PET studies in patients with PD-dementia have shown a pattern of fronto-temporo-parietal hypometabolism indistinguishable from that observed in patients with AD. [18]FDG studies in three of our patients that fulfilled clinical criteria for PD-dementia of DLBD type, also showed an AD metabolic pattern, although they only had a mild cognitive dysfunction. Further PET studies with postmortem confirmation are required to determine whether early frontal hypometabolism may help to distinguish PD-dementia of DLBD type from AD.

References

Alavi, A., Dann, R., Chawluk, J., Alavi, J., Kushner, M. & Reivich, M. (1986). Positron emission tomography imaging of regional cerebral glucose metabolism. *Semin. Nucl. Med.*, **16**, 2–34.

Brown, R.G. & Marsden, C.D. (1984). How common is dementia in Parkinson's disease? *Lancet*, **2**, 1262–5.

Byrne, J., Lennox, G., Lowe, J. & Godwin-Austen, R.B. (1989). Diffuse Lewy body disease: clinical features in 15 cases. *J. Neurol. Neurosurg. Psychiatry*, **52**, 709–17.

Chase, T.N., Foster, N.L., Fedio, P., Brooks, R., Mansi, L. & Di Chiro, G. (1984). Regional cortical dysfunction in Alzheimer's disease as determined by positron emission tomography. *Ann. Neurol.*, **15** (suppl), S170–4.

Costa, D.C., Ell, P.J., Philpot, M. & Levy, R. (1988). CBF tomograms with ^{99m}Tc-HM-PAO in patients with dementia (Alzheimer's type and HIV) and Parkinson's disease – Initial results. *J. Cereb. Blood Flow Metab.*, **8** (suppl 1), S109–15.

Crystal, H.A., Dickson, D.W., Lizardi, J.E., Davies, P. & Wolfson, L.I. (1990). Antemortem diagnosis of diffuse Lewy body disease. *Neurology*, **40**, 1523–8.

Eidelberg, D., Moeller, J.R., Dhawan, V. et al. (1990). The metabolic anatomy of Parkinson's disease: complementary [18F]Fluorodeoxyglucose and [18F]Fluorodopa positron emission tomographic studies. *Mov. Disord.*, **5**, 203–13.

Eidelberg, D., Moeller, J.R., Dhawan, V. et al. (1994). The metabolic topography of parkinsonism. *J. Cereb. Blood Flow Metab.*, **14**, 783–801.

Foster, N.L., Chase, T.N., Fedio, P., Patronas, N.J., Brooks, R.A. & Di Chiro, G. (1983). Alzheimer's disease: Focal cortical changes shown by positron emission tomography. *Neurology*, **33**, 961–5.

Frackowiak, R.S.J., Pozilli, C., Legg, N.J. et al. (1981). Regional cerebral oxygen supply and utilization in dementia. *Brain*, **104**, 753–8.

Friedland, R.P., Budinger, T.F., Ganz, E. et al. (1983). Regional cerebral metabolic alterations in dementia of the Alzheimer type: positron emission tomography with [18F]Fluorodeoxyglucose. *J. Comput. Assist. Tomogr.*, **7**, 590–8.

Garnett, E.S., Firnau, G. & Nahmias, C. (1984). Central dopaminergic pathways in hemyparkinsonism examined by positron emission tomography. *Can. J. Neurol. Sci.*, **11** [suppl 1], 174–9.

Goto, I., Taniwaki, T., Hosokawa, S., Otsuka, M., Ichiya, Y. & Ichimiya, A. (1993). Positron emission tomographic (PET) studies in dementia. *J. Neurol. Sci.*, **114**, 1–6.

Hansen, L., Salmon, D., Galasko, D. et al. (1990). The Lewy body variant of Alzheimer's disease: A clinical and pathologic entity. *Neurology*, **40**, 1–8.

Hughes, A.J., Daniel, S.E., Blankson, S. & Lees, A.J. (1993). A clinicopathologic study of 100 cases of Parkinson's disease. *Arch. Neurol.*, **50**, 140–8.

Karbe, H., Holthoff, V., Huber, M. et al. (1992). Positron emission tomography in degenerative disorders of the dopaminergic system. *J. Neural Transm. [Park. Dis. Dement. Sect.]*, **4**, 121–30.

Kennedy, A.M., Frackowiak, R.S.J., Newman, S.K. et al. (1995). Deficits in cerebral glucose metabolism demonstrated by positron emission tomography in individuals at risk of familial Alzheimer's disease. *Neurosci. Lett.*, **186**, 17–20.

Kosaka, K., Yoshimura, M., Ikeda, K. & Budka, H. (1984). Diffuse type of Lewy body disease: progressive dementia with abundant cortical Lewy bodies and senile changes of various degree – a new disease? *Clin. Neuropathol.*, **3**, 185–92.

Kuhl, D.E., Metter, E.J. & Riege, W.H. (1984a). Patterns of local cerebral glucose utilization determined in Parkinson's disease by the [18F]Fluorodeoxyglucose method. *Ann. Neurol.*, **15**, 419–24.

Kuhl, D.E., Metter, E.J., Riege, W.H. & Markham, C.H. (1984b). Patterns of cerebral glucose utilization in Parkinson's disease and Huntington's disease. *Ann. Neurol.*, **15**(suppl), S119–25.

Lennox, G., Lowe, J., Landon, M., Byrne, E.J., Mayer, R.J. & Godwin-Austen, R.B. (1989). Diffuse Lewy body disease: correlative neuropathology using anti-ubiquitin immunocytochemistry. *J. Neurol. Neurosurg. Psychiatry*, **52**, 1236–47.

McKeith, I., Fairbairn, A., Perry, R., Thompson, P. & Perry, E. (1992). Neuroleptic sensitivity in patients with senile dementia of Lewy body type. *BMJ*, **305**, 673–8.

Miletich, R.S., Chase, T., Gillespie, M., Di Chiro, G. & Stein, S. (1988). Contralateral basal ganglia glucose metabolism is abnormal in hemiparkinsonian patients: An FDG-PET study. *Neurology*, **38**(suppl 1), 260.

Molsa, P.K., Marttila, R.J. & Rinne, U.K. (1984). Extrapyramidal signs in Parkinson's disease. *Neurology*, **34**, 1114–16.

Okada, J., Peppard, R. & Calne, D.B. (1989). Comparison study of positron emission tomography, X-ray CT and MRI in parkinsonism with dementia. *Nippon Igaku Hoshasen Gakkai Zasshi*, **49**, 643–56.

Otsuka, M., Ichiya, Y., Hosokawa, S. et al. (1991). Striatal blood flow, glucose metabolism and ^{18}F-dopa uptake: difference in Parkinson's disease and atypical parkinsonism. *J. Neurol. Neurosurg. Psychiatry*, **54**, 898–904.

Peppard, R.F., Martin, W.R.W., Guttman, M. et al. (1988). The relationship of cerebral glucose metabolism to cognitive deficits in Parkinson's disease. *Neurology*, **38**(suppl 1), 364.

Perry, E.K., McKeith, I., Thompson, P. et al. (1991). Topography, extent, and clinical relevance of neurochemical deficits in dementia of Lewy body type, Parkinson's disease and Alzheimer's disease. *Ann. NY Acad. Sci.*, **640**, 197–202.

Piccini, P., Turjanski, N. & Brooks, D.J. (1995). PET studies of the striatal dopaminergic system in Parkinson's disease (PD). *J. Neural. Transm. [Gen. Sect.]*, **45**[suppl], 123–31.

Sawada, H., Udaka, F., Kamyama, M. et al. (1992). SPECT findings in Parkinson's disease associated with dementia. *J. Neurol. Neurosurg. Psychiatry*, **55**, 960–3.

Schapiro, M.B., Grady, C., Ball, M.J., DeCarli, C. & Rapoport, S.I. (1990). Reductions in parietal/temporal cerebral glucose metabolism are not specific for Alzheimer's disease. *Neurology*, **40**(suppl 1), 152.

Schmidt, M.L., Murray, J., Lee, VM-Y., Hill, W.D., Wertkin, A. & Trojanowski, J.Q. (1991). Epitope map of neurofilament protein domains in cortical and peripheral nervous system Lewy bodies. *Am. J. Pathol.*, **139**, 53–65.

Smith, F.W., Besson, J.A.O., Gemmell, H.G. & Sharp, P.F. (1988). The use of Technetium-99m-HM-PAO in the assessment of patients with dementia and other neuropsychiatric conditions. *J. Cereb. Blood Flow Metab.*, **8**(suppl 1), S116–22.

Tison, F., Dartigues, J.F., Auriacombe, S., Letenneur, L., Boller, F. & Alperovitch, A. (1995). Dementia in Parkinson's disease: A population-based study in ambulatory and institutionalized individuals. *Neurology*, **45**, 705–8.

Tyrrell, P.J., Sawle, G.V., Ibanez, V. et al. (1990). Clinical and positron emission tomographic studies in the 'extrapyramidal syndrome' of dementia of the Alzheimer type. *Arch. Neurol.*, **47**, 1318–23.

12

Clinical features of diffuse Lewy body disease in the elderly: analysis of 12 cases

S. KUZUHARA, M. YOSHIMURA,
T. MIZUTANI, H. YAMANOUCHI
and Y. IHARA

Summary

The clinical features of diffuse Lewy body disease (DLBD) in the elderly were retrospectively reviewed in 12 cases which had been diagnosed on pathological grounds. Their ages at onset and at death were between 60 and 85 years and between 76 and 92 years respectively. All of them had dementia of mild to severe degree, and eight presented with persistent severe hallucination-delusion psychosis with or without delirium. A single case presented with symptoms typical of Parkinson's disease including resting tremor, cogwheel rigidity and akinesia, while four of them showed no parkinsonian features. In the other seven, dementia or psychosis was followed by rigidity and akinesia at a late stage in the disease. Four had a history of orthostatic hypotension with syncope reminiscent of Shy–Drager syndrome. One can suspect DLBD when an elderly patient presents with atypical dementia of varying degrees, in combination with any of persistent delusion–hallucination psychosis, mild parkinsonism, and orthostatic syncope or dizziness.

12.1 Introduction

Diffuse Lewy body disease (DLBD) is a neuropathological entity in which abundant Lewy bodies (LBs) are found throughout the cerebral cortex, as well as in the brainstem nuclei in a manner identical to that seen in Parkinson's disease (Kosaka et al., 1980; Kosaka et al., 1984). Marked senile changes including abundant senile plaques and Alzheimer neurofibrillary tangles of diverse degree are also found in the elderly patients. As we reported previously (Kuzuhara et al., 1988; Kuzuhara & Yoshimura 1993), the clinical features of DLBD vary from case to case despite the rather uniform neuropathological findings; most patients present with progressive dementia with or without parkinsonism, while others showed persistent delusions or hallucinations, or progressive autonomic failure with or without dementia. The present paper describes the clinical features of 12 cases of neuropathologically verified DLBD, including the eight cases reported previously.

12.2 Materials and methods

Out of the 3,500 consecutive autopsy cases of the Tokyo Metropolitan Geriatric Hospital, a general hospital for the elderly patients in the Tokyo Metropolitan area, the neuropathological findings of 12 cases agreed with the criteria of DLBD (group A of Lewy body disease described by Kosaka et al., 1980). Lewy bodies are widely distributed not only in the brainstem and diencephalic nuclei but also in the cerebral cortex and basal ganglia, and senile changes of various degree are distributed in the cerebral cortex. Assessment of the medical history and clinical features were based on the medical records and information from the doctors, nurses and other therapists.

12.3 Results

Clinical features of the 12 cases are shown in Table 12.1. The mean age at onset of symptoms was 76.3 years (range: 60–85 years) and that at death, 82.8 years (range: 75–92 years). The mean duration of the illness was 6.6 years (range: 1–16 years).

12.3.1 Initial symptoms

As shown in Table 12.2 amnesia occurred in five cases (41.7%); dizziness/syncope, in four cases (33.3%); psychotic symptoms with visual hallucination in two cases (16.7%); and parkinsonian gait, in one case (8.3%) only.

12.3.2 Clinical signs and symptoms during the course of illness

The neuropsychiatric features, parkinsonism and autonomic symptoms are summarized in Table 12.3.

Neuropsychiatric features. All 12 cases (100%) presented with dementia of various degree, and nine of them (75%) were accompanied with

Table 12.1. *Clinical features of 12 cases of diffuse Lewy body disease in the elderly*

Case no	Sex	Age at onset	Age at death	Dur (yr)	Initial symp	Dementia	Psychosis	Parkinsonism Ri	Ak	Tr	Dizziness syncope
1*	M	80	83	3	Amnesia	+++	-	++	++	-	+
2*	M	82	84	2	Amnesia	+++	++	-	-	-	-
3*	F	82	92	10	Dizziness	+++	-	+	+	-	+
4*	M	72	75	3	Amnesia	+++	++	-	-	-	-
5*	F	75	80	5	Hallucination	+++	+++	++	+	+	-
6*	M	75	85	10	Hallucination	+	+++	-	-	-	+++
7*	M	60	75	15	Dizziness	++	+	++	+++	+++	+++
8*	M	81	85	4	Dizziness	+++	+	++	+	-	+++
9	F	64	80	16	Amnesia	+++	++	-	+	-	-
10	M	75	76	1	Akinesia	+++	+	++	++	-	-
11	M	85	90	5	Amnesia	+++	-	-	-	-	-
12	M	84	89	5	Syncope	+	+++	+	-	-	++

*Cases 1–8 were reported previously (Kuzuhara et al., 1988, 1993).

M:F = 9:3; Age at onset: 76.25 ± 7.8 years; Age at death: 82.8 ± 5.8 years; Duration of illness: 6.6 ± 5.0 (1–16) years

Dur: duration of illness, yr: year(s), Ri: rigidity, Ak: akinesia, Tr: tremor, −: none, +: mild, ++: moderate, +++: severe

Table 12.2. *Initial symptom of the 12 cases*

Amnesia	5 (41.7%)
Dizziness/syncope	4 (33.3%)
Psychosis and visual hallucination	2 (16.7%)
Parkinsonian gait	1 (8.3%)

Table 12.3. *Signs and symptoms of the 12 cases*

Neuropsychiatric features					
Dementia	12	(100%)	severe 3;	moderate 7;	mild 2
Psychosis with hallucination	9	(75%)	severe 6;		mild 3
Parkinsonism					
Typical parkinsonian feature	1	(8.3%)			
Rigidity and akinesia at the late stage	7	(58.3%)			
No parkinsonian features	4	(33.3%)			
Autonomic symptoms					
Orthostatic dizziness/ syncope	6	(50.0%)			
Confirmed orthostatic hypotension	5	(41.7%)			

psychotic-paranoiac symptoms with hallucinations. Three cases (25%) had very severe dementia, reminiscent of senile dementia of Alzheimer type (SDAT), without psychotic symptoms, while the remaining nine cases showed both dementia and psychotic symptoms. In the latter, dementia was severe to moderate in seven cases (58.3%) and four of them (33.3%) presented with delusions and hallucinations, reminiscent of schizophrenia or paranoia. The remaining two cases showed very severe delusions and hallucinations with minimal dementia and their antemortem diagnoses were organic delusional syndrome with hallucinations and atypical dementia with negativism. Antiparkinsonian drugs induced or aggravated the delusions and hallucinations.

Parkinsonian features. Eight cases (66.7%) presented with parkinsonian symptoms. Only one of them had symptoms and signs typical of Parkinson's disease including resting tremor, rigidity, akinesia, parkinsonian gait disturbance and masked face; whereas the other seven cases merely showed rigidity and bradykinesia at the late stage, and no tremor. Seven cases (58.3%) showed flexed posture with rigidity and gegenhalten at the terminal stage. Five of them were treated with antiparkinsonian drugs including levodopa, trihexyphenidyl and amantadine hydrochloride. Motor symptoms improved in one case only, while adverse psychotic symptoms including restlessness, confusion, delirium, visual hallucination, and delusion occurred in the remaining four cases and antiparkinsonian drugs were discontinued.

Autonomic symptoms. Six patients (50%) often complained of orthostatic dizziness, and four of them (33.3%) had a history of syncopal attacks when they stood up. Orthostatic hypotension was confirmed in five of them.

12.4 Discussion

Peculiar progressive dementia characterized neuropathologically by widely disseminated intracytoplasmic eosinophilic inclusions (cortical LBs) in the neurons in the cerebral cortex as well as brainstem nuclei was first described in two elderly white male Americans (Okazaki, Lipkin & Aronson 1961). Many similar cases have been reported since then, mostly from Japan (Ikeda et al., 1978; Kosaka et al., 1980; Yoshimura, 1983; Kuzuhara et al., 1988), then from North America and Europe. Kosaka et al. (1984) reviewed the clinical and neuropathological features of 12 cases of DLBD from Japan, Austria and Germany, and proposed that DLBD might be a new entity of presenile dementia. In recent years, more and more similar cases have been accumulated from Europe (Gibb et al., 1985, 1989; Byrne et al., 1989; Perry et al., 1990) and North America (Sima et al., 1986; Dickson et al., 1987; Burkhardt et al., 1988; Hansen et al., 1990; Crystal et al., 1990). Although it is a condition originally defined neuropathologically, antemortem diagnosis of DLBD has been attempted. In the previous clinical and neuropathological study of eight elderly cases of DLBD aged between 75–92 years at death (Kuzuhara et al., 1988; Kuzuhara & Yoshimura, 1993), we have found that DLBD of elderly patients presented with a variety of neuropsychiatric, parkinsonian and autonomic symptoms including dementia, delusions and hallucinations, parkinsonism and orthostatic hypotension. The present study of the clinical features of 12 cases of DLBD including the eight previous cases and four new ones has confirmed our previous findings. The cardinal clinical features were dementia (100%) with delusions and hallucinations in 75% of cases. Typical parkinsonian features were uncommon, though the neuropathological findings in the brainstem nuclei were similar to those of Parkinson's disease. Marked orthostatic hypotension showing syncope and dizziness was also characteristic and frequently the initial symptom, although very little attention had been paid to autonomic functions previously. Several cases with severe autonomic dysfunction resembling Shy–Drager syndrome were reported from Japan (Kono et al., 1976; Nagura et al., 1984; Kuzuhara et al., 1988 – cases 6, 7 and 8) and the USA (Burkhardt et al., 1988 – case 1), and neuropathological examination revealed severe involvement of the autonomic neurons of the brain, spinal cord, and autonomic ganglions and plexus of the peripheral nerves. Therefore, atypical dementia of mild to severe degree accompanied by psychotic symptoms of delusions and hallucinations, by mild to moderate parkinsonism with muscle rigidity and bradykinesia but no resting tremor, and by dizziness, syncope or orthostatic hypotension reminiscent of autonomic failure, seems to be the typical clinical features of patients associated with DLBD.

Crystal et al. (1990) reported on an analysis of the clinical symptoms of six patients with DLBD. Gait impairment with mild to moderate dementia was found in most patients, and muscle rigidity and resting tremor, agitation, hallucinations and delusions were frequent early symptoms. Although the findings of the present study basically agree with those of Crystal et al., parkinsonian features were far less prominent in the present series. This is probably partly because our patients were older than those of Crystal et al. (age at onset: 76.2 vs. 73.7 years, age at death: 82.8 vs. 81.3 years). The only one of the present series who presented with typical parkinsonian symptoms was 60 years old at onset. According to Kosaka and his colleagues (1984, 1990), parkinsonian features are prominent in patients of juvenile and presenile onset; whereas dementia is the main feature in those of senile onset.

Absent or very mild parkinsonian features despite brainstem pathology similar to that of typical Parkinson's disease are still a puzzling problem of DLBD in the elderly. Both the dopaminergic and cholinergic systems are severely affected in DLBD not only neuropathologically but also biochemically (Langlais et al., 1993). The clinical features and neuropathological findings of the pure form of DLBD, in which there are abundant LBs but no or few senile changes in the central nervous system (Kosaka, 1990; Kosaka et al., 1984), may in part account for the puzzling problem. Patients with the pure form present with the clinical feature of juvenile parkinsonism; most of them develop dementia later, but some never show dementia. These findings suggest that the presence or absence of senile changes affects the occurrence of parkinsonism, as well as of dementia, in the presence of abundant cortical and brainstem LBs. Marked depletion of the cholinergic activity of the brain in DLBD may counteract the dopaminergic dysfunction which produces parkinsonian symptoms.

Acknowledgements

The present study was supported in part by a Grant-in-Aid for Scientific Research (B-03454240) from the Ministry of Education, Science and Culture of Japan. We thank Mr Aikyo N. and Ms Saishoji J. for their technical assistance.

References

Burkhardt, C.R., Filley, C.M., Kleinschmidt-DeMasters, B.K., de la Monte S. et al. (1988). Diffuse Lewy body disease and progressive dementia. *Neurology*, **38**, 1520–8.

Byrne, E.J., Lennox, G., Lowe, J. & Godwin-Austen, R.B. (1989). Diffuse Lewy body disease: clinical features in 15 cases. *J. Neurol. Neurosurg. Psychiatry*, **52**, 709–17.

Crystal, H. A., Dickson, D.W., Lizardi. J.E., Davis, P. et al. (1990). Antemortem diagnosis of diffuse Lewy body disease. *Neurology*, **40**, 1523–8.

Dickson, D.W., Davies, P., Mayeux, R., Crystal, H. et al. (1987). Diffuse Lewy body disease. Neuropathological and biochemical studies of six patients. *Acta Neuropathol. (Berl.)*, **75**, 8–15.

Gibb, W.R.G., Esiri, M.M. & Lees, A.J. (1985). Clinical and pathological features of diffuse cortical Lewy body disease (Lewy body dementia). *Brain*, **110**, 1131–53.

Gibb, W.R.G., Luthert, P.J., Janota, I. & Lantos, P.L. (1989). Cortical Lewy body dementia: clinical features and classification. *J. Neurol. Neurosurg. Psychiatry*, **52**, 185–92.

Hansen, L., Salmon, D., Galasko, D., Masliah, E. et al. (1990). The Lewy body variant of Alzheimer's disease: a clinical and pathologic entity. *Neurology*, **40**, 1–8.

Ikeda, K., Ikeda, S., Yoshimura, T., Kato, H. et al. (1978). Idiopathic parkinsonism with Lewy-type inclusions in cerebral cortex. A case report. *Acta Neuropathol. (Berl.)*, **41**, 165–8.

Kono, C., Matsubara, M. & Inagaki, T. (1976). Idiopathic orthostatic hypotension with numerous Lewy bodies in the sympathetic ganglia. Report of a case. *Neurol. Med. (Tokyo)*, **4**, 568–70.

Kosaka, K. (1990). Diffuse Lewy body disease in Japan. *J. Neurol.*, **237**, 197–204.

Kosaka, K., Matsushita, M., Oyanagi, S. & Mehraein, P. (1980). A clinicopathological study of the 'Lewy body disease'. *Psychiat. Neurol. Jpn. (Tokyo)*, **82**, 292–311.

Kosaka, K., Yoshimura, M., Ikeda, K. & Budka, H. (1984). Diffuse type of Lewy body disease: progressive dementia with abundant cortical Lewy bodies and senile changes of varying degree – A new disease? *Clin. Neuropathol.*, **3**, 185–92.

Kuzuhara, S. & Yoshimura, M. (1993). Clinical and neuropathological aspects of diffuse Lewy body disease in the elderly. In *Advances in Neurology,* Vol. 60, ed. H. Narabayashi, T. Nagatsu, N. Yanagisawa & Y. Mizuno, pp. 464–9. New York: Raven Press.

Kuzuhara, S., Yoshimura, M., Nagura, H., Yamanouchi, H. et al. (1988). Clinical features of diffuse Lewy body disease. Report of 8 cases and review of the literature. *Clin. Neurol.* (*Toyko*), **28**, 1274–81.

Langlais, P.J., Thal, L., Hansen, L., Galasko, D. et al. (1993). Neurotransmitters in basal ganglia and cortex of Alzheimer's disease with and without Lewy bodies. *Neurology*, **43**, 1927–34.

Nagura, H., Yamanouchi, H., Yoshimura, M. & Tomonaga, M. (1984). Shy–Drager syndrome with extensive distribution of numerous Lewy bodies in the central nervous system. Report of a case. *Neurol. Med.* (*Toyko*), **20**, 157–65.

Okazaki, H., Lipkin, L.E. & Aronson, S.M. (1961). Diffuse intracytoplasmic ganglionic inclusions (Lewy type) associated with progressive dementia and quadriparesis in flexion. *J. Neuropathol. Exp. Neurol.*, **20**, 237–44.

Perry, R.H., Irving, D., Blessed, G., Fairbairn, A. & Perry, E.K. (1990). Senile dementia of Lewy body type. A clinically and neuropathologically distinct form of Lewy body dementia in the elderly. *J. Neurol. Sci.*, **95**, 119–39.

Sima, A.A.F., Clark, N.A., Sternberg, N.A. & Sternberger, L.A. (1986). Lewy body dementia without Alzheimer changes. *Can. J. Neurol. Sci.*, **13**, 490–7.

Yoshimura, M. (1983). Cortical changes in the parkinsonian brain: a contribution to the delineation of 'diffuse Lewy body disease'. *J. Neurol.*, **229**, 17–32.

13

Senile dementia of Lewy body type – clinical features and prevalence in neuropathological postmortems

L. M. D R A C H , S. W A C H and J. B O H L

Summary

Though the history of Lewy body related diseases started in Germany, German neurology and psychiatry still ignore the existence of dementias with cortical Lewy bodies (LB). In order to estimate the proportion of senile dementia of the Lewy body type (SDLBT) in neuropathological postmortems in Germany, we screened all brains ($n = 273$) of adult patients, who died in 1991 and were examined by one neuropathologist at the University Medical Center in Mainz, Germany. A multi-stage approach to detecting LBs was used with final detection by ubiquitin immunohistochemistry.

Four cases were discovered (1.5% of all cases and 4.3% of demented or confused patients). Thirty cases from the series had a neuropathological diagnosis of Alzheimer's disease (AD). All four cases with cortical LBs showed additional neurofibrillary pathology. In other years, independent of this study, solitary cases attracted attention in which no additional neurofibrillary pathology was detected. The clinical spectrum and its nosological implications are discussed and a diagnostic separation between a condition with 'pure' cortical Lewy bodies and one representing a combination with Alzheimer pathology is suggested.

13.1 Introduction

In 1912 the history of Lewy body (LB)-related diseases started in Germany with Friederich H. Lewy's contribution to Lewandowsky's *Handbuch der Neurologie* (Lewy, 1912). In this chapter, concerning the pathology of paralysis agitans, Lewy gave the first description of 'classical' ('brainstem-type') and 'serpiginous' LBs in the neurons of the dorsal

161

vagal nucleus. Lewy himself did not mention the substantia nigra in particular, even when he described the occurrence of LBs in other brain-stem nuclei in his famous book *Die Lehre vom Tonus und der Bewegung* (Lewy, 1923). The involvement of the substantia nigra in Parkinson's disease (PD) was described first by Trétiakoff, who coined the term Lewy body (Trétiakoff, 1919).

Only since the introduction of levodopa therapy of PD by Birkmayer and Barbeau (Barbeau et al., 1961; Birkmayer & Hornykiewicz, 1961), have German neurology and neuropathology focused on the substantia nigra in PD (Jacob & Kawagoe, 1984; Cervós-Navarro, 1991). In German neurology, PD with symptoms exceeding the classical range of rigidity, tremor, akinesia, autonomic disorders, and bradyphrenia is called Parkinson plus (Fischer, 1984). In German studies, up to 70% of PD patients are reported to suffer cognitive impairment in the course of the disease and up to 50% can be diagnosed as demented by various criteria (Martin et al., 1973; Schneider et al., 1982). By Fischer's defini-tion, a patient suffering from PD with dementia would be diagnosed Parkinson plus.

The first description of a dementia with numerous cortical LBs with-out parkinsonian features (Okazaki et al., 1961) and its confirmation by many other groups (Kosaka, 1978; Kosaka et al., 1984; Dickson et al., 1987; Gibb et al., 1987; Lennox et al., 1989a; Perry et al., 1990) after the introduction of ubiquitin immunohistochemistry into the detection of LBs (Lennox et al., 1989b) was ignored by German psychiatry. To our knowledge there has to date been no paper on senile dementia of the Lewy body type (SDLBT) in a German psychiatric journal.

This would be understandable if SDLBT was only another rare cause of degenerative dementia, and if the diagnosis had no important clinical implications. Since 1992, however, there have been indications that there is an increased neuroleptic sensitivity in SDLBT with fatal consequences for some patients (McKeith et al., 1992). In addition there are some hints, that SDLBT patients are in fact the responders to cholinergic replace-ment therapy with tacrine in putative Alzheimer's disease (AD) (Levy et al., 1994).

In the absence of classical parkinsonian symptoms it is very important to establish valid clinical diagnostic criteria for SDLBT, especially if the findings of increased neuroleptic sensitivity and better response to tacrine in SDLBT are confirmed in the future. Operational criteria have been proposed and evaluated (McKeith et al., 1994).

The proportion of SDLBT in brain banks of demented patients varies between 3.7% (Pollanen & Bergeron, 1989) and 26.3% (Lennox et al., 1989c). To our knowledge, no data on the proportion of SDLBT in German postmortems have been published so far.

The nosological status of SDLBT is uncertain. Cortical LBs have been found in 76% of cases in a postmortem series of PD patients (Hughes et al., 1992). On the other hand, most cases of SDLBT show some histological features of AD (Sima et al., 1986). As amyloid pathology in AD is not correlated with the severity of dementia, but neurofibrillary pathology is (Braak & Braak, 1991; Arriagada et al., 1992), the latter seems to be a more specific histological marker for AD. Though there are descriptions of SDLBT with diffuse amyloid plaques only and with no neurofibrillary tangles (Sima et al., 1986; Hansen et al., 1993), the relationship of SDLBT to both AD and PD is not clear. On neuropathological grounds, however, it is known that the combination of AD and PD has six times the frequency expected due to age (Boller et al., 1980).

We present data which estimates the prevalence of SDLBT in a series of neuropathological autopsies in Germany. In addition we wish to contribute to the discussion of the nosological status of SDLBT.

13.2 Proportion of cases of senile dementia of the Lewy body type in German postmortems

In order to estimate the proportion of SDLBT in neuropathological postmortems in Germany, we screened all the brains of adult patients for SDLBT, who died in 1991 and were prepared by one neuropathologist of the neuropathology service of the University Medical Center in Mainz (J.B.). We chose this particular neuropathology service because it served a number of general and mental hospitals in the region. Due to the broad spectrum of hospitals served by the service, its postmortems of adults probably is generally representative of typical German neuropathology services. (See Fig. 13.1).

The total number of brains of adult patients (> 18 years of age) was 273. One hundred and sixty-three patients were 65 years of age or older (59.7%). The vast majority of all brains (251) had been screened for amyloid plaques using the Campbell staining technique (Campbell et al., 1987); 145 cases showed some degree of plaque formation (53%). The available clinical information on 92 of these cases indicated dementia or delirium (33% of all adult cases and 63% of the cases with plaques). All the cases except one who suffered from Creutzfeldt–Jakob's disease

total: 273

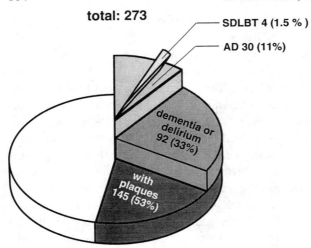

SDLBT 4 (1.5 %)

AD 30 (11%)

dementia or delirium 92 (33%)

with plaques 145 (53%)

Fig. 13.1 In order to estimate the proportion of senile dementia of Lewy body type (SDLBT) in neuropathological postmortems in Germany, we screened all brains ($n = 273$) of adult patients who died in 1991 and were prepared by one neuropathologist of the neuropathology service of the University Medical Center in Mainz (Germany) for cortical Lewy bodies. We used a multistage approach. In the first step, the vast majority of brains (251) were screened for amyloid plaques using the Campbell staining technique. One hundred and forty-five (53%) cases showed some degree of plaque formation. The available clinical information of 92 (33% of all) cases indicated dementia or delirium. These cases were examined with ubiquitin immunohistochemistry for cortical Lewy bodies. Four (1.5% of all) cases of SDLBT were detected. All four had Alzheimer pathology enough to warrant an additional diagnosis of Alzheimer's disease according to the CERAD protocol. In our sample only 13.3% of Alzheimer's disease cases showed cortical Lewy bodies at the same time. The 30 cases with Alzheimer's disease represent 11% of our sample.

were examined with ubiquitin immunohistochemistry (DAKO Z-458) for LBs in paraffin sections (Lennox et al., 1989b).

Four cases showed LBs in cortical areas in addition to insular cortex and cingular gyrus and thereby conformed to one definition of SDLBT (Lennox et al., 1989c). This represents 1.5% of all adult brains, 2.5% of all those 65 years of age or over, and 4.3% of cases with clinical information indicating dementia or delirium.

All four cases had AD pathology (neuritic plaques and neurofibrillary tangles) enough to warrant an additional diagnosis of AD according to the CERAD protocol (Mirra et al., 1991) or Braak's criteria (Braak & Braak, 1991). A total of 30 cases (11% of all adult cases) had a neuropathological diagnosis of 'definite' or 'probable' AD according to the CERAD protocol. In our sample only one (3% of all AD cases) showed

LB pathology at the same time. In 1991 all SDLBT cases had been detected by ubiquitin immunohistochemistry only, whereas in other years solitary cases had attracted attention by H and E staining only. In these cases, there was no neurofibrillary pathology at the same time.

These data show that, using appropriate methods, cases of SDLBT can be identified in neuropathological postmortems in Germany, but they are relatively rare compared with AD. One can speculate about a higher proportion of SDLBT cases in brains of demented patients from mental hospitals, but three of the four SDLBT cases in 1991 died in general hospitals.

13.3 Differences in clinical features between 'pure' Lewy body pathology and the combination with Alzheimer's disease

The debate concerning the nosological status of SDLBT is puzzling and the differences of nosological concepts are expressed in the variety of names adopted for the condition (e.g. SDLBT, Lewy body dementia, diffuse Lewy body disease, Lewy body variant of Alzheimer's disease). In order to illustrate the spectrum of clinical presentations, which can be associated with dementia with cortical LBs, two case reports follow.

Case report 1

A 62-year-old woman presented complaining of weakness in her hands and legs, as well as tremor of her right leg. A strumectomy had been performed 20 years ago. Repeatedly she refused to walk, but did so a few hours later. She appeared depressed and due to her mental state, a diagnosis of conversion neurosis with psychogenic gait disorder was made and she was treated as an inpatient on a psychiatric ward. She received antidepressive medication and was discharged with an improved mental state six weeks later.

One year later she was admitted to another mental hospital, because she again complained of a rapidly progressing weakness. On the day of admission she showed psychomotor retardation and was fully orientated, but memory deficits were obvious. Her mood was depressed and again she refused to walk. A monotonous and slightly slurred speech as well as a weak gag reflex was noted. A few hours after admission, she walked across the ward without needing help.

Over the next three weeks her physical state deteriorated and she had to be transferred to a medical ward due to bronchopneumonia. On return to the mental hospital, she was disorientated and bewildered. Difficulties of swallowing required tube-feeding. She developed contractures of her legs and muscular fasciculations occurred in both legs.

The patient was transferred to a neurological ward. There she was almost mute and did not cooperate with examination. Dysarthria and rigidity of neck, arms and legs were obvious. She showed a positive Babinsky's sign on the right side and muscular fasciculations of both legs. The small muscles of the hands were atrophic. High TSH and low T3 and T4 values were detected and L-thyroxine up to 100 μg was started. The bronchopneumonia was treated with antibiotics. The patient's mental state improved. She was speaking again and appeared to be orientated. Through this improvement it became obvious that the patient was hearing voices and had delusions of persecution. She behaved very aggressively and refused to participate in physiotherapy.

The rigidity was not improved by intravenous amantadine. CSF was normal. A MRI scan revealed a few white matter lesions in the right hemisphere. The EEG was slowed. The EMG confirmed muscular fasciculations and a cortical magnetic stimulation revealed a conduction block of the pyramidal tract.

In order to control hallucinations and aggressive behavior, neuroleptic therapy with haloperidol and promethazine was started but failed to control the hallucinations. After transfer back to the mental hospital her condition was continuously deteriorating. She needed tube-feeding again and became completely paralysed (quadriparesis in flexion). She lost orientation and died, aged 64 years, of central failure of circulatory regulation.

The postmortem examination showed numerous cortical LBs in all cortical areas examined and also LBs in the brainstem, especially in the substantia nigra. Though there had been numerous diffuse amyloid plaques, no neurofibrillary pathology was present.

Case report 2

This 90-year-old male patient lived together with his wife, who was five years younger, but not able to care for him anymore. Memory deficits had developed over several years and for the last years he became abusive towards his wife. He had a previous history of alcoholism, but no recent heavy drinking. Chronic gastritis, chronic bronchitis and an aneurysm of the aorta were known. Three months before admission, he became confused and agitated every evening. The family reported that he had not tolerated every attempted medication, especially neuroleptics.

At the time of admission to a psychogeriatric ward, the patient was not fully orientated for time and place. Recent memory and attention were poor, long-term memory well preserved. No delusions or hallucinations were found. He was cooperative and friendly. The neurological examination was normal, no parkinsonian features were found. Every evening he developed a confusional state with wandering and aggressive behavior. Neuroleptic medication was started and he calmed down. There was no description of side effects of neuroleptic drugs in the clinical notes. Two weeks later he was found dead, sitting in an armchair. The postmortem examination disclosed left ventricular hypertrophy of the heart and severe general arteriosclerosis with an infrarenal aneurysm of the aorta. The cause of death was right ventricular heart failure.

The brain showed slight fronto-temporal cortical atrophy and marked ventricular enlargement. Several small old cerebral contusions were found. Histologically the density of neuritic plaques and neurofibrillary tangles warranted a diagnosis of AD. Additionally, cortical LBs were found in all cortical areas examined. In the brainstem, including the substantia nigra, classical and serpiginous LBs were detected.

Comparing the two case reports, they are very different both from a clinical and neuropathological point of view. Clinically speaking, the first patient suffered from a very complex neurological and psychiatric disorder, clinically resembling a combination of PD, motor neuron disease, paranoid-hallucinatory psychosis, and dementia. The second patient, however, suffered from a degenerative dementia, putative AD, with fluctuating cognitive impairment and increased neuroleptic sensitivity. He did not show abnormal neurological features, especially no parkinsonian ones.

On neuropathological grounds both cases are also very different. The first case is a good example of 'pure' LB pathology, whereas the second is a combination of AD pathology with cortical and brainstem LBs. According to various studies (Braak & Braak, 1991; Arriagada et al., 1992) only neurofibrillary pathology is correlated with the severity of dementia and the diagnosis of AD requires a minimum of tangles, neuropil threads, and neuritic plaques. The first case presented did not fulfil these criteria for AD.

In the second case one can speculate, whether the LB pathology modified the clinical picture and lead to the increased neuroleptic sensitivity, but dementia can be explained by the AD pathology itself. One can also speculate, whether the condition of the second patient could be better described as a combination of AD and subclinical PD.

13.4 Conclusions

The data from neuropathological postmortems in Mainz, indicate that SDLBT is present in Germany, as it is in other countries. The proportion of SDLBT, however, is small compared with 'pure' AD. There are still no German data available, concerning the proportion of SDLBT in postmortems from demented patients, dying in mental hospitals or nursing homes. Additionally our study illustrates that one has to use ubiquitin immunohistochemistry to identify SDLBT cases properly.

The clinical and neuropathological spectrum of dementia with cortical LB shows two extremes:

1. There is a combination of AD pathology with cortical LB, which clinically is very similar to 'pure' AD except for possible additional symptoms, for example, increased neuroleptic sensitivity. A diagnostic separation of the disease characterized by the combination of AD and LB pathologies from 'pure' AD would be useful on clinical grounds, if the two groups could be separated by valid clinical diagnostic criteria and if the effort of separation could be shown to have consequences for subsequent management. In our opinion those cases deserve the names SDLBT or 'LB variant of AD'.
2. At the other end of the spectrum, there is 'pure' LB pathology with more complex neurological symptoms. There are some case reports of 'pure' LB pathology with exceptional clinical features as observed in our first case (Yoshimura et al., 1988; Fearnley et al., 1991; Reyes et al., 1993), which stress the necessity for making a nosological difference between the cases with 'pure' and 'mixed' LB pathology. Some of these cases, like our first case, occurred under the age of 65. For this reason the name SDLBT is misleading and 'diffuse LB disease' would be more accurate.

Acknowledgements

This work was supported by the Ludwig Edinger Foundation. The authors thank Prof. W. Schlote and Prof. H.-H. Goebel for their kind support and stimulating discussions as well as Mrs B. Lafferton and Mrs R. Ruhl for technical assistance. Above all we thank Drs H. Steinmetz and W. Oehl for their kind permission to use the clinical information of their patients.

References

Arriagada, P.V., Crowdon, J.H., Hedley-Whyte, E.T. & Hyman, B.T. (1992). Neurofibrillary tangles but not senile plaques parallel duration and severity of Alzheimer's disease. *Neurology*, **42**, 631–9.

Barbeau, A., Murphy, G.F. & Sourkes, T.L. (1961). Excretion of dopamine in diseases of basal ganglia. *Science*, **133**, 1706.

Birkmayer, W. & Hornykiewicz, O. (1961). Der L-3,4-Dioxyphenylalanin (=Dopa)-Effekt bei der Parkinson-Akinese. *Wien. Klin. Wschr.*, **73**, 787–8.

Boller, F., Mizutani, T., Roessmann, U. & Gambetti, P. (1980). Parkinson's disease dementia and Alzheimer's disease: clinicopathological correlations. *Ann. Neurol.*, **7**, 329–35.

Braak, H. & Braak, E. (1991). Neuropathological stageing of Alzheimer-related changes. *Acta Neuropathol.*, **82**, 239–59.

Campbell, S.K., Switzer, R.C. & Martin, T.L. (1987). Alzheimer's plaques and tangles: A controlled and enhanced silver staining method. *Soc. Neurosci. Abstr.*, **13**, 687.

Cervós-Navarro, J. (1991) Degenerative Krankheiten des Thalamus, der Stammganglien und des Mittelhirns. 5. Parkinsonismus. In *Spezielle pathologische Anatomie* Vol. 13/5 *Pathologie des Nervensystems – Degenerative und metabolische Erkankungen*. ed. W. Doerr & E Uehlinger, pp. 547–61. Springer: Berlin.

Dickson, D.W., Davies, P., Mayeux, R. et al. (1987). Diffuse Lewy body disease. Neuropathological and biochemical studies of six patients. *Acta Neuropathol.*, **75**, 8–15.

Fearnley, J.M., Revesz, T., Brooks, D.J., Frackowiak, R.S.J. & Lees, A.J. (1991). Diffuse Lewy body disease presenting with a supranuclear gaze palsy. *J. Neurol. Neurosurg. Psychiatry*, **54**, 159–61.

Fischer, P-A. (1984). Parkinson plus—Einleitung und definition. In *Parkinson Plus*. ed. P-A Fischer, pp. 1–3. Springer: Berlin.

Gibb, W.R., Esiri, M.M. & Lees, A.J. (1987). Clinical and pathological features of diffuse cortical Lewy body disease (Lewy body dementia). *Brain*, **110**, 1131–53.

Hansen, L.A., Masliah, E., Galasko, D. & Terry, R.D. (1993). Plaque-only Alzheimer's disease is usually the Lewy body variant and vice versa. *J. Neuropathol. Exp. Neurol.*, **52**, 648–54.

Hughes, A.J., Daniel, S.E., Blankson, S. & Lees, A.J. (1992). Accuracy of clinical diagnosis of idiopathic Parkinson's disease: A clinico-pathological study of 100 cases. *J. Neurol. Neurosurg. Psychiatry*, **55**, 181–4.

Jacob, H. & Kawagoe, T. (1984). Klinische Neuropathologie des Parkinson Syndroms. Proteintyp und Dopamintyp der Demyelinisierung. In *Parkinson Plus*. ed. P-A Fischer, pp. 18–31. Springer: Berlin.

Kosaka, K. (1978). Lewy bodies in cerebral cortex. Report of three cases. *Acta Neuropathol.*, **42**, 127–34.

Kosaka, K., Yoshimura, M., Ikeda, K. & Budka, H. (1984). Diffuse type of Lewy body disease: Progressive dementia with abundant cortical Lewy bodies and senile changes of varying degree. A new disease? *Clin. Neuropathol.*, **3**, 185–92.

Lennox, G., Lowe, J., Landon, M., Byrne, E.J., Mayer, R.J & Godwin-Austen, R.B. (1989a). Diffuse Lewy body disease: correlative neuropathology using anti-ubiquitin immunohistochemistry. *J. Neurol. Neurosurg. Psychiatry*, **52**, 1236–47.

Lennox, G., Lowe, J., Morrel, K., Landon, M. & Mayer, R.J. (1989b). Anti-ubiquitin immunohistochemistry is more sensitive than conventional techniques in the detection of diffuse Lewy body disease. *J. Neurol. Neurosurg. Psychiatry*, **52**, 67–71.

Lennox, G., Lowe, J.S., Godwin-Austen, R.B., Landon, M. & Mayer, R.J. (1989c). Diffuse Lewy body disease: An important differential diagnosis in dementia with extrapyramidal features. *Prog. Clin. Biol. Res.*, **317**, 121–30.

Levy, R., Eagger, S., Griffiths, M. et al. (1994). Lewy bodies and response to tacrine in Alzheimer's disease (Letter). *Lancet*, **343**, 176.

Lewy, F.H. (1912). Paralysis agitans. I. Pathologische Anatomie. In *Handbuch der Neurologie*. Vol. 3, ed. M. Lewandowsky, pp. 920–33. Berlin: Springer.

Lewy, F.H. (1923). *Die Lehre vom Tonus und der Bewegung*. Berlin: Springer.

Martin, W.E., Loewensen, R.B. & Resch, J.A. (1973). Parkinson's disease: Clinical analysis of 100 patients. *Neurology*, **23**, 783–90.

McKeith, L., Fairbairn, A., Perry, R.H., Thompson, P. & Perry, E.K. (1992). Neuroleptic sensitivity in patients with senile dementia of Lewy body type. *BMJ*, **305**, 673–8.

McKeith, I., Fairbairn, A., Bothwell. R. A. et al. (1994). An evaluation of the predictive validity and inter-rater reliability of clinical diagnostic criteria for senile dementia of Lewy body type. *Neurology*, **44**, 872–7.

Mirra, S.S., Heyman, A., McKeel, D. et al. (1991). The Consortium to Establish a Registry for Alzheimer's Disease (CERAD): II. Standardization of the neuropathological assessment of Alzheimer's disease. *Neurology*, **44**, 872–7.

Okazaki, H., Lipkin, L.E. & Aronson, S.M. (1961). Diffuse intracytoplasmatic ganglionic inclusions (Lewy type) associated with progressive dementia and quadriparesis in flexion. *J. Neuropathol. Exp. Neurol.*, **20**, 237–44.

Perry, R.H., Irving, D., Blessed, G., Fairbairn, A. & Perry, E.K. (1990). Senile dementia of the Lewy body type. A clinically and neuropathologically distinct form of Lewy body dementia in the elderly. *J. Neurol. Sci.*, **95**, 119–39.

Pollanen, M.S. & Bergeron, C. (1989). Morphometric analysis of Alzheimer's disease with Lewy bodies. *Prog. Clin. Biol. Res.*, **317**, 485–92.

Reyes, E., Gamboa, A. & Masliah, E. (1993). Atypical diffuse Lewy body disease with neuritic abnormalities. *Clin. Neuropathol.*, **12**, 330–4.

Schneider, F., Fischer, P-A., Jacobi, P. & Becker, H. (1982). Demenz beim Parkinson Syndrom. In *Psychopathologie des Parkinson Syndroms*. ed. P-A. Fischer, pp. 93–114. Basel: editiones Roche.

Sima, A.A.F., Clark, A.W., Sternberger, N.A. & Sternberger, L.A. (1986). Lewy body dementia with Alzheimer changes. *Can. J. Neurol. Sci.*, **13**, 490–7.

Trétiakoff, C. (1991). Contribution l'étude de l'anatomie pathologique du locus niger de Soemmering. Thèse de Paris.

Yoshimura, N., Yoshimura, I., Asada, M. et al. (1988). Juvenile Parkinson's disease with widespread Lewy bodies in the brain. *Acta Neuropathol.*, **77**, 213–18.

14

Lewy body dementia in clinical practice

D. COLLERTON, C. DAVIES and
P. THOMPSON

Summary

A clinical diagnosis of dementia of Lewy body type (DLT) was made in 10% of referrals to a clinical service providing psychogeriatric care to a locality based population of 18,000 people aged > 65 years. Thirty per cent of referrals received a diagnosis of Alzheimer's disease and 22% of multi-infarct dementia. Inter-rater agreement for the three different diagnoses was equally good (kappa = 0.67) and the profile of differential diagnosis was stable in two consecutively sampled years. We suggest that a cluster of symptoms exists which we can reliably define in clinical practice as dementia of Lewy body type. It may be useful to view a person with any three of the following features, cognitive impairment, extrapyramidal symptoms, fluctuating confusion and visual hallucinations, as most likely having DLT, regardless of coexisting cerebrovascular disease or other physical illnesses, both to avoid potentially hazardous treatments such as conventional neuroleptics and to select patients for future beneficial interventions.

14.1 Introduction

Does Lewy body dementia[*] exist in clinical practice? Can it be recognized in the routine work of an old age psychiatry service? In whom do we recognize Lewy body dementia, and what character does it have?

[*] We use the term Lewy body dementia to refer to a syndrome characterized by intellectual impairment, a fluctuating confusional state, extrapyramidal symptoms and visual hallucinations, and which is associated with cortical Lewy bodies. This is broadly consistent with the published criteria of McKeith et al. (1992b). However, we have found that, in

Our own interest in these questions began in the late 1980s when we were looking at cases of presumed Charles Bonnet syndrome. At the same time, colleagues in Newcastle were describing senile dementia of Lewy body type. We soon found the second diagnosis subsumed the first. In this chapter, we report on our subsequent experiences with the diagnosis of Lewy body dementia and attempt to answer our questions from the perspective of the sole service for elderly people with mental health problems within a geographically limited area. We compare our experiences with reports of cases from selected autopsy or research series. We hope that this comparison may illustrate some of the controversies which have developed in this area. Since some of these disagreements may reflect different referral, selection, and reporting biases, we will describe our own situation in some detail.

Gateshead is a socially homogenous community on the south bank of the river Tyne. It has a population of 208,000; 32,000 of whom are aged over 65. Most of the population is concentrated in a central urban area but smaller, more rural villages extend to the west. It was previously a heavy industrial area, though little of this remains. It scores highly on indices on deprivation and health need; more so in the central area. The population is relatively stable, with little inward or outward migration, particularly amongst the elderly, and it has the smallest proportion of ethnic minority groups of any urban district in England.

Specialized services for elderly people in Gateshead who have mental health problems are primarily provided by two psychogeriatric teams. Each covers a sector which is defined by geographically clustered primary care practices. We work within the Western sector (population aged over 65 of 18,190) and therefore report results from only that area.

The psychogeriatric services staff consists of psychiatrists, clinical psychologists, community and ward-based nurses, occupational therapists and physiotherapists and administrative staff, who work as a multi-disciplinary team.

Referrals come from primary care practices; from physicians, particularly specialists in old age medicine; and from general adult psychiatrists.

---

clinical practice, a history of falls and transient changes in consciousness is difficult to establish, and have therefore tended not to use them. This would agree with Shergill et al. (1994) who also found that these factors did not distinguish DLT patients. We are agnostic as to the relationship of this to the other reports of Lewy body associated syndromes, and to other dementing illnesses, particularly Alzheimer's disease. We have used these criteria rather than those of Byrne et al. (1991) because their validity has been examined in a second sample (McKeith et al., 1994a,b). Arguments in this area are well rehearsed in this book and elsewhere (for example, Byrne, 1995; McKeith, 1995).

Neurological services are mostly provided in a different district, but there is a limited local service which refers people with presenile dementia. The psychogeriatric service deals with virtually all people over 65 who are referred with dementing illnesses; the majority of people under 65 who have pre-senile dementia (others being dealt with by a variety of differing services); and 85% of people over 65 who have functional illnesses – mainly those with *de novo* disorders (others being dealt with by general adult psychiatric services). By no means all people with dementia or functional problems will be referred; our samples are therefore probably biased towards more severe and problematic illnesses.

Routine investigations include a full medical and mental state examination and blood screen (full blood count, erythrocyte sedimentation rate, urea, electrolytes, glucose, liver and thyroid function tests, bone chemistry, syphilis serology, vitamin B12 and red cell folate levels). Supplementary investigations including chest X-rays, ECGs, CT scans, EEGs and psychometric assessments are performed as clinically indicated.

14.2 Subjects and methods

14.2.1 The case series

We report preliminary data and analyses from two retrospective case series: those referrals received in 1993, and those in 1994. Full details of the data are being prepared for publication and are available from the authors.

We first made a postmortem confirmed clinical diagnosis of Lewy body dementia in 1990; previous cases had been identified as dementia with superimposed confusional states, multi-infarct dementia or Charles Bonnet syndrome. With a newly described disorder, there is an understandable learning process amongst referrers and specialized services which has implications for sample biases. We therefore selected 1993 and 1994 to allow us to look at data for patients with Lewy body dementia once the diagnosis was well established.

In constructing the case series we used an audit database to select all referrals from 1993 and 1994 who received diagnoses at first contact with our service (initial diagnosis) of dementia Alzheimer type (DAT), multi-infarct type dementia (MID), dementia Lewy body type (DLT), dementia not otherwise specified (DNOS) or depression (DEP). We excluded cases with an initial diagnosis of personality disorder, bipolar affective disorder, paraphrenia, schizophrenia, a single stroke or single episode of delir-

ium due to a physical cause, or no mental disorder. We also excluded
mixed initial diagnoses (6% of all referrals). There were 566 people with
our selected diagnoses – 79% of referrals. Case notes were available for
478 of these patients, although not all contained full information. These
formed the case series.

The case notes were then independently reviewed and re-diagnosed by
two of the authors using a standard proforma. The proforma was con-
structed on the basis of expected symptomatology and other features of
dementing illness. Agreement at this stage was over 90%. Disagreements
were reviewed by a third author, and a consensus decision taken on
diagnoses. Seventy per cent of disagreements were resolved at this stage
giving an overall agreement of 97%. The remaining cases were analysed
within the 'other' category. At this stage, all patients were assigned one of
the following categories of diagnosis: DAT ($n = 142$), DLT ($n = 48$), MID
($n = 105$), DEP ($n = 98$), mixed DAT/MID ($n = 24$), DNOS ($n = 25$) or
other ($n = 39$). The 'other' category included diagnoses we had previously
excluded, as well as those cases for which the authors were unable to
reach a consensus decision.

Criteria for the various diagnoses were based on published guidelines;
DSM-IV (American Psychiatric Association, 1994), NINCDS–ADRDA
(McKhann et al., 1984), and for DLT the Newcastle criteria (McKeith et
al., 1992). However, since we are reporting clinical series, we based our
diagnoses upon our best clinical judgement rather than strict adherence
to research diagnostic criteria, the application of which would have substantially increased the proportion of unclassified or multiply classified
cases. In conjunction with colleagues in Newcastle, cases are being followed up neuropathologically where possible but as yet too few cases
have been examined to allow agreement to be analysed. Three cases
have been reported, one each of DAT, DLT and MID; all had the
same clinical and pathological diagnoses.

14.3 Results

In this section we report on the characteristics of patients who received a
consensus diagnosis of DLT. We draw out significant differences, and
similarities between the various diagnostic groups. We also compare our
findings with those of other studies.

We now return to the questions we asked at the beginning of this
chapter.

14.3.1 Can we recognize DLT in clinical practice?

14.3.1.1 Diagnosis

In both the 1993 and 1994 case series', we classified 10% of the referrals as having DLT, 30% as DAT and 22% as MID. The remainder of the cases were classified as suffering from depression, mixed DAT/MID or other diagnoses. The 10% of referrals diagnosed as having DLT by our criteria is comparable to the 10% of dementia referrals to old-age psychiatry services reported by Ballard et al. (1995), though is lower than the 23% previously reported by the same authors (Ballard et al., 1993) and the 26% reported by Shergill et al. (1994).

Overall, initial and consensus diagnoses were in agreement in approximately two-thirds of cases. The percentages diagnosed as having DLT and other diagnoses were consistent for both years, suggesting both that it is consistently diagnosed, and that it is consistently referred. For this reason, we will report the combined series from now on unless otherwise indicated. Where reclassification did take place, most cases reclassified as DLT at consensus diagnosis were initially diagnosed as DAT or DNOS, while most who were reclassified from an initial diagnosis of DLT received a consensus diagnosis of MID or DNOS. The kappa values for initial and consensus diagnosis for all dementia groups are equally good (0.67 for DLT, DAT and MID; 0.88 for DEP), suggesting that DLT, MID, and DAT can be clinically diagnosed with equal reliability.

We also analysed referral source and reason for referral by consensus diagnosis. There is a significant relationship between reason for referral and consensus diagnosis ($\chi^2 p < 0.05$). DLT patients were more likely to be referred because of hallucinations (39%) and, as expected, DEP patients because of mood problems (81%). One implication of this is that if a service does not receive referrals for hallucinations, there may be a lower prevalence of DLT within that service.

The majority of referrals (72–82%) in all groups came from primary care settings. The highest proportion of referrals from secondary care came in the DEP group. Most of these patients had depression secondary to physical illness. However, overall, symptomatology and consensus diagnosis did not differ by source of referral.

We classified the duration of the history at referral into three bands, under 1 year, 1–2 years and over 2 years. Our data shows that this does not differ between DLT and DAT, with half of the people referred with both these conditions having a 2-year plus history of difficulties. In contrast, more people who received a consensus diagnosis of MID or DEP tended to have shorter histories with 40% under one year ($\chi^2 p < 0.05$).

In answer to our question, we have shown that we can diagnose DLT in a significant minority of our patients on the basis of routine clinical examinations. This diagnosis is, in our hands, as stable as the diagnosis of DAT or MID.

Although referrals came from different sources, in our setting we found no significant variations between these.

14.3.2 In whom do we recognize DLT?

14.3.2.1 Demographic characteristics

These are shown in Table 14.1. The average age of all patients is in the late seventies to early eighties with no significant differences between groups. Similar age ranges have been reported in other case series (Crystal et al., 1990; Hansen et al., 1990; Perry et al., 1990; Förstl et al., 1993; Galasko et al., 1994; McKeith et al., 1994a), although some series have reported patients to be slightly younger, ranging in age from the late sixties to seventies (Dickson et al., 1987; Byrne et al., 1989). The youngest cases, reported by Gibb et al. (1985) were from a neurology rather than psychogeriatric setting.

There is a significant overall difference in sex ratios between the four groups and DLT patients are more likely than those with DAT to be male in all age bands ($\chi^2 p < 0.001$). This is consistent with other series which have reported equal numbers or an excess of males with Lewy body symptomatology (e.g. Dickson et al., 1992; Mayeux et al., 1992). In contrast to other reports (see e.g., Ballard et al., 1993), all groups reported very low rates of family history, possibly reflecting unsystematic questioning and a failure of family members to survive to high risk ages.

We also analysed consensus diagnosis by geographical location of those patients living at home. Although this approached significance for the 1993 series ($\chi^2 0.05 < p < 0.1$), there was no relationship for the 1994 series or both combined.

14.3.3 When we do recognize DLT, what character does it have?

14.3.3.1 Symptomatology

Symptomatology at referral by consensus diagnosis is shown in Table 14.2. As required by our diagnostic criteria, and in common with reports

Table 14.1. *Demographic characteristics by consensus diagnosis*

	DLT	DAT	MID	DEP
% male[*]	58	14	46	32
Male/total *n*	28/48	20/142	48/105	31/98
Mean age	78	82	79	78
Standard deviation	7	7	5	8
% male by age range				
66–70	0	25	45	54
71–75	50	19	65	44
76–80	78	9	33	27
81–85	29	12	41	20
86–90	82	11	29	14
91–95	67	33	100	67

[*]at least two of the groups differ significantly; χ^2 $p < 0.001$

from other series (Gibb et al., 1985; Dickson et al., 1987; Byrne et al., 1989; Gibb et al., 1989; Crystal et al., 1990; Perry et al., 1990; Förstl et al., 1993; Lippa et al., 1994; McKeith et al., 1994a) our DLT cases have high levels of cognitive impairment, fluctuating confusion and extrapyramidal symptoms, although none of these symptoms are present in 100% of cases at referral. Comparisons with DAT suggest fewer cases with cognitive impairment, which is also milder when present as measured by Blessed Mental Test Score at referral. Fluctuating confusion is common in the DAT and MID groups, though less so than in DLT. A high proportion of DLT cases have visual hallucinations, more so than most postmortem derived series (Dickson et al., 1987; Byrne et al., 1989; Gibb et al., 1989; Hansen et al., 1990; Perry et al., 1990; Förstl et al., 1993), but equal to that previously reported from this area (McKeith et al., 1994b). This could reflect several potential factors; a lack of recognition in life of hallucinations or exclusion from initial samples because of these, differential referral patterns of people with hallucinations, or that we have classified DLT cases without hallucinations into another category. Compared with other groups, people who received a diagnosis of DLT also had higher rates of auditory hallucinations (which always coexisted with visual hallucinations), delusions, falls and clouding of consciousness.

Of course, all of these symptoms are common in a population of older adults with dementing illnesses, and all have multiple possible aetiologies.

Table 14.2. *Symptom prevalence by consensus diagnosis*

Symptom	Consensus diagnosis								s.p. (%)
	DLT		DAT		MID		DEP		
	n	%	*n*	%	*n*	%	*n*	%	
Disabling cognitive impairment[*1]	37	77	141	99	98	93	11	11	71
Blessed MTS at referral† (mean and standard deviation)	25±7		19±8		23±8		30±5		–
Fluctuating confusion[*2]	36	75	35	25	58	55	11	11	36
Extrapyramidal symptoms[*3] (including neuroleptic associated)	39	81	11	8	7	7	7	7	14
Visual hallucinations[*4]	41	85	9	6	10	10	2	2	17
Auditory hallucinations[*5]	12	25	3	2	4	4	5	5	7
Delusions[*6]	17	35	7	5	5	5	4	4	10
Clouding of consciousness[*7]	9	19	3	2	7	7	1	1	6
Unexplained falls[*8]	22	46	16	11	25	24	1	1	18
Depression[*9]	7	15	14	10	14	13	97	99	30

s.p. = sample prevalence
[*] significant overall differences between groups by χ^2. Subsequent analyses showed:
[1]DAT > MID > DLT > DEP; [2]DLT > MID > DAT > DEP; [3]DLT > DAT = MID = DEP; [4]DLT > DAT = MID = DEP; [5]DLT > DAT = MID = DEP; [6]DLT > DAT = MID = DEP; [7]DLT > MID > DAT = DEP; [8]DLT > MID > DAT > DEP; [9]DEP > DLT = DAT = MID
† MTS significantly differed between DLT and DAT, DEP and MID, and DEP and DAT by t-test.

However, using the population base rates of the prevalence of each symptom, it is possible to calculate the probability that these symptoms would co-exist purely by chance. This calculation† would suggest that, by

† For the whole case series: probability of cognitive impairment × probability of extrapyramidal symptoms × probability of fluctuating confusion × probability of visual hallucinations × sample size = 0.71 × 0.14 × 0.36 × 0.17 × 478 = 3 cases.

chance, three patients out of the 478 in the study sample would have all four symptoms. We found fourteen – more than four times as many (χ^2 $p < 0.02$), suggesting a nonchance grouping. These results, of course, do not confirm that this grouping is necessarily due to the presence of DLT.

An analysis of medications taken by consensus diagnosis indicated that people diagnosed as having DLT were more likely than the others to be taking both a combined levodopa preparation (28% vs $1-4\%$ χ^2 $p < 0.05$) and neuroleptic medication (30% vs $14-21\%$ $\chi^2 p < 0.05$). Our analyses also indicated that within the DLT group there is a significant association between extrapyramidal symptoms and levodopa use (spearman phi 0.30 $p < 0.05$) and significant negative associations between neuroleptics and fluctuating confusion (spearman phi -0.37 $p < 0.02$) and clouding of consciousness (spearman phi -0.32 $p < 0.05$); raising the possibility that they may have a specific effect on these symptoms, or are avoided in people with such symptoms.

We looked at relationships between the major symptoms within the total sample. The most interesting findings are reported here, the figure in brackets representing spearman's phi coefficient. Disabling cognitive impairment correlated with unexplained falls (0.12) and fluctuating confusion (0.10). Extrapyramidal symptoms correlated with a diagnosis of Parkinson's disease (0.44), visual hallucinations (0.34), clouding of consciousness (0.20) and use of neuroleptics (0.10). Visual hallucinations correlated with delusions (0.40), infections (0.15), clouding of consciousness (0.14) and Parkinson's disease (0.11). Fluctuating confusion correlated with delusions (0.17), infections (0.15), clouding of consciousness (0.14) and Parkinson's disease (0.11).

14.3.3.2 Physical disorders

Physical disorders by consensus diagnosis are shown in Table 14.3. This shows that total physical diagnoses do not distinguish the four groups. Patients in the DLT group are more likely to have received diagnoses at referral of Parkinson's disease than those in the other groups (χ^2 $p < 0.05$). Patients who received a consensus diagnosis of DLT were also less likely to have documented cardiac disease, a cardiovascular accident, a transient ischaemic attack, hypertension, infection or airways disease ($\chi^2 p < 0.05$). This lower frequency of infections is particularly significant in view of the general association between infection and fluctuating confusion.

Table 14.3. *Documented physical disorders by consensus diagnosis*

	DLT $n=48$		DAT $n=142$		MID $n=105$		DEP $n=98$	
Average number of diagnoses per patient	2.2		1.7		2.7		2.3	
Standard deviation	2.0		1.5		1.7		1.5	
Documented physical conditions	n	%	n	%	n	%	n	%
Parkinson's disease[*1]	10	21	2	1	0	0	3	3
Eye disease	10	21	22	15	17	16	9	9
Impaired hearing	7	15	22	15	9	9	8	8
Cardiac disease[*2]	7	15	22	15	38	36	33	34
Cerebrovascular accident[*3]	4	8	1	1	25	24	7	9
Transient ischaemic attack[*4]	3	6	0	0	13	12	4	4
Infection[*5]	2	4	24	17	14	13	8	8
Airways disease[*6]	1	2	4	3	12	11	16	16
Hypertension[*7]	1	2	12	8	16	15	6	6

[*]significant differences for at least two groups by χ^2 $p<0.05$. Analyses showed:
[1]DLT > DAT = MID = DEP; [2]MID = DEP > DLT = DAT; [3]MID > -
DEP = DLT > DAT; [4]MID > DLT = DAT = DEP; [5]DAT = MID = DEP > DLT;
[6]MID = DEP > DLT = DAT; [7]MID > DLT = DAT = DEP
No other concurrent diagnosis was reported in more than 10 per cent of patients in any group, and these were therefore not further analysed.

14.3.3.3 Mortality and institutionalization

An analysis of the proportion of people in institutional care indicated no differences between the various diagnostic groups. Total mortality to June 1995 did not differ between people with diagnoses of DLT (21%), MID (16%) or DEP (20%). A significantly smaller proportion of those diagnosed with DAT died within the same timescale (10%, $p<0.05$). There is also an excess of total mortality in the DLT 1994 series compared with other groups within the 1994 series ($p<0.05$). However, when mortality is analysed separately for each sex, there are no differences between groups, suggesting that the higher mortality in the DLT group is due to its higher proportion of males with their shorter life expectancy. Because of the suggestion of life threatening side effects of neuroleptic medication in DLT (McKeith et al., 1992a), we separately analysed mortality by use of neuroleptic medication in this group. We found no significant relationship, possibly because, being alert to this possibility, we avoided or minimized its use. In contrast to the other diagnostic groups, mortality in the DLT 1993 and 1994 series are equal, suggesting the possibility that a subgroup of patients may rapidly die, with the remainder having a longer life expectancy. We have not as yet analysed dates of death within the 1993 series, and so are unable to confirm this trend for patients referred in 1993.

14.4 The clinical diagnosis of Lewy body dementia

The cases we report reflect the biases operating in our own area, both in terms of who refers, why they refer to us and how we then diagnose different disorders. Particularly in the case of Lewy body disease, where there is as yet no agreement on definitive diagnostic criteria, the symptomatology we report obviously reflects the criteria we use. The data was also collected in the course of clinical work rather than as a structured research study with consequent variability and incomplete ascertainment.

However, this would only be important if these factors systematically varied by diagnosis. Therefore, despite the limitations outlined above, we believe that there are several conclusions that we can draw.

14.4.1 The archetypal case

We can consistently diagnose a group of patients with fluctuating confusion, visual hallucinations, extrapyramidal symptoms and cognitive impairment. This symptom cluster occurs more often than chance would suggest and makes up 8% of all our referrals, 14% of all referrals with dementia. Our archetypal case is a man in his late seventies. He usually lives at home, and is referred from primary care because of visual hallucinations or confusion after a one year plus history. He may have a previous diagnosis of Parkinson's disease, but usually will not, and may be taking levodopa or neuroleptics but usually not. He will be unlikely to have cardiac or cerebrovascular disease or a current infection. He stands a one in five chance of dying within a year of the first contact with our service, but thereafter will probably survive the second year. We will change our minds about his diagnosis about one time in four.

Although prescriptions of dopaminergic drugs are frequent in this group, they do not consistently relate to the symptomatology, and other factors which might account for the symptomatology (concurrent infections, other diseases or other classes of medication) are rare. These clinically diagnosed patients with DLT have similar age, sex ratio and symptomatology to pathologically derived series and, although the clinical criteria may be less rigidly applied than in research studies, the fact that we have actually reported lower prevalences than most other studies suggests that we are cautious in applying this diagnosis.

What is the relationship of this symptom cluster to other definitions of Lewy body disease? We believe that we are reporting one section of a continuum, though a consistent and important part of that spectrum. Elucidation of the relationship of this to other parts of the spectrum awaits systematic and unselective neuropathological follow-up (Brayne, 1993).

Undoubtedly, our DAT, MID and other diagnostic groups include patients with Lewy body pathology. In common with others (Shergill et al., 1994), we have found that the Newcastle and Nottingham criteria do not identify the same patients. There are, for example, 11 DAT, 6 DNOS and 7 MID cases with the combination of disabling cognitive impairment and extrapyramidal symptoms suggested in the Nottingham criteria for DLT (Byrne et al., 1991). Conversely, only 28 of our DLT cases have both these features.

14.4.2 Predictive validity

Ultimately, the clinical utility of a diagnosis depends upon whether it can be made in life. Table 14.4 indicates how the relationships between diagnoses may vary according to the number of symptoms used to categorize them.

For example, a cut-off of three out of four symptoms from cognitive impairment, extrapyramidal symptoms, fluctuating confusion and visual hallucinations agrees with a consensus diagnosis in 89% of DLT cases, 95% of DAT cases, and 91% of MID cases. A looser criteria of two out of four symptoms would include all cases diagnosed as having DLT, but also include a third of cases who currently receive a diagnosis of DAT and just over half of those with MID. Although negative predictive values are uniformly high due to the low prevalence of DLT in this population, positive predictive values vary more than threefold and there is a strong inverse relationship between sensitivity and specificity. Where the division is ultimately drawn will depend upon both clinical and neuropathological correlations and the clinical utility of DLT.

Table 14.4. *Illustrative relationships of consensus diagnosis, sensitivity, specificity, and positive and negative predictive value of DLT diagnosis by number of symptoms, using consensus diagnosis as gold standard*

No. of symptoms	Consensus diagnosis					Accuracy			
	DLT	DAT	MID	DEP	DNOS + Mixed	Sensitivity	Specificity	Pos. Predictive Value	Neg. Predictive Value
0/4	0	2	0	71	1	–	–	–	–
1/4	0	91	47	23	33	–	–	–	1.00
2/4	5	43	48	4	21	1.00	0.66	0.24	0.99
3/4	29	6	9	0	5	0.90	0.94	0.63	0.93
4/4	14	0	1	0	0	0.29	1.00	0.93	0.93
EPS + DCI*	–	–	–	–	–	0.58	0.93	0.49	0.95

*EPS = Extrapyramidal symptoms, DCI = Disabling cognitive impairment

14.5 Conclusion

To return to our initial question, we would suggest that in clinical practice, something exists which we can recognize as dementia of Lewy body type. We would suggest that it may be useful to view a person with three out of four symptoms as most likely having DLT, regardless of coexisting cerebrovascular disease or other physical illnesses, both to avoid potentially hazardous treatments such as conventional neuroleptics and to select patients for future beneficial interventions.

Acknowledgements

We would like to thank all of our colleagues in the Lewy body Body, especially Dorothy Irving, for their help, support and stimulation. We would also like to thank all those staff and patients in Gateshead who have participated in our studies, especially Sarah Black and Isabel Moloney for helpful comments on earlier drafts of this article.

References

American Psychiatric Association (1994). *Diagnostic Criteria from DSM-IV*. Washington: Psychiatric Association.

Ballard, C.G., Mohan, R.N.C., Patel, A. & Bannister, C. (1993). Idiopathic clouding of consciousness—do the patients have cortical Lewy body disease? *Int. J. Geriatr. Psychiatry*, **8**, 571–6.

Ballard, C.G., Saad, K., Patel, A. et al. (1995). The prevalence and phenomenology of psychotic symptoms in dementia sufferers. *Int. J. Geriatr. Psychiatry*, **10**, 477–85.

Brayne, C. (1993) Clinicopathological studies of the dementias from an epidemiological viewpoint. *Br. J. Psychiatry*, **162**, 439–46.

Byrne, E.J. (1995). Cortical Lewy body disease: an alternative view. In *Developments in Dementia and Functional Disorders in the Elderly*, ed. R. Levy & R. Howard, pp. 21–30, Petersfield, UK: Wrightson.

Byrne, E.J., Lennox, G., Lowe, J. & Godwin-Austen, R.B. (1989). Diffuse Lewy body disease: clinical features in 15 cases. *J. Neurol. Neurosurg. Psychiatry*, **52**, 709–17.

Byrne, E.J., Lennox, G.G., Godwin-Austen, R.B. et al. (1991). Dementia associated with cortical Lewy bodies: proposed clinical diagnostic criteria. *Dementia*, **2**, 283–4.

Crystal, H.A., Dickson, D.W., Lizardi, J.E., Davies, P. & Wolfson, L.I. (1990). Antemortem diagnosis of diffuse Lewy body disease. *Neurology*, **40**, 1523–8.

Dickson, D.W., Davies, P., Mayeux, R. et al. (1987). Diffuse Lewy body disease. *Acta Neuropathol.*, **75**, 8–15.

Dickson, D.W., Wu, E., Crystal, H. A. et al. (1992). Alzheimer's disease and age-related pathology in diffuse Lewy body disease. In *Heterogeneity in Alzheimer's Disease*, ed. Boller et al., pp. 169–86. Berlin: Springer-Verlag.

Förstl, H., Burns, A., Luthert, P., Cairns, N. & Levy, R. (1993). The Lewy-body variant of Alzheimer's disease. Clinical and pathological findings. *Br. J. Psychiatry*, **162**, 385–92.

Galasko, D., Hansen, L.A., Katzman, R. et al. (1994). Clinical-neuropathological correlations in Alzheimer's disease and related dementias. *Arch. Neurol.*, **51**, 888–95.

Gibb, W.R.G., Esiri, M.M. & Lees, A.J. (1985). Clinical and pathological features of diffuse cortical Lewy body disease (Lewy body dementia). *Brain*, **110**, 1131–53.

Gibb, W.R.G., Luthert, P.J., Janota, I. & Lantos, P.L. (1989). Cortical Lewy body dementia: clinical features and classification. *J. Neurol., Neurosurg. Psychiatry*, **52**, 185–92.

Hansen, L., Salmon, D., Galasko, D. et al. (1990). The Lewy body variant of Alzheimer's disease: A clinical and pathological entity. *Neurology*, **40**, 1–8.

Lippa, C.F., Smith, T.W. & Swearer, J.M. (1994). Alzheimer's disease and Lewy body disease: A comparative clinicopathological study. *Ann. Neurol.*, **35**, 81–8.

Mayeux, R., Denaro, J., Hemenegildo, N. et al. (1992). A population-based investigation of Parkinson's disease with and without dementia. *Arch. Neurol.*, **49**, 492–7.

McKeith, I.G. (1995). Cortical Lewy body disease: the view from Newcastle. In *Developments in Dementia and Functional Disorders in the Elderly*, ed. R. Levy & R. Howard ed., pp. 9–20. Wrightson: Petersfield, UK.

McKeith, I. G., Fairbairn, A.F., Perry, R.H., Thompson, P. & Perry, E.K. (1992a). Neuroleptic sensitivity in patients with senile dementia of Lewy body type. *BMJ*, **305**, 673–8.

McKeith, I.G., Perry, R.H., Fairbairn, A.F., Jabeen, S. & Perry, E.K. (1992b). Operational criteria for senile dementia of Lewy body type (SDLT). *Psychol. Med.*, **22**, 911–22.

McKeith, I.G., Fairbairn, A.F., Bothwell, R.A. et al. (1994a). An evaluation of the predictive validity and inter-rater reliability of clinical diagnostic criteria for senile dementia of Lewy body type. *Neurology*, **44**, 872–7.

McKeith, I.G., Fairbairn, A.F., Perry, R.H. & Thompson, P. (1994b). The clinical diagnosis and misdiagnosis of senile dementia of Lewy body type (SDLT). *Br. J. Psychiatry*, **165**, 324–32.

McKhann, G., Drachman, D., Folsten, M., Katzman, R., Price, D. & Stadlan, E.M. (1984). Clinical diagnosis of Alzheimer's disease: report of the NINCDS–ADRDA Work Group under the auspices of Department of Health and Human Services Task Force on Alzheimer's disease. *Neurology*, **34**, 939–44.

Perry, R., Irving, D., Blessed, G., Fairbairn, A. & Perry, E.K. (1990). Senile dementia of Lewy body type – A clinically and neuropathologically distinct form of Lewy body dementia in the elderly. *J. Neurol. Sci.*, **95**, 119–39.

Shergill, S., Mullan, E., D'Ath, P. & Katona. C. (1994). What is the clinical prevalence of Lewy body dementia? *Int. J. Geriatr. Psychiatry*, **9**, 907–12.

Résumé of clinical workshop sessions

I. G. McKEITH, D. GALASKO and N. QUINN

The clinical workshop adopted a two-stage approach to the challenging task of agreeing clinical diagnostic criteria for dementia with Lewy bodies (DLB).

Session one – Where does DLB fit within the diagnostic framework?

The first step was to define the scope of the new criteria, in particular whether they ought to be part of a unifying diagnostic category covering the whole spectrum of clinical presentations of LB disorders, or whether they should restrict themselves to only one part of this. The subsequent task would then be to select and operationally define the specific items of diagnostic importance. Two existing sets of clinical diagnostic criteria (the Newcastle criteria for senile dementia of Lewy body type (SDLT) (McKeith et al., 1992) and the Nottingham criteria for dementia associated with cortical Lewy bodies (Byrne et al., 1991)) were tabled for consideration, as were supplementary data from other participants (all to be found in the preceding clinical chapters).

Preliminary discussion centred on the principle that diagnostic criteria should be framed in the way most relevant to established clinical procedures. It was agreed that a single set of clinical criteria encompassing the whole spectrum of LB disorders, ranging from motor Parkinson's disease (PD) to primary cognitive failure, would produce a diagnostic category containing enormous clinical heterogeneity. Such a system would be difficult to apply in clinical practice and would have low face validity. The approach recommended was to concentrate upon describing the constellation of neuropsychiatric manifestations thought to be associated with cortical LB – namely fluctuating cognitive impairment, attentional deficits and perceptual disturbances – and to position this correctly in

187

relation to existing clinical diagnostic systems, in particular those for Alzheimer's disease (AD) and for PD. This clinical syndrome, designated as dementia with LB (DLB), could either occur de novo, in which case the important diagnostic discrimination would be from other causes of dementia, particularly AD, or could occur as a later development in a patient already diagnosed as having Parkinson's disease. In these latter circumstances, workshop participants felt that the term PD with dementia should be used to describe the general clinical category. Within this appellation, subgroups such as PD with LB dementia or PD with AD, might be distinguished using clinical and neuropsychological criteria. The group acknowledged that very little data yet exists regarding the practical aspects of accuracy of these finer clinical distinctions, although it was thought that the hallmark features of primary DLB should be helpful in identifying those PD patients in whom dementia is due to cortical progression of LB pathology.

Two areas of potential diagnostic uncertainty emerged from these early discussions. First, elderly patients often present a complex admixture of extrapyramidal and mental symptoms of almost simultaneous onset. How should such cases be categorized? The consensus view was that if dementia occurred within 12 months of the onset of motor PD, the patient should be classified as having a primary diagnosis of dementia with LB – if the clinical history of PD is longer than this, PD with dementia will usually be a more appropriate diagnostic label. Secondly, the role of anti-parkinsonian medication in precipitating and perpetuating the confusional and hallucinatory symptoms considered to be typical of DLB, was debated. The group discussed these symptoms in the setting of PD, based more upon collective clinical experience than on formal studies. The impression of many participants was that when these symptoms do not recede or clear only slowly after withdrawal of medication in PD patients, they may be harbingers of subsequent progressive cognitive decline and dementia.

In defining the boundaries of DLB, the potential overlap with other conditions causing dementia, notably Alzheimer's disease (AD) and vascular dementia (VaD) was noted. Prevailing concepts of clinical heterogeneity have extended the diagnostic boundaries of AD sufficiently that the majority of DLB patients may be included within them. This is particularly so for the NINCDS–ADRDA 'possible AD' criteria (McKhann et al., 1984). When these were proposed, it was acknowledged that amendments would be required in the light of new developments. Revisions of the existing diagnostic systems for AD and VaD are now underway and those engaged working on them must be kept informed by our endeavours to delineate patients with DLB.

Session two – Which features can be used to discriminate DLB from dementias of other aetiology?

In the continuing absence of disease-specific biological markers, precise operational definitions of the key symptoms of DLB will need to form the basis of accurate clinical discrimination between it and other pathological causes of dementia. The second phase of the clinical workshop moved to consider which individual symptoms and symptom clusters possess sufficient discriminatory power to warrant inclusion in diagnostic criteria.

Preliminary discussions had predetermined dementia as a mandatory requirement for diagnosis. When applied strictly, most existing criteria for the dementia syndrome pose problems, because, having been developed in relation to AD, they list delirium as an exclusionary feature. Fluctuation resembling delirium is common in DLB and in the earliest stages, patients may show deficits of attention, cognitive function and global performance alternating with periods of normal or near-normal performance. A broader definition of dementia is therefore required.

It was agreed that a demonstration of impaired cognition by formal testing of mental status is essential to establishing the diagnosis of DLB. The participants concurred that symptoms of prominent or persistent memory impairment were not essential early in the course of DLB, but were likely to develop with progression. This again is not entirely consistent with most standard definitions of the dementia syndrome. Some studies suggest that DLB patients are impaired in memory retrieval, in contrast to AD patients whose major deficit lies in memory acquisition and consolidation. The presence of prominent deficits on tests of attention and of frontal-subcortical skills and visuospatial ability may be useful clinical diagnostic markers of DLB (see Chapters 8 and 9).

Fluctuation in cognitive function and global performance was agreed by most participants to be an important and common characteristic of LB disorders, and one which is mandatory for a diagnosis of senile dementia of LB type using the Newcastle criteria. However, some DLB patients (perhaps 10–20% of all cases) may not show these variations, and there are considerable difficulties inherent in defining and quantifying fluctuation, particularly later in the illness when it becomes submerged in the progressive cognitive deterioration. Caregiver reports via diary keeping was felt to be the most productive approach to identifying a fluctuating state, a strategy which has been successfully employed to measure motor fluctuations in PD. It was eventually agreed that fluctuation should be retained as a core feature of DLB, that is, one with considerable diagnostic weight, but should not be mandatory, because of the difficulty in adequately operationalizing it.

Visual hallucinations, typically recurrent, formed and detailed have been described by most groups investigating DLB, and there was no dissent to their inclusion as a core feature. Clinicians with considerable experience of DLB patients commented on the overlap between true hallucinatory symptoms and other perpetual disorders including misidentification syndromes and visual agnosias. It was suggested that a new descriptive phenomenology needs to be developed to sufficiently describe the full range of these symptoms, although no one present volunteered to take up the challenge. The precise descriptions of the visual hallucinations are similar to those described in association with delirium due to systemic disturbance and also to those caused by anticholinergic toxicity, but dissimilar to hallucinations produced by other hallucinogens (e.g. LSD). Hallucinations in other modalities may also occur, but do so much less frequently. Delusions in DLB often have a bizarre content and well systematized nature, based as they often are upon these hallucinatory experiences.

Spontaneous motor features of parkinsonism were agreed to be the third core feature of DLB, rigidity and bradykinesia being the usual extrapyramidal manifestations, with tremor less common, especially in older individuals. Levodopa responsiveness is present in an as yet undetermined proportion of cases. The role of antiparkinsonian treatments in provoking psychiatric symptoms has already been discussed, as has the nosological relationship between DLB and PD.

The group tried to achieve consensus on the number of core features which 'are essential' for a clinical diagnosis of DLB, when they occur in conjunction with the dementing syndrome already described. The use of two or more core features was suggested to have high specificity for the diagnosis of 'probable AD' and may be suitable for most research, while a requirement for only one core feature would have higher sensitivity in generating a diagnosis of 'possible DLB' more applicable in routine clinical practice.

A variety of other candidates for core symptom status were considered, six of which were eventually considered of sufficient importance to warrant mention as 'supportive of' the diagnosis of DLB. There was lengthy debate about the importance of recurrent falls as a useful diagnostic item. Although groups in the UK and Japan identified falling as a presenting symptom in up to one-third of DLB cases, the consensus view was that there is a high background rate of falling in the cognitively impaired elderly, making it a relatively nonspecific symptom and therefore supportive of, rather than a core symptom of DLB.

Syncopal attacks in DLB with complete loss of consciousness and muscle tone have been described by several investigators and may represent the extension of LB associated pathology to involve the autonomic nervous system. Focal neurological signs and symptoms do not generally appear in conjunction with these episodes, aiding in their discrimination from transient ischaemic attacks. The associated phenomena of transient episodes of unresponsiveness without loss of muscle tone may represent the extreme of fluctuating attentional impairment due to perturbations in central nervous system cholinergic function. The workshop felt that the preliminary nature of these descriptions of syncope and transient disturbances in consciousness in DLB patients did not yet warrant their inclusion in clinical diagnostic criteria.

A severe adverse reaction to standard neuroleptic medication (neuroleptic sensitivity) was considered to be an important indicator of underlying LB disorder, but one of limited clinical application in the diagnostic process, especially if neuroleptic prescribing is routinely and desirably avoided in patients suspected of having DLB. Systematized delusions were felt usually to be secondary to hallucinations and other perceptual disturbances as previously described. Auditory, olfactory, and tactile hallucinations, although substantially less common than visual perceptual disturbances, were considered to be important features in some DLB cases.

Summary

The first important outcome of the clinical workshop was agreement about the guiding principles to be adopted in formulating clinical diagnostic categories suitable for use across the spectrum of LB disorders. The general approach advocated in the first session was first to define the cognitive and neuropsychiatric aspects of the DLB syndrome, and then to additionally consider the significance of extrapyramidal motor features with particular regard to the temporal sequence of presentation. This strategy is more consistent with the previous attempts of the Newcastle group to focus upon the atypical dementia syndrome, than with the encompassing approach of the Nottingham criteria which incorporate both motor and psychiatric presentations within one common diagnostic category. Comparative studies now need to establish the relative performance of these different diagnostic approaches.

Another important outcome of the workshop was to identify clinical research priorities. Fluctuating cognition, syncope, transient disturbances of consciousness, recurrent falls and characterization of extrapyramidal features in DLB all require intensive cross-sectional and longitudinal comparative studies. The significance of delirium, induced in PD by anti-parkinsonian medication, as an indicator of cortical LB involvement also needs to be examined. Finally, the workshop brought together clinicians and other scientists from around the globe who share major clinical and research interests in the overlap between dementia and parkinsonism and between Alzheimer and LB pathology. The excitement and commitment of common purpose was reflected in the discussions both formal and informal, and will, we hope, bear fruit in future research collaborations.

The consensus diagnostic clinical criteria are included in Appendix 1.

References

Byrne, E.J., Lennox, G., Godwin Austen, R.B., Jefferson, D., Lowe, J., Mayer, R.J., Landon, M. & Doherty, F.J. (Nottingham Group for the study of Neurodegenerative Disorders) (1991). Diagnostic criteria for dementia associated with cortical Lewy bodies. *Dementia*, **2**, 283–4.

McKeith, I.G., Perry, R.H., Fairbairn, A.F., Jabeen, S. & Perry, E.K. (1992). Operational criteria for senile dementia of Lewy body type (SDLT). *Psychol. Med.*, **22**, 911–22.

McKhann, G., Drachman, D., Folstein, M., Katzman, R., Price, D. & Stadlan, E. M. (1984). Clinical diagnosis of Alzheimer's disease: report of the NINCDS–ADRDA Work Group under the auspices of Department of Health and Human Services Task Force on Alzheimer's disease. *Neurology*, **34**, 939–44.

Part two

Pathological issues

15

Pathological significance of Lewy bodies in dementia

J. S. LOWE, R. J. MAYER and M. LANDON

Summary

Lewy bodies are an important histological feature of several neurodegenerative diseases typified by idiopathic Parkinson's disease. With the increasing recognition of dementia associated with Lewy bodies in cortical neurons it is desirable to have a better understanding of the biogenesis and function of these neuronal inclusions. There is considerable indirect evidence, based on immunohistochemical identification of constituent proteins, that the Lewy body is a structural manifestation of a cytoprotective cell response. When encountered in diagnostic practice a distinction is presently made between primary Lewy body disorders, where the Lewy body is felt to be closely related to the pathogenesis of disease, and coincidental Lewy body disorders where Lewy bodies are inconsistently associated with other pathological processes. This division is still arbitrary and based on relative ignorance about the functional biology of the Lewy body phenomenon.

15.1 Introduction

An important histological characteristic of idiopathic Parkinson's disease is the presence of intraneuronal inclusions termed Lewy bodies. Recent morphological and cell biological studies have also characterized Lewy bodies in a variety of disorders, particularly in the cerebral cortex in association with dementia. These observations have prompted important considerations as to the biological function of the Lewy body and whether the presence of Lewy bodies can be used to define specific types of neurodegenerative disease.

15.2 Functional biology of Lewy bodies

There are two distinctive morphological types of Lewy body, the classical (brainstem) type and the cortical type (Lowe, 1994). In addition, so-called pale bodies are felt to be a possible precursor of Lewy bodies (Dale et al., 1992; Hayashida et al., 1993). Using immunohistochemical techniques, many proteins have been demonstrated in Lewy bodies and it is now possible to suggest that the presence of the Lewy body is a reflection of a neuronal cytoprotective response.

Several groups have confirmed that neurofilament proteins are an important component of Lewy bodies (Goldman et al., 1983; Forno et al., 1986; Galloway et al., 1988; Pollanen et al., 1992). The incorporated neurofilament proteins are phosphorylated and truncated by proteolysis (Bancher et al., 1989; Hill et al., 1991; Schmidt et al., 1991) Neurofilaments are also probably cross-linked to form insoluble filaments (Pollanen et al., 1993a,b).

Lewy bodies also contain ubiquitin, ubiquitin carboxyl-terminal hydrolase (PGP9.5), the multicatalytic protease (MCP), and α B crystallin, all of which are involved in the elimination of abnormal or damaged proteins. Their presence can be considered as part of a cell stress response to eliminate damaged proteins from cells. Lewy bodies have also been shown to contain tubulin, microtubule-associated proteins, β-amyloid precursor protein and $Ca2^+$/calmodulin-dependent protein kinase II (Galloway et al., 1988; Kuzuhara et al., 1988; Lowe et al., 1988; Bancher et al., 1989; Lennox et al., 1989; Lowe et al., 1990a,b; Ito et al., 1991; Iwatsubo et al., 1991; Kwak et al., 1991; Schmidt et al., 1991; Arai et al., 1992; Love & Nicoll, 1992; Lowe et al., 1992, 1993).

Lewy bodies represent one form of a more generalized pathological phenomenon, filament/ubiquitin/crystallin inclusions, which include hepatic Mallory's hyaline, Rosenthal fibres, and Crooke's hyaline (Lowe et al., 1988; Manetto et al., 1988). This perspective suggests that the Lewy body is the manifestation of a cytoprotective response and therefore a beneficial phenomenon (Pollanen et al., 1993; Lowe, 1994).

The substances demonstrated in Lewy bodies can be divided into two groups: those that might be intrinsic to the biological function of Lewy bodies in degrading proteins, and the damaged proteins themselves. The presence of APP, synaptophysin and chromogranin-A in Lewy bodies possibly represent damaged cell components undergoing elimination (Nishimura et al., 1994). Ubiquitin has important roles in targeting abnormal or damaged proteins for breakdown, being one of the cell stress proteins (Mayer et al., 1991; Lowe et al., 1993). The fact that Lewy bodies contain enzymes associated with the ubiquitin-mediated proteolytic pathway, PGP9.5, and MCP suggests that Lewy bodies are a structural rearrangement designed to eliminate damaged cellular elements. α B crystallin is known to be an intermediate-filament associated protein and has roles as a molecular chaperone. It is possible that the assembly of neurofilaments to form a Lewy body is mediated through α B crystallin, which is present in about 10% of cortical Lewy bodies (Lowe et al., 1990a; Lowe et al., 1992).

An equally distinctive process which is present in association with Lewy body disorders is ubiquitin-immunoreactive neuritic degeneration. This is seen in substantia nigra, hippocampal region CA2/CA3, the dorsal vagal nucleus, and the nucleus basalis of Meynert. Immunohistochemical studies show that these 'Lewy neurites' have variable neurofilament immunoreactivity and contain the ubiquitin C-terminal hydrolase PGP9.5 (Dickson et al., 1991; Dickson et al., 1994). The association with Lewy bodies and similar patterns of immunoreactivity suggest that this distinctive neuritic degeneration should be regarded as part of the Lewy body phenomenon.

15.3 Hypothetical scheme for Lewy body biogenesis

Lewy bodies presumably form from an interplay between environmental stimuli and intrinsic responsiveness of neurons (see Fig 15.1). The first stage is probably associated with a cell stress response in neurons. The intermediate filament network is known to collapse in cell stress and this may be an initial response (Lowe et al., 1988). The molecular motor involved in this response is uncertain but a strong candidate is α B crystallin, known to associate with intermediate filaments and itself a cell stress protein. Once collapsed, neurofilaments become phosphorylated and truncated by proteolysis. Ubiquitin and enzymes of the ubiquitin system then become associated with the Lewy body. It is possible that some of the neurofilament modification is brought about through ubiquitin-mediated proteolysis, but this is uncertain. At present the proteins which are ubiquitinated in Lewy bodies are uncertain, however in the biologically similar Rosenthal fibres one has been found to be α B crystallin (Goldman & Corbin, 1991).

This scheme is at best speculative. There is a pressing need to understand the functional biology of the Lewy body and important aspects of their formation remain to be elucidated.

Function biology of ubiquitin-IF inclusions

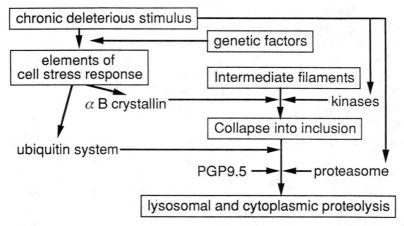

Fig. 15.1 Functional biology of ubiquitin-intermediate filament inclusions.

15.4 Diagnostic grouping of Lewy body disorders

Most neuropathologists would consider Lewy bodies distinctive enough to be used to define disease processes. An emerging consensus is that it is possible to consider a family of primary Lewy body disorders in which Lewy body pathology is believed to be closely related to the fundamental biology of the disease (Table 15.1). The key pathological feature of these disorders is neuronal loss associated with Lewy body and Lewy neurite formation, in the absence of other defined neuropathological lesions. There are good clinical correlates between the sites of neuritic or Lewy body pathology, neuronal loss and clinical features. Pure clinical syndromes occur when Lewy pathology is restricted to one site, with a mixed clinical picture being seen with involvement of several sites. The fact that these disorders may be grouped on the basis of a histological finding does not necessarily imply a common aetiology, however the frequent finding of overlap between these conditions argues for such a case.

Lewy bodies may also be seen in association coincidental with other neurological diseases (Table 15.2). The characteristic of these coincidental Lewy body diseases is the inconsistent presence of Lewy bodies in association with another, more dominant, pathological process.

One important point of debate is the significance of Lewy bodies in association with pathological changes of Alzheimer's disease. It is

Table 15.1. *Primary Lewy body disorders*

Region affected	Clinical syndrome	Name
Nigro-striatal system	Extrapyramidal movement disorder	Parkinson's disease
Cerebral cortex	Cognitive decline	Dementia with cortical Lewy bodies
Sympathetic neurons in spinal cord	Autonomic failure	Primary autonomic failure
Dorsal vagal nuclei	Dysphagia	Lewy body dysphagia

uncertain whether this represents a coincidental association or is a primary process. The inconsistency of association of Lewy bodies with Alzheimer changes is at present unexplained. It may indicate a common susceptibility to formation of Lewy bodies, plaques and tangles due to deleterious stimuli distinct from those causing Alzheimer's disease. Alternatively, the association may be due to the propensity of certain individuals to mount a cytoprotective response thereby modifying what would otherwise be 'straight' Alzheimer's disease. In view of the interplay of several genetic factors in the development of Alzheimer's disease it is likely that the association of Lewy bodies and Alzheimer's changes is a reflection of the interplay of several factors common to Alzheimer's disease and Parkinson's disease (Fig 15.2).

The association between cortical Lewy bodies and Alzheimer pathology

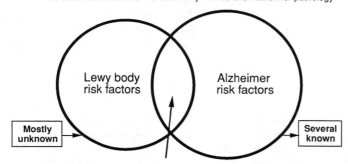

Hypothesis: dementia with cortical Lewy bodies associated with Alzheimer pathology represents the **intersection** of two sets of risk factors

Fig. 15.2 Genetic risk factors explaining dementia with cortical Lewy bodies.

Table 15.2. *Coincidental Lewy body disorders*

Condition	References
Multiple system atrophy	(Morin et al., 1980; Gibb, 1986; Sima et al., 1987)
Progressive supranuclear palsy	(Gibb, 1986; Mori et al., 1986)
Corticobasal degeneration	(Paulus & Selim, 1990; Wakabayashi et al., 1994; Horoupian & Chu, 1994)
Motor neuron disease	(Hedera et al., 1995; Williams et al., 1995)
Hallervorden-Spatz disease	(Helfand, 1935; Defendini et al., 1973; Dooling et al., 1974; Kalyanasundaram et al., 1980; Williamson et al., 1982; Gaytan-Garcia et al., 1990)
Neuroaxonal dystrophy	(Vuia, 1977; Sugiyama et al., 1993)
Ataxia telangiectasia	(DeLeon et al., 1976; Monaco et al., 1988).
Subacute sclerosing panencephalitis	(Gibb et al., 1990)
Sporadic Alzheimer's disease	(Joachim et al., 1988; Gibb, 1989)
Familial Alzheimer's disease	(Lantos et al., 1992)
Down's syndrome	(Raghavan et al., 1993; Bodhireddy et al., 1994)

15.5 Conclusion

Full understanding of the pathological significance of Lewy bodies will only be achieved with full understanding of their biogenesis and function. Until then we have indirect evidence that the Lewy body is a structural manifestation of a cytoprotective cell response. When encountered in diagnostic practice a distinction is presently made between apparently primary Lewy body disorders and presumed coincidental Lewy body disease. This division is still arbitrary and based on relative ignorance about the neuronal responses to injury.

References

Arai, H., Lee, V. M., Hill, W. D., Greenberg, B. D. & Trojanowski, J.Q. (1992). Lewy bodies contain beta-amyloid precursor proteins of Alzheimer's disease. *Brain Res.*, **585**(1–2), 386–90.
Bancher, C., Lassmann, H., Budka, H. et al. (1989). An antigenic profile of Lewy bodies: immunocytochemical indication for protein phosphorylation and ubiquitination. *J. Neuropathol. Exp. Neurol.*, **48**, 81–93.
Bodhireddy, S., Dickson, D. W., Mattiace L., Weidenheim, K. M. (1994). A case of Down's syndrome with diffuse Lewy body disease and Alzheimer's disease. *Neurology*, **44**, 159–61.

Dale, G. E., Probst, A., Luthert, P., Martin, J., Anderton, B. H. & Leigh, P. N. (1992). Relationships between Lewy bodies and pale bodies in Parkinson's disease. *Acta Neuropathol. (Berl.)*, **83**(5), 525–9.

Defendini, R., Markesbury, W., Mastri, A. & Duffy, P. (1973). Hallervorden–Spatz disease and infantile neuroaxonal dystrophy. *J. Neurol. Sci.*, **20**, 7–23.

DeLeon, G., Grover, W. & Huff, D. (1976). Neuropathological changes in ataxia telangiectasia. *Neurology*, **26**, 947–51.

Dickson, D., Ruan, D., Crystal, H. et al. (1991). Hippocampal degeneration differentiates diffuse Lewy body disease (DLBD) from Alzheimer's disease: light and electron microscopic immunohistochemistry of Ca2-3 neurites specific to DLBD. *Neurology*, **41**, 1402–9.

Dickson, D. W., Schmidt, M. L., Lee, V. M., Zhao, M. L., Yen, S. H. & Trojanowski, J. Q. (1994). Immunoreactivity profile of hippocampal CA2/3 neurites in diffuse Lewy body disease. *Acta Neuropathol. (Berl.)*, **87**(3), 269–76.

Dooling, E., Schoene, W. & Richardson, E. (1974). Hallervorden–Spatz syndrome. *Arch. Neurol.*, **30**, 70–83.

Forno, L. S., Sternberger, L., Sternberger, N., Strefling, A., Swanson, K. & Eng, L. (1986). Reaction of Lewy bodies with antibodies to phosphorylated and non-phosphorylated neurofilaments. *Neurosci. Lett.*, **64**, 253–8.

Galloway, P., Grundke-Iqbal, I., Iqbal, K. & Perry, G. (1988). Lewy bodies contain epitopes both shared and distinct from Alzheimer's neurofibrillary tangles. *J. Neuropath. Exp. Neurol.*, **47**, 654–63.

Gaytan-Garcia, S., Kaufmann, J. C. & Young, G. (1990). Adult onset Hallervorden–Spatz syndrome or Seitelberger's disease with late onset: variants of the same entity? a clinico-pathological study. *Clin. Neuropathol.*, **9**(3), 136–42.

Gibb, W. R. G. (1986). Idiopathic Parkinson's disease and the Lewy body disorders. *Neuropathol. Appl. Neurobiol.*, **12**: 223–34.

Gibb, W. (1989). Dementia and Parkinson's disease. *Br. J. Psychiatry*, **154**, 596–614.

Gibb, W., Scaravilli, F. & Michaud, J. (1990). Lewy bodies and subacute sclerosing panencephalitis. *J. Neurol. Neurosurg. Psychiatry*, **53**, 710–11.

Goldman, J. & Corbin, E. (1991). Rosenthal fibres contain ubiquitinated α B crystallin. *Am. J. Pathol.*, **139**, 933–8.

Goldman, J., Yne, S.-H., Chiu, F. & Peress, N. (1983). Lewy bodies of Parkinson's disease contain neurofilament antigens. *Science*, **221**, 1082–4.

Hayashida, K., Oyanagi, S., Mizutani, Y. & Yokochi, M. (1993). An early cytoplasmic change before Lewy body maturation: an ultrastructural study of the substantia nigra from an autopsy case of juvenile parkinsonism. *Acta Neuropathol. (Berl.)*, **85**(4), 445–8.

Hedera, P., Lerner, A., Castellani, R. & Frieland, R. (1995). Concurrence of Alzheimer's disease, Parkinson's disease, diffuse Lewy body disease and amyotrophic lateral sclerosis. *J. Neurol. Sci.*, **128**, 219–24.

Helfand, M. (1935). Status pigmentatus: its pathology and relation to Hallervorden–Spatz disease. *J. Nerv. Ment. Dis.*, **81**, 662–75.

Hill, W. D. V., Lee, M.-Y., Hurtig, H. I., Murray, J. M. & Trojanowski, J. Q. (1991). Epitopes located in spatially separated domains of each neurofilament subunit are present in Parkinson's disease Lewy bodies. *J. Comp. Neurol.*, **309**, 150–60.

Horoupian, D. & Chu, P. (1994). Unusual case of corticobasal degeneration with tau/Gallyas-positive neuronal and glial tangles. *Acta Neuropathol. (Berl.)*, **88**, 592–8.

Ito, H., Ii, K., Hirano, A. & Dickson, D. (1991). Immunohistochemical identification of the proteasome in ubiquitin reactive abnormal structures of the nervous system (Abstract). *J. Neuropathol. Exp. Neurol.*, **50**, 360.

Iwatsubo, T., Nakano, I., Fukunaga, K. & Miyamoto, E. (1991). $Ca2^+$/calmodulin-dependent protein kinase II immunoreactivity in Lewy bodies. *Acta Neuropathol. (Berl.)*, **82**, 159–63.

Joachim, C., Morris, J. & Selkoe, D. (1988). Clinically diagnosed Alzheimer's disease: autopsy results in 150 cases. *Ann. Neurol.*, **24**(1), 50–6.

Kalyanasundaram, S., Srinivas, H. V. & Deshpande, D. H. (1980). An adult with Hallervorden–Spatz disease: Clinical and pathological study. *Clin. Neurol. Neurosurg.*, **82**(4), 245–9.

Kuzuhara, S., Mori, H., Izumiyama, N., Yoshimura, M. & Ihara, Y. (1988). Lewy bodies and ubiquitin. A light and electron microscopic immunocytochemical study. *Acta Neuropathol. (Berl.)*, **75**, 345–53.

Kwak, S., Masaki, T., Ishiura, S. & Sugita, H. (1991). Multicatalytic proteinase is present in Lewy bodies and neurofibrillary tangles in diffuse Lewy body disease brains. *Neurosci. Lett.*, **128**, 21–4.

Lantos, P., Luthert, P., Hanger, D., Anderton, B., Mullan, M. & Rossor, M. (1992). Familial Alzheimer's disease with the amyloid precursor protein position 717 mutation and sporadic Alzheimer's disease have the same cytoskeletal pathology. *Neurosci. Lett.*, **137**, 221–4.

Lennox, G., Lowe, J., Morrell, K., Landon, M. & Mayer, R. (1989). Antiubiquitin immunocytochemistry is more sensitive than conventional techniques in the detection of diffuse Lewy body disease. *J. Neurol. Neurosurg. Psychiatry*, **52**, 67–71.

Love, S. J. & Nicoll, A. (1992). Comparison of modified Bielschowsky silver impregnation and anti-ubiquitin immunostaining of cortical and nigral Lewy bodies. *Neuropathol. Appl. Neurobiol.*, **18**(6), 585–92.

Lowe, J. (1994). *Lewy Bodies. Neurodegenerative Diseases.* pp. 51–69, Philadelphia: WB Saunders.

Lowe, J., Blanchard, A., Morrell, K. et al. (1988). Ubiquitin is a common factor in intermediate filament inclusion bodies of diverse type in man, including those of Parkinson's disease, Pick's disease, and Alzheimer's disease as well as Rosenthal fibres in cerebellar astrocytomas, cytoplasmic bodies in muscle and Mallory's bodies in alcoholic liver disease. *J. Pathol.*, **155**, 9–15.

Lowe, J., Landon, M., Pike, I., Spendlove, I., McDermott, H. & Mayer, R. (1990a). Dementia with b-amyloid deposition: involvement of α B crystallin supports two main diseases. *Lancet*, **336**, 515–16.

Lowe, J., McDermott, H., Landon, M., Mayer, R. & Wilkinson, K. (1990b). Ubiquitin carboxyl-terminal hydrolase (PGP9.5) is selectively present in ubiquitinated inclusion bodies characteristic of human neurodegenerative diseases. *J. Pathol.*, **161**, 153–60.

Lowe, J., McDermott, H., Pike, I., Spendlove, I., Landon, M. & Mayer, R. J. (1992). Alpha B crystallin expression in non-lenticular tissues and selective presence in ubiquitinated inclusion bodies in human disease. *J. Pathol.*, **166**(1), 61–8.

Lowe, J., Mayer, R. J. & Landon, M. (1993). Ubiquitin in neurodegenerative diseases. *Brain Pathol.*, **3**(1), 55–65.

Manetto, V., Perry, G., Tabaton, M. et al. (1988). Ubiquitin is associated with abnormal cytoplasmic filaments characteristic of neurodegenerative disease. *Proc. Natl. Acad. Sci. (USA)*, **85**, 4501–5.

Mayer, R., Arnold, J., Laszlo, L., Landon, M. & Lowe, J. (1991). Ubiquitin in health and disease. *Biochim. Biophys. Acta*, **1089**, 141–57.

Monaco, S., Nardelli, E., Moretto, G., Cavallaro, T. & Rizzuto, N. (1988). Cytoskeletal pathology in ataxia telangiectasia. *Clin. Neuropathol.*, **7**, 44–5.

Mori, H., Yoshimura, M., Tomonaga, M. & Yamanouchi, H. (1986). Progressive supranuclear palsy with Lewy bodies. *Acta Neuropathol. (Berl.)*, **71**, 344–6.

Morin, P., Lechevalier, B. & Bianco, C. (1980). Cerebellar atrophy associated with lesions of the pallidum and Luys' body and presence of Lewy bodies. Relationships with degenerative disorders of the pallidum, substantia nigra and Luys' body. *Rev. Neurol.*, **136**(5), 381–90.

Nishimura, M., Tomimoto, H., Suenaga, T. et al. (1994). Synaptophysin and chromogranin A immunoreactivities of Lewy bodies in Parkinson's disease brains. *Brain Res.*, **634**(2), 339–44.

Paulus, W. & Selim, M. (1990). Corticonigral degeneration with neuronal achromasia and basal neurofibrillary tangles. *Acta Neuropathol. (Berl.)*, **81**(1), 89–94.

Pollanen, M.S., Bergeron, C. & Weyer, L. (1992). Detergent-insoluble cortical Lewy body fibrils share epitopes with neurofilament and tau. *J. Neurochem*, **58**(5), 1953–6.

Pollanen, M.S., Bergeron, S. C. & Weyer, L. (1993a). Deposition of detergent-resistant neurofilaments into Lewy body fibrils. *Brain Res.*, **603**(1), 121–4.

Pollanen, M. S., Dickson, D. W. & Bergeron, C. (1993b). Pathology and biology of the Lewy body. *J. Neuropathol. Exp. Neurol.*, **52**(3), 183–91.

Raghavan, R., Khin, N. C., Brown, A. et al. (1993). Detection of Lewy bodies in Trisomy 21 (Down's syndrome). *Can. J. Neurol. Sci.*, **20**(1), 48–51.

Schmidt, M. L., Murray, J., Lee, V. M.-Y., Hil, W. D., Wertkin, A. & Trojanowski, J. Q. (1991). Epitope map of neurofilament protein domains in cortical and peripheral nervous system Lewy bodies. *Am. J. Pathol.*, **139**, 53–65.

Sima, A. A., Hoag, G. & Rozdilsky, B. (1987). Shy-Drager syndrome: the transitional variant. *Clin. Neuropathol.*, **6**(2), 49–54.

Sugiyama, H., Hainfellner, J. A., Schmid, S. B. & Budka, H. (1993). Neuroaxonal dystrophy combined with diffuse Lewy body disease in a young adult. *Clin. Neuropathol.*, **12**(3), 147–52.

Vuia, O. (1977). Neuroaxonal dystrophy: a juvenile adult form. *Clin. Neurol. Neurosurg.*, **79**, 305–15.

Wakabayashi, K., Oyanagi, K., Makifuch, T. et al. (1994). Corticobasal degeneration: etiopathological significance of the cytoskeletal alterations. *Acta Neuropathol. (Berl.)*, **87**(6), 545–53.

Williams, T., Shaw, P., Lowe, J., Bates, D. & Ince, P. (1995). Parkinsonism in motor neuron disease: case report and literature review. *Acta Neuropathol. (Berl.)*, **89**, 275–83.

Williamson, K., Sima, A., Curry, B. & Ludwin, S. (1982). Neuroaxonal dystrophy in young adults: a clinicopathological study of two unrelated cases. *Ann. Neurol.*, **11**, 335–43.

16

Tautological tangles in neuropathologic criteria for dementias associated with Lewy bodies

L. A. HANSEN

Summary

Only a minority of Lewy body dementia brains lack concomitant Alzheimer disease pathology, but the percentages of combined Lewy body disease and Alzheimer disease versus pure Lewy body disease vary depending upon what neuropathological criteria are employed to make a diagnosis of Alzheimer disease. Using criteria from the Consortium to Establish a Registry for Alzheimer Disease, nearly 90% of all Lewy body dementia brains have definite or probable Alzheimer disease. Such Lewy body variants of Alzheimer disease also show medial temporal lobe neurofibrillary pathology intermediate in severity between that seen in pure Alzheimer disease and that encountered in elderly nondemented controls or pure Lewy body disease patients. Like Alzheimer disease, but unlike pure Lewy body disease, Lewy body variants of Alzheimer disease have an increased apolipoprotein $\epsilon4$ allelic frequency. If myriads of neocortical neurofibrillary tangles are deemed requisite for a diagnosis of Alzheimer disease, the percentage of mixed Alzheimer disease and Lewy body disease falls from 89% of all Lewy body dementia brains to 32%. Even in the absence of concomitant Alzheimer disease pathology, nosologic uncertainty persists in Lewy body disease since no established neuropathologic criteria can reliably distinguish pure Parkinson's disease from so-called diffuse Lewy body disease.

16.1 Introduction

'When I use a word', Humpty Dumpty said in a rather scornful tone 'It means just what I choose it to mean – neither more nor less.' 'The question is,' said Alice, 'Whether you can make words mean so many different things.' 'The question,' said Humpty Dumpty, 'Is which is to be master – that's all.'

No fewer than 15 competing pathological appellations have been employed to describe dementia associated with Lewy bodies (Hansen & Galasko, 1992). Each label puts a different spin on what are apparently the same, or at least closely related, clinico-neuropathologic entities. The resulting nosologic Tower of Babel is illustrated in Fig. 16.1. These terminological discrepancies stem from underlying tautologies about neuropathologic and clinical criteria for the diagnoses of Alzheimer disease, Parkinson's disease, and Lewy body disease.

16.2 Alzheimer disease in Lewy body dementia

An occasionally heated controversy has been raging for several years over whether or not Lewy body dementia brains typically have concomitant Alzheimer disease. Some authorities contend that most so-called diffuse Lewy body disease is in fact Alzheimer disease with an incidental Lewy body flavoring. On the opposite side of the issue, other investigators hold that it is the Alzheimer disease pathology in Lewy body dementia which is incidental, constituting mere 'pathologic aging'. Proponents on both sides can muster supporting tautologic arguments. Those who emphasize concomitant Alzheimer disease cite diagnostic criteria from both the National Institute on Aging (NIA) (Khachaturian, 1985), and the Con-

Tower of Babel - Lewy Body Type

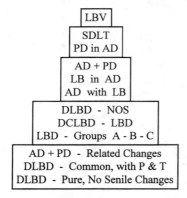

Fig. 16.1 Competing diagnostic appellations in dementias associated with Lewy bodies. DLBD = diffuse Lewy body disease, AD = Alzheimer disease, PD = Parkinson's disease, LBD = Lewy body disease, DCLBD = diffuse cortical Lewy body disease, NOS = not otherwise specified, LB = Lewy bodies, SDLT = senile dementia of the Lewy body type, LBV = Lewy body variant of Alzheimer disease.

sortium to Establish a Registry for Alzheimer disease (CERAD) (Mirra et al., 1993). According to these criteria, most Lewy body dementia brains qualify as Alzheimer disease, definite Alzheimer disease, or probable Alzheimer disease. A minority remain which can be construed as either diffuse Lewy body disease, or Parkinson's disease, according to clinical context. The NIA and CERAD criteria, however, are based on neocortical plaque densities, either diffuse and neuritic (NIA), or exclusively neuritic (CERAD). Those who argue that most dementia with Lewy bodies does not involve Alzheimer disease contend, again tautologically, that a diagnosis of Alzheimer disease requires numerous neocortical neurofibrillary tangles. Since Alzheimer disease in Lewy body dementia is typically 'neocortical plaque only or plaque predominant', then according to this perspective, most dementia with Lewy bodies does not show concomitant Alzheimer disease. As is so often the case with such controversies, the truth probably lies somewhere in between these polar extremes.

Figure 16.2 diagrammatically depicts this explanation for nosologic divergence in dementia with Lewy bodies. If cases falling into the gray-shaded crescent (neocortical plaque only or plaque predominate Alzheimer disease, and CERAD probable Alzheimer disease) are interpreted as Alzheimer disease, then most dementia with Lewy bodies includes con-

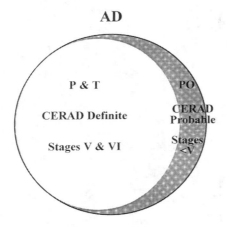

AD

P & T

CERAD Definite

Stages V & VI

PO

CERAD Probable

Stages <V

Fig. 16.2 This diagram illustrates the disputatious 'gray zone' in neuropathologic criteria for a diagnosis of Alzheimer disease. P and T = neocortical plaque and tangle Alzheimer disease, PO = neocortical plaque only Alzheimer disease, CERAD = Consortium to Establish a Registry for Alzheimer Disease, Stages refers to Braak and Braak, Alzheimer-related changes Neuropathology Staging Protocol.

comitant Alzheimer disease. This is the diagnostic conclusion dictated by NIA and CERAD criteria. Out of 71 Lewy body dementia brains received at our San Diego Alzheimer Disease Research Center over the past 10 years, 89% meet these criteria for concomitant Alzheimer disease; and so we refer to them as Lewy body variants of Alzheimer disease. Of these Lewy body variants, 68% are CERAD-definite Alzheimer disease, and 32% are CERAD-probable Alzheimer disease. We have previously shown that most Lewy body variants of Alzheimer disease have 'neocortical plaque-only or plaque predominate' Alzheimer disease pathology (Hansen et al., 1993).

On the other hand, if the diagnosis of Alzheimer disease is thought to require greater pathologic severity, as represented by the smaller inner circle in Fig. 16.2 (neocortical plaque and tangle Alzheimer disease and CERAD-definite Alzheimer disease), then the Alzheimer disease pathology in most Lewy body dementia brains falls short of the diagnostic threshold. If myriads of neocortical neurofibrillary tangles are considered requisite for the diagnosis of Alzheimer disease, only 32% of the 71 Lewy body dementia brains referred to above would have concomitant Alzheimer disease, rather than the 89% which would be so designated by CERAD and NIA criteria. Figure 16.3 illustrates the various nosologic implications of shifting threshold criteria for the diagnosis of Alzheimer disease with overlapping Lewy body disease.

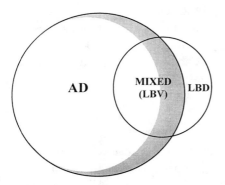

Fig. 16.3 The most nosologically contentious category in dementias associated with Lewy bodies is the combination of Lewy body disease (LBD) and neocortical 'plaque only or plaque predominate' 'Alzheimer disease (AD), represented by the gray shaded crescent. LBV = Lewy body variant of Alzheimer disease.

16.3 Neuropathological staging of Alzheimer disease in Lewy body dementia

Any neuropathological criteria for the diagnosis of Alzheimer disease are necessarily artificial, since they imply a threshold above which Alzheimer disease exists and below which it does not. However we know that Alzheimer disease does not appear full blown in a frothy instant, like Venus arising from the Cypriot sea. Rather, Alzheimer disease commences and progresses insidiously, as diffuse plaques in the neocortex evolving first to neuritic forms lacking paired helical filaments, and then eventually to tau-positive dense cored neuritic plaques accompanied by neurofibrillary tangles. Medial temporal lobe neurofibrillary pathology is even more stereotyped in its evolution. Braak and Braak (1991) have delineated six developmental stages in advancing Alzheimer disease, from the transentorhinal (I and II) to the limbic (III and IV), and eventually the isocortical (V and VI). Alzheimer disease neurofibrillary pathology in dementia with Lewy bodies is typically confined to the limbic system, occupying stages III or IV of the Braak scheme (Hansen et al., 1994). Figure 16.4 depicts the results of Alzheimer disease neuropathologic staging using a modification of the Braak and Braak protocol. Lewy body dementia brains with enough neuritic plaques to meet CERAD criteria for definite or probable Alzheimer disease are designated Lewy body variants of Alzheimer disease (LBV) in Fig. 16.4. Pure Alzheimer disease is typically associated with an advanced modified Braak stage V or VI. Age-matched nondemented elderly controls typically are at stage 0 or I, the same stages occupied by pure Lewy body disease brains. Brains with the Lewy body variant of Alzheimer disease are predominately at neuropathologic stages III and IV. These 'limbic stages' of Alzheimer disease correspond nicely to the categories of 'neocortical plaque only or plaque predominant' Alzheimer disease and CERAD-probable Alzheimer disease.

16.4 Apolipoprotein ε in Alzheimer disease and Lewy body dementias

Physical evidence implicating complicit Alzheimer disease in most Lewy body dementia includes diffuse plaques, neuritic plaques and medial temporal lobe neurofibrillary pathology, as detailed above. All this is much, and yet there is more. Numerous investigations have shown that possession of one or more apolipoprotein ε4 (APOE-4) alleles is a risk factor for Alzheimer disease (Strittmatter et al., 1993). APOE-4 allelic frequency is

Percent in AD Pathology Stages

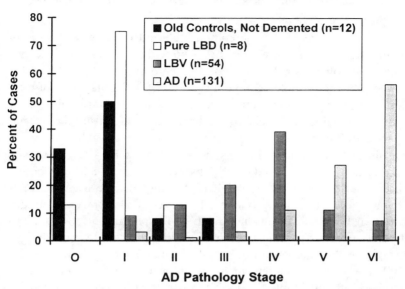

Fig. 16.4 The extent of Alzheimer disease (AD) neurofibrillary pathology in four different disease categories is expressed using a modification of Braak and Braak, Alzheimer Related Changes Neuropathology Staging Scheme. LBV = Lewy Body Variant of Alzheimer Disease, LBD = Pure Lewy Body Disease. The differences in neurofibrillary pathology stages are expressed as percentage of cases in each stage from each diagnostic category.

not, however, increased in pure Lewy body disease, either in the form of diffuse Lewy body disease with dementia (Galasko et al., 1994), or as neuropathologically pure idiopathic Parkinson's disease (Nalbantoglu et al., 1994). When the neuropathological hallmarks of Alzheimer disease are seen in brains with Lewy body disease, however, APOE-4 allelic frequency is again increased, as has been reported in the Lewy body variant of Alzheimer disease (Galasko et al., 1994), combined Alzheimer disease and Parkinson's disease (Nalbantoglu et al., 1994), and senile dementia of the Lewy body type (Harrington et al., 1994). One rather pedestrian interpretation of this convergence of neuropathological and genotypical data is that when the lesions of Alzheimer disease are present, so is Alzheimer disease, *sui generis*.

16.5 Lewy body dementia, Parkinson's disease and Parkinson's disease with dementia

Setting aside, momentarily, the complicated and controversial issue of concomitant Alzheimer disease in Lewy body disease, we encounter yet another tautological tangle when considering only pure Lewy body diseases. There is no pathological 'gold standard' for the diagnosis of idiopathic Parkinson's disease, but neurodegenerative changes and Lewy bodies in the pigmented nuclei of the brainstem and substantia innominata are certainly necessary, if not in and of themselves sufficient for the diagnosis. A neuropathological distinction between Parkinson's disease and Lewy body disease based on the absence of neocortical Lewy bodies in the former is untenable, since all Parkinson's disease brains have at least some neocortical Lewy bodies (Hughes et al., 1992). A clinical differentiation between Parkinson's disease with parkinsonism and Lewy body disease with dementia is more appealing, but this too is compromised by over-lapping Parkinson's disease with dementia syndromes and variable parkinsonism in demented patients with Lewy body disease. In the absence of clinical information, brains with subcortical and neocortical Lewy bodies can often not be meaningfully categorized as either Parkinson's disease or Lewy body disease.

16.6 Summary and conclusions

Depending upon which diagnostic criteria are employed, between 32% and 89% of all Lewy body dementia is mixed with Alzheimer disease. The results of APOE-4 genotyping and medial temporal lobe neurofibrillary pathology staging imply that the higher percentage of mixed Alzheimer disease and Lewy body disease versus pure Lewy body disease is probably the more accurate figure. Nevertheless, to reduce profitless nosologic acrimony, it might facilitate communication among dementia investigators if diagnostic categories could, for research purposes, be eschewed altogether, and descriptive profiling and Alzheimer disease Braak staging utilized in their stead. If specific diagnoses must be assigned, the criteria employed in arriving at a diagnosis of Alzheimer disease in Lewy body disease should be specified, that is, Alzheimer disease, definite or probable, according to CERAD criteria. At present, no neuropathologic 'gold standard' exists to distinguish Parkinson's disease from so-called diffuse Lewy body disease, although the former may have greater loss of pigmented neurons in the substantia nigra and the latter may have more neocortical Lewy bodies. Although it is a humbling admission, at present the neuropathologist requires the assistance of the clinician to meaningfully distinguish between Parkinson's disease and Lewy body dementia when assigning a final diagnosis.

Acknowledgements

The author wishes to express his gratitude to Pam Zuniga for her competence and efficiency in preparing this manuscript. The research reported in this paper was supported by a grant from the National Institutes of Health #2P50-AGO53131-11, Alzheimer's Disease Research Center.

References

Braak, H. & Braak, E. (1991). Neuropathological stageing of Alzheimer-related changes. *Acta Neuropathol.*, **82**, 239–59.

Galasko, D., Saitoh, T., Xia, Y. et al. (1994). The apolipoprotein E allele ∊4 is over-represented in patients with the Lewy body variant of Alzheimer's disease. *Neurology*, **44**, 1950–3.

Hansen, L. A. & Galasko, D. (1992). Lewy body disease. *Curr. Opin. Neurol. Neurosur.*, **5**, 889–94.

Hansen, L. A., Masliah, E., Galasko, D. & Terry, R. D. (1993). Plaque only Alzheimer disease is usually the Lewy body variant, and vice versa. *J. Neuropath. Exper. Neurol.*, **52**, 648–54.

Hansen, L. A., Galasko, D., Samuel, W., Xia, Y., Chen, X. & Saitoh, T. (1994). Apolipoprotein-E ∊-4 is associated with increased neurofibrillary pathology in the Lewy body variant of Alzheimer disease. *Neurosci. Lett.*, **182**, 63–5.

Harrington, C. R., Louwagie, J., Rossau, R. et al. (1994). Influence of apolipoprotein E genotype on senile dementia of the Alzheimer and Lewy body types. *Am. J. Pathol.*, **145**, 1472–84.

Hughes, A. J., Daniel, S. E., Kilford, L. & Lees, A. J. (1992). Accuracy of clinical diagnosis of idiopathic Parkinson's disease: A clinicopathologic study of 100 cases. *J. Neurol. Neurosurg. Psychiatry*, **55**, 181–4.

Khachaturian, Z. S. (1985). Diagnosis of Alzheimer's disease. *Arch. Neurol.*, **42**, 1097–105.

Mirra, S. S., Hart, M. N. & Terry, R. D. (1993). Making the diagnosis of Alzheimer's disease. *Arch. Pathol. Lab. Med.*, **117**, 132–44.

Nalbantoglu, J., Gilfix, B. M., Bertrand, P. et al. (1994). Predictive value of apolipoprotein E genotyping in Alzheimer's disease: Results of an autopsy series and an analysis of several combined studies. *Ann. Neurol.*, **36**, 889–95.

Strittmatter, W. J., Saunders, A. M., Schmechel, D. et al. (1993). Apolipoprotein E: High-avidity binding to β-amyloid and increased frequency of type 4 allele in late-onset familial Alzheimer disease. *Proc. Natl. Acad. Sci. USA*, **90**, 1977–81.

17

What is the neuropathological basis of dementia associated with Lewy bodies?

R. H. PERRY, E. B. JAROS, D. IRVING[†],
D. J. SCOONES, A. BROWN,
W. M. McMEEKIN, E. K. PERRY,
C. M. MORRIS, P.J. KELLY and P. G. INCE

Summary

Two alternative hypotheses – that there is either a unitary or a multiple neuropathological basis for dementia in diseases associated with Lewy bodies – are considered in relation to Parkinson's disease (PD) and Lewy body dementia (LBD including senile dementia of Lewy body type, SDLT). Densities of limbic (cingulate) cortical Lewy bodies, neocortical Lewy bodies, neocortical plaques, neocortical tangles, Braak staging, and Apo E frequency have been quantified in PD (demented and nondemented), SDLT, and Alzheimer's disease (AD with presenile and senile onset). Of these parameters the mean density of cingulate Lewy bodies is significantly greater in SDLT compared with all PD cases. There is no obvious correlation between Lewy body density and cognitive impairment assessed using a simple test of mental ability, and other measures of mental function in LBD may need to be considered. Since there is no absolute density of limbic Lewy bodies that clearly differentiates SDLT or demented PD cases from all nondemented PD cases, neuropathological criteria may need to incorporate severity of Alzheimer-type pathology as an additional optional factor. Mean neocortical plaque density is significantly lower in SDLT compared with AD cases but it is also significantly higher than in demented and nondemented PD cases, and higher than densities in normals. Even so, neocortical plaque density does not itself differentiate all SDLT cases from the normal. It is likely that the biological basis for dementia or psychoses in LBD, a cardinal feature of which is fluctuating symptomatology, is in part a functional or neurochemical abnormality.

[†] Deceased.

17.1 Introduction

Dementia associated with Lewy bodies (cortical and subcortical) occurs in idiopathic Parkinson's disease (PD); cases presenting primarily with dementia (Lewy body dementia – LBD described variously as Diffuse Lewy body disease, senile dementia of Lewy body type, and Lewy body variant of Alzheimer's disease); in a minority of cases of classical Alzheimer's disease (AD) including familial AD; in a small proportion of Down's syndrome; and in a number of other rare disorders such as Hallervorden–Spatz disease (see also Chapter 23). In Parkinson's disease with dementia and LBD there is no consensus on the neuropathological basis for the dementia. Since Boller and others originally described an increased frequency of Alzheimer pathology in Parkinson's disease in 1980, at least ten different potential correlates have been identified (Table 17.1).

In the present exploration of the neuropathological basis for dementia in senile dementia of Lewy body type (SDLT) and PD, a variety of quantitative histopathological indices together with apolipoprotein ϵ allele frequencies have been examined in different clinical groups. Key comparisons, likely to highlight important correlates of dementia, include those between nondemented and demented PD subgroups; and between age-matched SDLT and normal groups. It is suggested that differences common to these two comparisons are likely to be important. The validity of this strategy depends on a close relation between the disease process in PD and SDLT. Such a relation is indicated neuropathologically by several features including the distribution of Lewy bodies in cortical areas and subcortical nuclei; loss of dopaminergic substantia neurons; and increased β-amyloidosis in the absence of neurofibrillary tangles in the neocortex.

The hypothesis that there is a unitary basis for dementia in these disorders is considered in conjunction with the alternative – that the dementia has a multifactorial basis. Potential neuropathological criteria for SDLT/LBD are proposed on the basis of the present neuropathological analysis.

17.2 Observations

The demographic data are summarized in Tables 17.2 and 17.3. Clinical and pathological criteria used for group allocation are described in detail elsewhere (Perry et al., 1990). The SDLT group was defined clinically by presentation with dementia or dementia concurrent (1–2 years) with mild

Table 17.1. *Potential correlates of dementia associated with Lewy bodies in Lewy body dementia or Parkinson's disease*

- Cortical Lewy bodies
- Degeneration of cortically projecting nuclei with Lewy bodies (nucleus of Meynert, raphé nuclei, ventral tegmental nucleus, pedunculopontine nucleus, locus coeruleus)
- Lewy neurites (hippocampus and limbic cortex)
- Cortical B-amyloidosis/neuritic plaques
- Cortical neurofibrillary tangles/abnormal tau
- Hirano bodies (hippocampus)
- Cortical synapse loss
- Intrinsic cortical neuron loss (e.g. somatostatin positive neurons) in archi-, limbic, and neocortex
- Nigro-striatal dopaminergic degeneration and disruption of frontal-striatal 'loop' circuitry
- Apolipoprotein E4 allele
- Increasing age

For references see: Boller et al., 1980; Dickson et al., 1987, 1991; Gibb et al., 1987; Harrington et al., 1994; Ince et al., 1991; Kosaka, 1993; Leake et al., 1991; Lennox et al., 1989; Mitake et al., 1995; Paulus & Jellinger, 1991; Perry et al., 1990; Whitehouse et al., 1983; Yoshimura, 1988; Zweig et al., 1993

extrapyramidal symptoms, but not with typical PD symptoms alone. The PD cases were defined as cases showing a typical extrapyramidal disorder for many years (minimum 3 years) and were further subdivided into those with and without dementia on the basis of mental test scores (MTS) (obtained within six months of death and below or equal to 26 out of 37, Blessed et al., 1968). In all of the PD and SDLT cases there were brainstem, including substantia nigra, Lewy bodies. In the PD group there was also extensive substantia nigra neuron loss, although neuron loss was moderate and variable in SDLT (Perry et al., 1990; Chapter 34). Histopathological analysis included: quantification of neuritic plaques and neurofibrillary tangles in the 4 neocortical lobes (von Braunmühl and Palmgren staining); quantification of ubiquitin positive Lewy bodies in anterior cingulate; and staging of Alzheimer type pathology according to the procedure of Braak and Braak (1991) based on the density of tangles in the hippocampus, parahippocampal gyrus and in entorhinal, transentorhinal, and occipital cortices.

There was no difference in mean age of onset between the SDLT and AD groups although duration of illness was significantly shorter in the SDLT group (2.5 versus 4.9 years). The PD group had a significantly earlier mean age of onset and a significantly longer duration than both the SDLT and AD groups. In the PD subgroups, age of onset was significantly lower in the nondemented compared with demented cases. In the nondemented PD cases onset age (mean 58 years) was also significantly lower than in SDLT (mean 76 years). There was a tendency for the demented PD and SDLT groups to consist of more male than female cases (the reverse trend being apparent in AD) although this may reflect case ascertainment bias.

Histopathologically, Lewy bodies were present in one or more regions of the limbic cortex (including parahippocampal gyrus, amygdaloid nucleus, anterior cingulate and insular gyri) in all of the SDLT and PD cases, and absent in the normal group. The mean anterior cingulate Lewy body density was significantly greater (twofold) in SDLT compared to PD cases, as a whole (Table 17.2) but not compared with either of the PD subgroups separately (Table 17.3). In the demented PD subgroup the mean Lewy body density was more than twofold that in the nondemented PD cases but this difference did not quite reach significance reflecting the overlap in cingulate Lewy body density between the two subgroups (Table 17.3). Although mean neocortical plaques were significantly higher than normal in the SDLT group as a whole, there was a substantial subgroup (17/61, 28%) in which neocortical plaques were absent or within the normal range for that age. In PD, neocortical plaque density was generally low and not significantly higher in the demented compared with nondemented subgroup. Neocortical tangles were absent or sparse in PD and SDLT, being on average only slightly, and not significantly, above the normal and over tenfold lower than the average density in AD (Tables 17.2 and 17.3). In terms of Braak staging based on archicortical and occipital cortical tangles (Tables 17.2 and 17.3) this was more advanced in the SDLT group as a whole: in 21% of SDLT cases staging exceeded 4, compared to normal cases none of which exceeded stage 4. Braak staging also tended to be more advanced in the demented compared to nondemented PD cases, although in neither subgroup stage 4 was exceeded. The frequency of the Apo E 4 allele (Tables 17.2) was, as reported elsewhere (Harrington et al., 1994), higher in SDLT compared with the normal: 58% of SDLT cases had 1 (or 2) alleles compared with 28% of the normal. This contrasts with 64.2% in a combined group of presenile and senile AD. It should be noted, however, that homozygosity for Apo E 4 allele (ϵ 4/4) was not detected in any normal or PD case, in only 8% of SDLT but in 21% of AD cases (Table 17.2). In the SDLT group, a higher proportion of cases sharing numerous neocortical tangles

Table 17.2. *Demographic, quantitative neuropathological and genetic data in PD, SDLT and AD*

	Female	Male	Total	Age at death (mean years± SD)	Age at onset (mean years ±SD)	Duration (mean years ±SD)	Neocortical plaques[b] per mm² (mean ±SD)	Neocortical tangles[b] per mm² (mean ±SD)	Lewy bodies[c] per cm² (mean ±SD)	Braak stage[d] (mean ±SD)	APoE Status (%) 2:2	2:3	3:3	2:4	3:4	4:4
Normal controls	64	74	138	75.4±13.3	NA[e]	NA[e]	2.0±3.3[h]	0.07±0.58[i]	NA[e]	2.6±1.1	0	10.0	62.0	6.0	22.0	0
PD all cases[a]	19	27	46	74.2±8.9	64.5±11.7[f]	9.2±6.3[g]	4.1±6.6[h]	0.08±0.18[i]	56.5±64.1[j]	1.8±1.4	0	15.6	43.8	3.1	37.5	0
SDLT all cases	26	35	61	78.6±6.4	76.0±6.7[f]	2.5±2.0[g]	12.4±9.2[h]	1.52±3.2[i]	110.3 ±134.9[j]	3.22±1.8	0	5.3	36.8	10.5	39.5	7.9
AD all cases	68	45	113	77.5±9.3	73.5±9.0[f]	4.9±2.7[g]	19.6±13.4[h]	23.3±17.3[i]	NA[e]	NA[e]	0	1.9	34.0	1.9	41.5	20.8

[a] PD with and without dementia and 9 PD cases unassessed for dementia

[b] Neocortical plaques and tangles given as the mean of the 4 neocortical lobes

[c] Anterior cingulate Lewy body density established in ubiquitin stained 10 μm section

[d] Braak staging established by assessing tangle load in the hippocampal formation, parahippocampal gyrus, occipitotemporal gyrus, and occipital cortex

[e] Not assessed

[f] to [j] refer to Tukey's pairwise comparisons between groups (significance level $p < 0.05$)

[f] significantly earlier in PD than in SDLT and AD; no difference between SDLT and AD

[g] significantly longer in PD than in SDLT and AD; significantly shorter in SDLT than in AD

[h] in SDLT significantly lower than in AD but significantly higher than in PD and normal controls; the difference between PD and controls is not significant

[i] no difference between SDLT, PD, and controls; AD cases are significantly higher than SDLT, PD and controls

[j] in SDLT significantly higher than in PD

Table 17.3. *Demographic, quantitative neuropathological and genetic data in PD, SDLT and AD subgroups*

	Female	Male	Total	Age at death (mean years ±SD)	Age at onset (means years ±SD)	Duration (mean years ±SD)	Neocortical plaques[c] per mm² (mean ±SD)	Neocortical tangles[c] per mm² (mean ±SD)	Lewy body density[d] per cm² (mean ±SD)	Braak stage[e] (%)							ApoE status (%)					
										0	1	2	3	4	5	6	2:2	2:3	3:3	2:4	3:4	4:4
Normal controls	64	74	138	75.4 ±13.3	NA[f]	NA[f]	2.0 ±3.3	0.07 ±0.58	NA[f]	8.0	4.0	32.0	36.0	20.0	0	0	0	10.0	62.0	6.0	22.0	0
PD without dementia	8	7	15	70.0 ±11.1	57.9 ±13.2[g]	11.9 ±7.3[h]	2.7 ±4.5[i]	0.02 ±0.07[i]	34.5 ±50.1[k]	33.3	26.7	13.3	13.3	13.3	0	0	0	0	44.4	0	55.6	0
PD with dementia	5	17	22	75.0 ±7.3	67.6 ±9.3[g]	7.7 ±5.0[h]	5.9 ±8.4[i]	0.13 ±0.23[i]	80.6 ±73.2[k]	22.7	13.7	18.2	22.7	22.7	0	0	0	11.8	52.9	0	35.3	0
SDLT <4 tangles/mm²	21	33	54	78.6 ±6.7	76.0 ±6.9[g]	2.5 ±2.0[h]	12.1 ±9.5[i]	0.55 ±1.22[i]	118.1 ±139.9[k]	16.3	4.1	14.3	20.4	30.6	14.3	0	0	6.3	37.5	9.4	43.8	3.1
SDLT >4 tangles/ mm²	5	2	7	79.0 ±4.3	75.7 ±4.8[g]	2.9 ±2.0[h]	15.0 ±7.0[i]	8.9 ±3.8[i]	54.4 ±76.1[k]	0	0	0	0	28.6	0	71.4	0	0	33.3	16.7	16.7	33.3
AD presenile[a]	11	13	24	63.8 ±5.3	59.2 ±5.0	5.4 ±3.7[h]	29.9 ±16.2[i]	32.6 ±18.6[i]	NA[f]	NA[f]							0	0	76.9	7.7	7.7	7.7
AD senile[b]	57	32	89	81.2 ±6.0	76.5 ±6.4[g]	4.8 ±2.4[h]	17.0 ±11.3[i]	20.8 ±16.1[i]	NA[f]	NA[f]							0	2.5	20.0	0	52.6	25.0

[a] Alzheimer's disease cases presenting with dementia and dying before the age of 70 years

[b] Alzheimer's disease cases presenting with dementia and dying after the age of 70 years

[c] Neocortical plaques and tangles given as the mean of the 4 neocortical lobes

[d] Anterior cingulate Lewy body density established in ubiquitin stained 10 μm section

[e] Braak staging established by assessing tangle load in the hippocampal formation, parahippocampal gyrus, occipitotemporal gyrus, and occipital cortex

[f] Not assessed

[g to k] refer to Tukey's pairwise comparisons between subgroups (significance level $p < 0.05$)

[g] significantly earlier in PD without dementia than in PD with dementia, and than in both SDLT subgroups, and than in AD with senile onset

[h] significantly shorter in SDLT <4 tangles/mm² subgroup than in AD with senile onset, and than in PD with dementia; significantly longer in PD without dementia than in all the other disease subgroups

[i] no difference between SDLT subgroups; significantly lower in SDLT <4 tangles/mm² subgroup than in AD with senile and presenile onset, in both SDLT subgroups significantly higher than in normal controls, and than in PD without dementia, and than in PD with dementia; no difference between controls and PD with or without dementia; AD with presenile onset is significantly higher than AD with senile onset

[j] SDLT and PD subgroups are not different from normal controls; both AD subgroups were significantly higher than normal controls, and than all the other disease subgroups; AD with presenile onset subgroup is significantly higher than AD with senile onset

[k] the differences between subgroups are not significant

($>4/mm^2$) were homozygous for APO E4 allele than cases with no or minimal tangle density ($<4/mm^2$ – Table 17.3). In the presenile AD group only 8% of cases were homozygous for the APO E4 allele, compared with 25% in the senile AD group. As previously reported (Harrington et al., 1994) the presence or absence of the E4 allele did not distinguish the SDLT subgroups on the basis of mean plaque, mean tangle, or mean Lewy body density (see also Table 17.4). However, when the SDLT, PD and AD disease groups were analysed together a group of 18 cases with the E 4/4 genotype had the median of the neocortical tangle density more than 10 fold higher than the remaining Apo E genotypic groups (Figure 17.1). There was no interaction of ApoE genotype with age of onset of symptoms in SDLT – mean ($\pm$SD) ages of onset were 76.6 ± 6 and 78 ± 6 y in 18 cases having E4 compared with 15 cases with no E4.

Since the extent of Alzheimer-type pathology within the SDLT group varied from absent or minimal to that encountered in moderately affected patients with AD, cases were subdivided on the basis of mean neocortical tangle densities into four subgroups: none; less than 1; 1–4; and $> 4\,mm^2$. Only the last group (>4) would be considered as fulfilling the criteria for AD based on Newcastle criteria for tangle density, although the last three subgroups would be classified as AD based on the CERAD criteria for plaque densities. Mean neocortical plaque densities were higher than

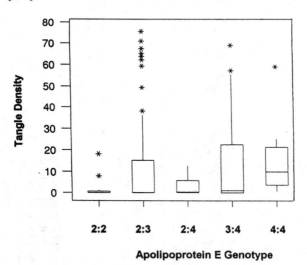

Fig. 17.1 Relationship between neocortical tangle density and apolipoprotein E genotype. Data expressed as median (lower or central box horizontal line) and quartiles (upper box and vertical line); * represent individual cases which fall outside these ranges.

Table 17.4. *Comparison of SDLT subgroups with varying degrees of Alzheimer-type pathology*

Subgroup	Tangles per mm²	Case number	Plaques per mm²	Lewy bodies per cm²	Onset age	Duration (y)	Gender M:F	ApoE4 alleles (%) 0	1	2
1	0	13	4.7±1.9	39.9±40.0	73.4±8.6	2.2±1.5	11:2	56	44	0
2	<1	28	14.6±9.5	127.2±133.4	76.9±6.6	2.5±2.4	17:11	44	50	6
3	1–4	7	17.9±8.5	148.3±184.4	76.0±6.0	3.5±1.5	5:2	25	75	0
4	>4	7	16.9±4.0	50.4±78.4	75.7±4.8	2.9±2.0	3:4	33	33	33

ApoE genotype assessed in 37 cases in the four subgroups
Plaque and tangle density given as the mean of four neocortical lobes
Lewy body density calculated in the anterior cingulate gyrus using ubiquitin immunohistochemistry

normal in all three groups with neocortical tangles, even in that with a mean tangle density of < 1 per mm^2. Lewy body densities in the four subgroups were highly variable with a trend towards lower numbers in the subgroups with no neocortical tangles and high tangle densities, compared with the intermediate subgroups. There were no differences in age of onset or duration of illness between the four subgroups. In terms of gender there were relatively more males (11/13, 85%) in the tangle free group compared with the other groups (25/42, 60%). In SDLT with an increase in mean neocortical tangle density there was a trend towards higher frequency of E4 allele.

In terms of clinico-pathological interaction, this was examined in the PD cases in relation to mental test scores obtained within a year of death. Scores ranged from 1–33 (maximum 37) in 17 cases tested. Within this group there was no significant correlation between MTS and densities of cingulate Lewy bodies ($n = 17$, $r = -0.25$), neocortical plaques or age of onset of extrapyramidal symptoms. Similar clinical pathological relations have not yet been analysed in the SDLT group although whether this particular mental test, originally developed for application in AD, is entirely appropriate to assessing the fluctuating mental function and psychoses which characterize SDLT and LBD is uncertain.

17.3 Discussion

This analysis does not immediately suggest a unitary neuropathological basis for dementia in SDLT and PD. Plaque densities are significantly elevated in the demented groups as a whole but not in all cases. Lewy bodies are evident (by definition) in all cases and in limbic cingulate cortex their mean density progressively increases from nondemented PD to demented PD, to SDLT cases but the distributions show large degrees of overlap, and hence, in the cingulate gyrus at least, intergroup differences just fail to reach statistical significance. There is no obvious relation between Lewy body density in the limbic cortex and severity of dementia in PD as noted in a previous analysis (Perry et al., 1990). It should also be noted that in a small minority of Lewy body cases Lewy bodies may not be demonstrated in the anterior cingulate gyrus using ubiquitin antisera, despite the predilection of this gyrus for cortical Lewy body formation and the sensitivity of ubiquitin analysis.

Clinico-pathological correlations are further complicated by the question of which clinical measure is the most appropriate. Assessing severity of dementia with cognitive testing instruments originally designed for AD may not be appropriate for investigating Lewy body diseases, although results are likely to parallel the extent of cognitive decline. Indices of fluctuating cognitive impairment or psychotic features such as hallucinations may be as, if not more, relevant than the MTS. Previous analyses (Perry et al., 1990) have however not demonstrated a differentiation of hallucinating and non-hallucinating SDLT cases on the basis of, for example, cortical Lewy body densities. Neurochemical analyses (see also Chapter 30) indicate that loss of neocortical (temporal and parietal) cholinergic activities is an invariant feature of SDLT and PD with dementia. Of the many potential correlates of dementia (Table 17.1), this neurobiological abnormality may be the most consistent. Neuropathology in the region of the nucleus of Meynert needs to be examined in more detail to explore the hypothesis that degeneration of the basal forebrain cholinergic system provides a unitary basis for the mental abnormalities. However, neither Meynert neuron loss nor reductions in choline acetyltransferase in the temporal cortex, for example, would distinguish all SDLT cases from AD.

The lack of consistent correlation between Lewy body density and dementia may reflect the fact that the presence of Lewy bodies in the cortex represents a 'tip of the iceberg' phenomenon – the remainder of the iceberg consisting of as yet unidentified cell loss in a select but critical population of cortical neurons. In PD cases the presence of Lewy bodies in the substantia nigra and locus coeruleus is associated with a mean of over 60% loss of dopaminergic and noradrenergic neurons (Perry et al., 1990) and there is no reason to expect a different scenario in the cortex. There may be a distinct subpopulation of cortical neurons which degenerates in SDLT/PD with dementia which leads to disruption of cortical connectivity and mental function. Quantitative assessment of neuronal populations and synaptic connectivity in key cortical areas should address this issue. Which areas in neo- or limbic cortex should be examined is a major question which may need to depend on current theories of anatomical function and parallel investigations of imaging in living subjects. The fluctuating nature of clinical features in SDLT suggests that cross sectional clinico-pathological correlations at the end of life will be challenging, to say the least.

The influence of ApoE4 genotypes on neuropathological phenotype is unclear. There is no obvious relation between the presence or absence of E4 on the presence of density of limbic Lewy bodies, neocortical plaques, or neocortical tangles, although the group of cases with ApoE 4/4 genotype appears to be associated with about more than ninefold higher median neocortical tangle density than the remaining ApoE genotypic groups (Figure 17.1). It has been suggested that in AD E4 allele number is directly related to age of onset of dementia but no such relation is apparent in the present SDLT series. The group of AD with presenile onset had a lower frequency of E 4/4 and E 3/4 genotypes than AD cases with senile onset. A more interesting relation in the present series may be the greater predominance of males in the SDLT subgroup with no neo-cortical Alzheimer type pathology (either plaques or plaques and tangles). This trend is consistent with a parallel analysis of elderly normal and AD cases in which female compared to male subgroups are more affected by Alzheimer pathology (Perry et al., submitted).

17.4 Conclusion

In the scientific doctrine of reductionism the goal of a unitary explanation for complex biological phenomena is predominant. To provide a satisfactory explanation of Lewy body dementia, it may however be necessary to consider a variety of co-correlates of different clinical features, genetics, cerebral abnormalities, brain regions and even different points in time. From this may emerge an interacting framework which, in some respects, may be unique to each individual. At present individuality or subjectivity in Lewy body dementia research arises as much from the focus of the different research groups as from differences in the types of patients being examined. Interactions between research groups and exchange of data should be one of the most productive strategies in the immediate future.

Acknowledgements

Acknowledgements are due to J. Hardy, and C. Harrington for Apo E typing.

References

Blessed, G., Tomlinson, B. E. & Roth, M. (1968). The association between quantitative measuring of dementia and of senile change in cerebral grey matter of elderly subjects. *Br. J. Psychiatry*, **114**, 797–811.

Boller, F., Mizutani, T., Roessman, U. & Gambetti, P. (1980). Parkinson's disease, dementia and Alzheimer disease: clinicopathological correlation. *Ann. Neurol.*, **7**, 329–36.

Braak, H. & Braak, E. (1991). Neuropathological staging of Alzheimer-related changes. *Acta Neuropathol.*, **82**, 239–59.

Dickson, D. W., Davies, P., Mayeux, R. et al. (1987). Diffuse Lewy body disease. Neuropathological and biochemical studies of six cases. *Acta Neuropathol.*, **75**, 8–15.

Dickson, D. W., Ruan D., Crystal H. et al. (1991). Hippocampal degeneration differentiates diffuse Lewy body disease (LBD) from Alzheimer's disease: light and electron microscopic immunocytochemistry of CA2–3 neurites specific to LBD. *Neurology*, **41**, 1402–9.

Gibb, W. R. G., Esiri, M. M. & Lees, A. J. (1987). Clinical and pathological features of diffuse cortical Lewy body disease (Lewy body dementia). *Brain*, **110**, 1131–53.

Harrington, C. R., Louwagie, J., Rossau, R. et al. (1994). The influence of apolipoprotein E genotype on senile dementia of the Alzheimer and Lewy body types: significance for etiological theories of Alzheimer's disease. *Am. J. Pathol.*, **145**, 1472–84.

Ince, P. G., Irving, D., MacArthur, F. & Perry, R. H. (1991). Quantitative neuropathological study of Alzheimer-type pathology in the hippocampus: comparison of senile dementia of Alzheimer type, senile dementia of Lewy body type, Parkinson's disease and non-demented elderly control patients. *J. Neurol. Sci.*, **106**, 142–52.

Kosaka, K. (1993). Dementia and neuropathology in Lewy body disease. *Adv. Neurol.*, **60**, 456–63.

Leake, A., Perry, E. K., Perry, R. H. et al. (1991). Neocortical concentrations of neuropeptides in senile dementia of the Alzheimer and Lewy body type. Comparison with Parkinson's disease and severity correlations. *Biol. Psychiatry*, **29**, 357–64.

Lennox, G., Lowe, J., Landon, M., Byrne, E. J., Mayer, R. J. & Godwin-Austen, R. B. (1989). Diffuse Lewy body disease, correlative neuropathology using anti-ubiquitin immunocytochemistry. *J. Neurol. Neurosurg. Psychiatry*, **52**, 1236–47.

Mitake, S., Ojika, K., Katada, E., Otsuka, Y., Matsukawa, N. & Fujimon, O. (1995). Accumulation of hippocampal cholinergic neurostimulating peptide (HCNP) – related components in Hirano bodies. *Neuropathol. Appl. Neurobiol.*, **21**, 35–40.

Paulus, W. & Jellinger, K. (1991). The neuropathological basis of different clinical subgroups of Parkinson's disease. *J. Neuropathol. Exp. Neurol.*, **50**, 743–55.

Perry, R. H., Irving, D., Blessed, G., Fairbairn, A. & Perry, E. K. (1990). Senile dementia of Lewy body type: a clinically and neuropathologically distinct form of Lewy body dementia in the elderly. *J. Neurol. Sci.*, **95**, 119–35.

Perry, E. K., McKeith, I. G., Thompson, P. et al. (1991). Topography, extent and clinical relevance of cholinergic and monoaminergic deficits in dementia of Lewy body, Parkinson and Alzheimer types. *Ann. NY Acad. Sci.*, **640**, 197–202

Whitehouse, P. J., Hedreen, J. O., White, C. L. & Price, D. L. (1983). Basal forebrain neurons in the dementia of Parkinson's disease. *Ann. Neurol.*, **13**, 243–5.

Yoshimura, M. (1988). Pathological basis for dementia in elderly patients with idiopathic Parkinson's disease. *Eur. Neurol.*, **28**, 29–35.

Zweig, R. M., Cardillo, J. E., Cohen, M., Giere, S. & Hedreen, J. C. (1993). The locus ceruleus and dementia in Parkinson's disease. *Neurology*, **43**, 986–91.

18

Cytoskeletal and Alzheimer-type pathology in Lewy body disease

D. W. DICKSON, H. A. CRYSTAL,
P. DAVIES and J. HARDY

Summary

Lewy bodies are neuronal cytoskeletal inclusions that contain ubiquitin and neurofilament proteins. Lewy bodies are found in a wide range of clinical settings, ranging from clinically normal people to those with various extrapyramidal movement disorders to those with a progressive dementia. There is a rough correlation between the number and distribution of Lewy bodies and the degree of cognitive impairment. People with numerous and widespread Lewy bodies are inevitably demented. The frequency of both Lewy bodies and senile changes of the Alzheimer type increase in frequency with age, and not surprisingly coexist in some patients. This has lead to controversy as to whether Lewy body disease (LBD) may actually be a variant of Alzheimer's disease (AD). It is our working hypothesis, on the other hand, that the two disorders are independent, and that when AD pathology is present in LBD, it represents an independent disease process. Qualitative differences in cytoskeletal pathology in LBD and AD associated with senile plaques and in certain regions of the limbic lobe support this hypothesis. Specific molecular markers for LBD do not currently exist, but recent studies suggest that frequency of apolipoprotein E ϵ4 allele may be increased in Lewy body disorders with coexistent AD, but apparently not in LBD without AD type pathology.

18.1 Neuropathology of aging

18.1.1 Insights from prospective clinicopathological studies

Prior to the 1980s there was a paucity of hard scientific information about the pathological correlates of cognitive changes that accompany normal aging. Most of the pathological studies prior to that time were based on small case studies or retrospective analyses for which longitudinal quantitative neuropsychological data were usually not available. Given the increasing awareness of the socioeconomic consequences of late life neurodegenerative diseases, increased attention has focused on this topic. A number of centers have instituted prospective, longitudinal studies of elderly humans. The discussion on aging in the following paragraphs is based upon information gained from longitudinal studies conducted at our institution over the last 13 years.

In aging humans amyloid deposition is a frequent and possibly inevitable finding. In a study of 20 centarians, all cases had at least some amyloid (Delaere et al., 1993). On the other hand, in our series of only slightly younger (average age over 85 years) prospectively studied elderly people, we have seen a few patients with no evidence of amyloid in the cortex, even though virtually every case had at least a few neurofibrillary tangles (NFT) in the entorhinal cortex (Dickson et al., 1992a). In contrast, some normal elderly people have extensive amyloid deposits in the cortex, sufficient to suspect a diagnosis of Alzheimer's disease (AD). We refer to this condition as pathological aging (Dickson et al., 1992a). These elderly subjects have had no apparent cognitive deficits on repeated neurological and neuropsychological evaluations over many years (Dickson et al., 1992a). Recent analysis of change measures based upon the longitudinal neuropsychological data also fails to reveal distinguishing features between those cases with amyloid compared with those without amyloid (unpublished). The reason for emphasizing this point is that when amyloid deposits are detected in Lewy body disease (LBD), it is not reasonable to assume that these deposits, in the absence of neuronal alterations (e.g. synaptic loss, dystrophic neurites, LBs or NFT), are related to the cognitive deficits in LBD or that they are sufficient to warrant a diagnosis of AD.

The most common type of amyloid deposit in the brains of cognitively normal elderly people is the diffuse or non-neuritic amyloid plaque. Diffuse amyloid deposits are not accompanied by synaptic loss (Masliah et al., 1990). Although they may contain a few ubiquitin-immunoreactive dystrophic neurites (Dickson et al., 1990), they lack argyrophilic, PHF-type neuritic degeneration. Immunocytochemical studies have further demonstrated a general dissociation between amyloid deposition and neurofibrillary pathology (Braak et al., 1989), indicating that amyloid deposition can occur independent of neurofibrillary pathology.

Increasing evidence supports the notion that the presence of numerous senile plaques is a necessary, but not sufficient pathological feature for the diagnosis of AD. It should be noted, however that senile plaques in AD are also accompanied by extensive neuronal alterations in the form of PHF formation in both neuronal perikarya (NFT) and neuritic processes (neuropil threads) (Braak et al., 1986), as well as with synaptic loss. Neuropil threads may be the major site for accumulation of abnormal tau protein in the AD brain.

Attempts to develop a rational pathological staging system for Alzheimer type pathology (Braak & Braak, 1991) are in accord with results from clinicopathological studies. These studies show that neurofibrillary degeneration is a better correlate of cognitive impairment than amyloid deposits (Arriagada et al., 1992; Crystal et al., 1993; Dickson et al., 1995). Likewise, the progression of neurofibrillary pathology is rather stereotypic, in contrast to the far less predictable patterns of amyloid deposition, which are influenced by age, genotype and the presence of amyloid angiopathy.

In addition to qualitative observations based upon examination of morphological differences, AD can also be differentiated from pathological aging by quantitative and sensitive enzyme-linked immunoassays for PHF protein (abnormal tau protein) (Dickson et al., 1995). In pathological aging levels of abnormal tau protein are very low to undetectable. Similar analyses in LBD with Alzheimer type pathology have also shown increased PHF proteins (Vermersch et al., 1993), but such an analysis has not been performed on LBD lacking Alzheimer type pathology.

18.1.2 Ubiquitin in age-related neuropathology

Ubiquitin is a highly conserved 76 amino protein that is involved in ATP-dependent nonlysosomal proteolytic degradation. It can be considered a heat shock or stress protein since its expression is increased in stressed cells. At least some ubiquitinated proteins are degraded by a multimeric protein complex called the proteasome. One of the major subunits of this complex is a multicatalytic proteinase, which incidentally also has been associated with Lewy bodies (LBs) (Pollanen et al., 1993). With increasing age there are an increasing number of ubiquitin-immunoreactive structures in the human brain (Dickson et al., 1990). The most consistent finding is fine granular staining in the white matter. At the electron microscopic level this granular degeneration of myelin is characterized by ubiquitin in electron dense pleomorphic bodies within expansions of

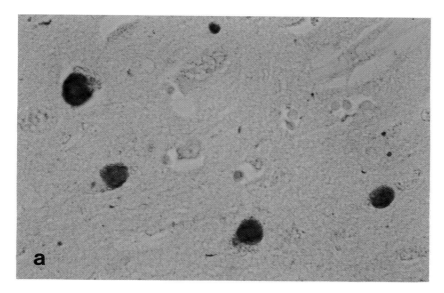

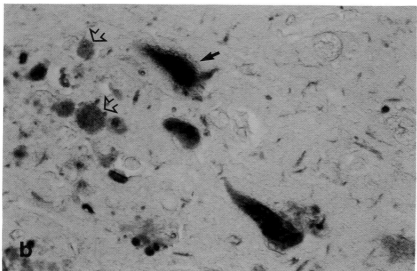

Plate 3
(a) Ubiquitin immunostaining of LBD cortex shows intense immunoreactivity of cortical Lewy bodies, but very little staining of anything else in the neuropil (×600);
(b) Double immunostaining with an antibody to ubiquitin (peroxidase method – brown) and with Alz-50 (β-galactosidase method – blue). An intracellular NFT (solid arrow) is stained with Alz-50, but extracellular NFT and granular dystrophic neurities in senile plaque (open arrows) are positive only for ubiquitin (×600);

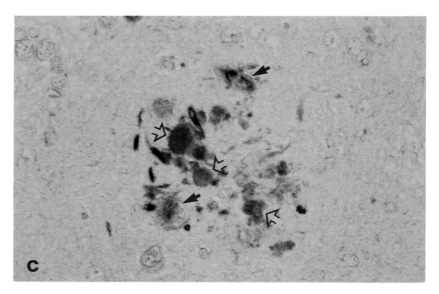

c

d

(c) Same staining methods as (b). Note that in this case of combined LBD/AD neurites in the senile plaque are heterogeneous. Some contain only ubiquitin immunoreactivity (open arrows), a type of dystrophic neurite that is common in aged brains, while others contain abnormal tau protein (solid arrows) as indicated by immunoreactivity with Alz-50. Using methods such as this it is possible to discern qualitative differences between senile plaques in aging and AD ($\times$600);

(d) The CA2/3 region of the hippocampus in LBD stained with an antibody to NFT. There is no immunoreactivity to be seen ($\times$150);

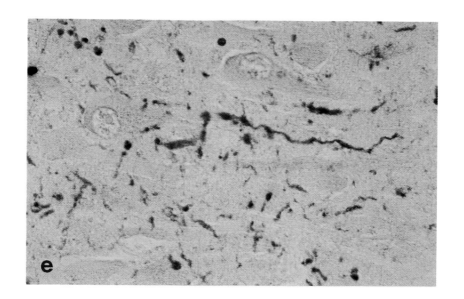

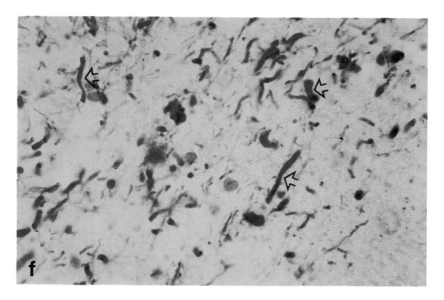

(e) The same region of the hippocampus stained with an antibody to ubiquitin shows a dense plexus of abnormal neurites (×600);

(f) The neurites in CA2/3 are double stained for neurofilament (alkaline phosphatase method – red) and ubiquitin (peroxidase method – brown). Note that many (open arrows), but not all, of the CA2/3 neurites are also reactive for phosphorylated neurofilaments (×600).

myelin lamellae, a feature of aging myelin first noted in brain biopsies many years ago. The advent of ubiquitin immunocytochemistry permitted an assessment of the extent of this change in aging. Granular degeneration is first detected in the third and fourth decades of life. It increases steadily with age and is accelerated in conditions that affect myelin, such as ischemic injury to the white matter.

In the gray matter, dystrophic neuronal processes are also common in aging. They occur in the dorsal column nuclei, pars reticularis of the substantia nigra and the globus pallidus. Axonal spheroids are consistently reactive with antibodies to ubiquitin. In addition, ubiquitin immunocytochemistry reveals neuritic dystrophy that is more extensive and widespread than apparent with routine histological techniques. In particular, granular dystrophic neurites are detected in the aging limbic gray matter, especially the entorhinal cortex and the amygdala. Similar dystrophic neurites are also detected around amyloid deposits, especially those with compact amyloid cores, in pathological aging and in LBD. In these lesions the ubiquitin is also localized to electron dense pleomorphic bodies, possibly of lysosomal origin.

Ubiquitin also immunostains a variety of neuronal inclusions, some of which are disease-specific and others which are found in normal elderly control subjects. Among the former are NFT and LBs. A clear distinction between LBs and NFT is not always easy; however, double immunocytochemical staining usually permits differentiation, since LBs do not contain tau protein. Furthermore, ubiquitin labels only a small proportion of NFT in routinely processed tissue sections. In contrast, it is the most sensitive marker for LBs (Lennox et al., 1989). (Plate 3a).

18.2 Lewy body disease

18.2.1 AD type pathology in LBD

Alzheimer type pathology occurs more frequently in Parkinson's disease than in an age-matched population (Hughes et al., 1993). Conversely, LBs have been detected with increased frequency in AD (Ditter & Mirra, 1987). Although the increased frequency of Alzheimer type pathology in Parkinson's disease has been noted previously, awareness of the frequency of cortical LBs and use of sensitive methods to detect cortical LBs were not features of studies prior to 1988 (Kuzuhara et al., 1988), which makes it difficult to evaluate these results in the context of current knowledge. Furthermore, it is only recently that attention has been devoted to qualitative differences among senile plaques in aging and AD (Dickson et al., 1989, 1992a; Crystal et al., 1993). (Plate 3b and c). It is likely that some of the cases of combined AD and Parkinson's disease described in the literature represent LBD with associated pathological aging (see below). Only retrospective analysis of such cases with sensitive methods for detecting cortical LBs and analysis of the type of senile plaques will answer this question.

18.2.2 Senile plaques in aging, AD and LBD

Many cases of LBD, especially those older than 60 years of age, have cortical senile plaques (Kosaka et al., 1984; Gibb et al., 1987; Dickson et al., 1989; Perry et al., 1990; Hansen et al., 1994a). Since some cases of LBD lack senile plaques, we would suggest that it is currently untenable to consider LBD with diffuse senile plaques (and lacking neurofibrillary tangles) as a variant of AD (Hansen et al., 1990). Such cases differ little from cases without amyloid deposits by all other currently available means of assessment. Given the fact that some clinically normal elderly people may have many amyloid plaques, we restrict our diagnosis of AD to cases that have both neocortical senile plaques and NFT as suggested by Tomlinson (1989) and are particularly careful to note the presence or absence of neuritic plaques and to place less emphasis on diffuse amyloid deposits. This approach has recently been adopted by a large multicenter study, the CERAD study (Mirra et al., 1991), and is a departure from previous pathological criteria for AD (Khachaturian, 1985).

There are sound reasons for this approach since clinicopathological studies have demonstrated that diffuse senile plaques have little or no correlation with clinical measures of cognitive function, but neuritic plaques correlate with presence of cognitive impairment typical of AD (Crystal et al., 1993).

Studies of qualitative differences in senile plaques in AD, LBD and pathological aging demonstrate that senile plaques in most cases of LBD are similar to those in pathological aging and different from those in AD. In most cases of LBD the senile plaques are diffuse deposits of β-protein (Aβ) with few or no neuritic components (Dickson et al., 1989, 1992a, b). In contrast, senile plaques in AD and those cases of LBD with concomitant AD (LBD/AD) are of the neuritic type with tau-positive, argyrophilic and thioflavin-S fluorescent neurites. (Plate 3c). A recent morphometric analysis of the density of neuropil threads in LBD cases clearly distinguished LBD from AD and another disorder associated with neurofibrillary pathology, progressive supranuclear palsy (Davis et al., 1992).

18.2.3 Hippocampal pathology in LBD

Neurofibrillary pathology in the hippocampus is an invariant feature of AD. On the other hand, it is frequently absent in LBD (Dickson et al., 1989). In our studies of cholinergic markers in AD and LBD, deficits were inconsistent in the hippocampus in LBD reflecting the heterogeneity of hippocampal pathology in LBD; in contrast, cholinergic deficits were consistent in AD (Dickson et al., 1987). The CA1 region of Ammon's horn and the subiculum appear to be particularly vulnerable to neurofibrillary degeneration in AD, but those sectors are frequently spared in LBD. On the other hand, ubiquitin-immunoreactive neuritic degeneration is more common in CA2/CA3 in LBD (Dickson et al., 1991). (Plate 3e). These neurites contain neurofilament immunoreactivity (Plate 3f) and are sometimes weakly reactive with Alz-50, a monoclonal antibody that binds to abnormal tau protein in AD, but not with antibodies specific to NFT. (Plate 3d). At the electron microscopic level they contain intermediate sized filaments that are sometimes partially invested in myelin.

Neurites similar to those in the CA2/CA3 region of the hippocampus are also found in other regions of the brain in LBD, including the amygdala (Braak et al., 1994), basal forebrain, substantia nigra, pedunculopontine nuclei, raphe nuclei and dorsal motor nuclei of the vagus. Recent studies have failed to demonstrate co-localization of tyrosine hydroxylase, a marker for dopaminergic neurons, with ubiquitin-immunoreactive CA2/CA3 neurites (Dickson et al., 1994). This indicates that the CA2/CA3 neurites are probably not derived from dopaminergic projections to the hippocampus. In a continuing study of LBD cases, we have noted that the extent of CA2/CA3 neuritic degeneration correlates with the density of cortical LB (Pollanen et al., 1993). To date we have not detected CA2/CA3 neurites in corticobasal ganglionic degeneration, striatonigral degeneration or dementia lacking distinctive histopathology.

The parahippocampal and entorhinal cortex has been the focus of increased study in recent years since it has been recognized that this region of the brain is unusually susceptible to neurofibrillary pathology in aging and AD. In patients with LBD the parahippocampal cortex usually has more NFT than age-matched controls, but fewer than advanced AD (Ince et al., 1991).

18.2.4 Combined AD and LBD

Some brains have unequivocal pathology of both AD and LBD. Although a minority of cases have extensive cortical NFT, the majority of cases have few NFT. A form of AD that has been increasingly recognized in recent years – 'limbic AD' (Mizutani et al., 1990) – appears to be especially frequent in LBD (Hansen et al., 1994a). In limbic AD there is severe neurofibrillary degeneration in the medial temporal lobe structures including the amygdala and hippocampus, but very little 'spread' beyond the temporal lobe. Such cases have many cortical SP, and many of the plaques are of the neuritic-type. These cases represent a form of plaque-predominant AD. They differ from pathological aging by the presence of neocortical plaques and severe temporal lobe neurofibrillary degeneration, as well as by the fact that the patients are demented. It is currently unclear whether these cases merely represent an early stage of Alzheimer type pathology or a distinct subtype of AD. In any event further studies are indicated to determine the reason this form of the Alzheimer type pathology should be more frequent in LBD.

18.2.5 Apolipoprotein E and amyloidosis in LBD

An uncommon allele for apolipoprotein E (Apo E), $\epsilon 4$, has been recently discovered to be linked to, or a marker for, risk for familial and sporadic late-onset AD (Saunders et al., 1993). Because of the interest in the AD pathology that occurs in LBD, it is of interest to determine if Apo E is associated with AD type pathology in LBD. We analyzed 21 cases of LBD (Table 18.1), including three cases of pure LBD, seven LBD with pathological aging and 11 LBD/AD. None of the pure cases were positive for $\epsilon 4$, while 2/7 of LBD with pathological aging and 4/11 LBD/AD were positive for $\epsilon 4$ (Table 18.2). The frequency of $\epsilon 4$ in the general population is only 10–15% so the 28.6% frequency in LBD with pathological aging and 36.4% frequency in LBD/AD is greater than expected. Similar increased frequency of $\epsilon 4$ allele in LBD cases with coexistent AD has recently been reported (Hansen et al., 1994b; Harrington et al., 1994; Pickering-Brown et al., 1994; Lippa et al., 1995). On the other hand, dementia in Parkinson's disease does not appear to be linked to $\epsilon 4$ allele (Koller et al., 1995). Further studies are needed to determine the significance of these observations, but the initial interpretation is that the Apo E may influence AD-type pathology (Table 18.3), and in particular the presence of amyloid deposits in LBD, but not be specific to LBD. We

Table 18.1. *Clinical features of LBD cases use for Apo-E genotyping*

Case	Apo-E	Age	Sex	Clinical manifestations
LBD				
4027	3,3	73	M	Dementia, mild; minimal EPS (familial PD)
4353	3,3	74	F	Parkinsonism; minimal cognitive change
4940	3,3	72	F	Dementia; mild EPS (rigidity, tremors)
		73 ± 0.8	1:2	
LBD/PA				
4046	2,2	81	M	Dementia; psychosis; parkinsonism
8828	2,2	85	F	Dementia; rigidity
4210	3,3	92	M	Dementia, mild; minimal EPS
4492	3,3	89	M	Dementia; mild EPS (rigidity)
4570	3,3	71	M	Dementia, rapid; rigidity; myoclonus
4714	4,3	63	F	Parkinsonism; mild dementia
4593	4,4	79	M	Parkinsonism; mild dementia
		80 ± 9.5	5:2	
LBD/AD				
4817	3,3	84	F	Dementia; no history of EPS
4213	3,3	71	M	Dementia; mild EPS
3939	3,3	85	M	Dementia; no history of EPS
4746	3,3	89	F	Dementia; no history of EPS
4475	3,3	82	M	Dementia; parkinsonism, mild
4719	3,3	81	M	Dementia; no history of EPS
9333	3,3	62	M	Dementia; no history of EPS
4774	3,3	62	M	Dementia; parkinsonism
4811	4,3	70	F	Dementia; parkinsonism, mild
4688	4,3	72	M	Dementia; no history of EPS
4622	4,4	90	F	Dementia; mild EPS
		80 ± 9.2	6:5	

LBD = Lewy body disease; PA = pathological aging (see text); AD = Alzheimer's disease; EPS = extrapyramidal signs

have found the same to be true for a series of vascular dementia cases, namely, that Apo E genotype influences the frequency with which amyloid is detected in these brains (unpublished). This would seem to add further support to the idea that AD and LBD are separate disease processes that may (and often do) coexist and that possibly distinct genetic factors may play a role in the expression of each disease process.

Table 18.2. *Pathological markers with respect to DLBD subtype*

Case	Frontal SP	Frontal NFT	Temporal SP	Temporal NFT	Parietal SP	Parietal NFT	Occipita 1 SP	Hippocampus SP	Hippocampus NFT	APO-E
LBD										
4027	0	0	0	0	0	0	0	0	0	3,3
	0	0	6	0	0	0	6	0	1	
4940	17	0	8	0	4	0	2	1	0	3,3
	5.6 ± 8.0*†	0	4.7 ± 3.4*†	0	1.3 ± 1.9*†	0	2.7 ± 2.5*	0.3 ± 0.5*	0.3 ± 0.5*	
LBD/PA										
4046	50	0	50	0	50	0	35	23	11	2,2
8828	50	0.5	20	0	28	0	1	6	14	2,2
4210	45	0	27	0	30	0	11	0	5	3,3
4492	50	0	13	0	50	0	2	0	0.5	3,3
4570	50	0	47	1	50	0	11	6	1.5	3,3
4714	50	0	50	0	50	0	16	21	0	4,3
4593	50	0	50	0.5	50	0	3	7	4.5	4,4
	49 ± 1.7	0.1 ± 0.2[f]	37 ± 15	0.2 ± 0.4†	44 ± 9.5	0†	11 ± 11†	9 ± 8.7	5.2 ± 5.0†	

Table 18.2 Cont'd

Case	Frontal SP	Frontal NFT	Temporal SP	Temporal NFT	Parietal SP	Parietal NFT	Occipita 1 SP	Hippocampus SP	Hippocampus NFT	APO-E
LBD/AD										
4817	50	0	50	2	50	1.5	43	17	14	3,3
4213	50	0.5	50	1.5	50	1	45	18	9	3,3
3939	10	0.5	21	2.5	20	0	7	14	8	3,3
4746	50	0.5	50	6	50	5.5	26	4	16	3,3
4475	50	1	50	7	50	2	40	8	23	3,3
4719	50	1	50	8	50	7	30	10	25	3,3
9333	50	0.5	34	15	36	0.5	20	8	3.5	3,3
4774	50	2	50	5.5	50	4	24	3.5	27	4,2
4811	50	1	42	0.5	50	5.5	28	12	6	4,3
4688	50	0.5	50	1.5	50	3	34	22	7	4,3
4622	50	5.5	50	1.5	50	3.5	50	5	15	4,4
	46±12	1.2±1.5	45±9.1	4.6±4.1	46±9.1	3.1±2.2	32±12	11±5.8	14±7.7	

*p < 0.05 (compared with DLBD/PA)
†p < 0.05 (compared with DLBD/AD)
‡p < 0.1 (compared with DLBD/AD)

Note. SP and NFT were counted in low power (100×) and high power (400×) fields from the indicated areas. The LBD cases differed from the LBD/PA and the LBD/AD cases by having fewer SP and only rare NFT. The LBD/PA cases differed from LBD/AD by having only rare NFT in the cortex and fewer NFT in the hippocampus. Note increasing frequency of apolipoprotein E ε4 allele in cases with increasing AD type pathology.

Table 18.3. *Pathological markers with respect to Apo-E genotype*

	Frontal		Temporal		Parietal		Occipital	Hippocampus	
	SP	NFT	SP	NFT	SP	NFT	SP	SP	NFT
e4(−)	38±19	0.3±0.4*	32±18*	2.9±4.2	35±19	1.2±2.1	19±16	7.7±7.2	8.8±8.0
e4(+)	50±0	1.5±1.9	49±3	1.6±1.8	50±0	2.7±2.0	26±15	12±7.4	9.9±8.8

(+) compared with 34   vith respect to AD ty]   iology the difference   in the pres   of more SP and NF', ...
all LBD cases are stra
e4(+) than in e4(−) in virtually every anatomical region. The differences reach statistical significance in the frontal and temporal lobes, again suggesting that apo-E influences AD type pathology in LBD, not LBD itself.

References

Arriagada, P. V., Growdon, J. H., Hedley-White, T. & Hyman, B. T. (1992). Neurofibrillary tangles but not senile plaques parallel duration and severity of Alzheimer disease. *Neurology*, **42**, 631–9.

Braak, H. & Braak, E. (1991). Neuropathological stageing of Alzheimer-related changes. *Acta Neuropathol.*, **82**, 239–59.

Braak, H., Braak, E., Grundke-Iqbal, I. & Iqbal, K. (1986). Occurrence of neuropil threads in the senile human brain and in Alzheimer's disease: a third location of paired helical filaments outside of neurofibrillary tangles and neuritic plaques. *Neurosci. Lett.*, **65**, 351–5.

Braak, H., Braak, E., Ohm, T. & Bohl, J. (1989). Alzheimer's disease: mismatch between amyloid plaques and neuritic plaques. *Neurosci. Lett.*, **103**, 24–8.

Braak, H., Braak, E. Yilmazer, D. et al. (1994). Amygdala pathology in Parkinson's disease. *Acta Neuropathol.*, **88**, 493–500.

Crystal, H. A., Dickson, D. W., Sliwinski, M. et al. (1993). Pathological markers associated with normal aging and dementia in the elderly. *Ann. Neurol.*, **34**, 566–73.

Davis, D. G., Wang, H. Z. & Markesbery, W. R. (1992). Image analysis of neuropil threads in Alzheimer's, Picks's and diffuse Lewy body disease and in progressive supranuclear palsy. *J. Neuropathol. Exp. Neurol.*, **51**, 594–600.

Delaere, P., He, Y., Fayet, G., Duyckaerts, C. & Hauw, J. J. (1993). Beta A4 deposits are constant in the brain of the oldest old: an immunocytochemical study of 20 French centenarians. *Neurobiol. Aging*, **14**, 191–4.

Dickson, D. W., Davies, P., Mayeux, R., Crystal, H. A., Thompson, D. & Goldman, J. E. (1987). Diffuse Lewy body disease: neuropathological and biochemical studies of six patients. *Acta Neuropathol.*, **75**, 8–15.

Dickson, D. W., Crystal, H. A., Mattiace, L. A. et al. (1989). Diffuse Lewy body disease: light and electron microscopic immunocytochemistry of senile plaques. *Acta Neuropathol.*, **78**, 572–84.

Dickson, D. W., Wertkin, A., Kress, Y., Ksiezak-Reding, H. & Yen, S.-H. (1990). Ubiquitin-immunoreactive structures in normal brains: distribution and developmental aspects. *Lab. Invest.*, **63**, 87–99.

Dickson, D. W., Ruan, D., Crystal, H. et al. (1991). Hippocampal degeneration differentiates diffuse Lewy body disease (LBD) from Alzheimer's disease: light and electron microscopic immunocytochemistry of CA2-3 neurites specific to LBD. *Neurology*, **41**, 1402–9.

Dickson, D. W., Crystal, H. A., Mattiace, L. A. et al. (1992a). Identification of normal and pathological aging in prospectively studied nondemented elderly humans. *Neurobiol. Aging*, **13**, 179–89.

Dickson, D. W., Wu, E., Crystal, H. A., Mattiace, L. A., Yen, S.-H. & Davies, P. (1992b). Alzheimer and age-related pathology in diffuse Lewy body disease. In *Heterogeneity of Alzheimer's Disease*, ed. F. Boller, F. Forcette, Z. Khachaturian, M. Poncet & Y. Christen, pp. 168–86. Berlin: Springer-Verlag.

Dickson, D. W., Schmidt, M. L., Lee, V.M.-Y., Trojanowski, J. Q. & Yen, S. H. (1994). Hippocampal neurites in diffuse Lewy body disease: immunocytochemical characterization and local origin. *Acta Neuropathol.*, **87**, 269–76.

Dickson, D. W., Crystal, H. A., Bevona, C., Honer, W., Vincent, I. & Davies, P. (1995). Correlations of synaptic markers with cognitive status in prospectively studied elderly humans. *Neurobiol. Aging*, **16**, 285–98.

Ditter, S. M. & Mirra, S. S. (1987). Neuropathologic and clinical features of Parkinson's disease in Alzheimer's disease patients. *Neurology*, **37**, 754–60.

Gibb, W. R. G., Esiri, M. M. & Lees, A. J. (1987). Clinical and pathological features of diffuse cortical Lewy body disease (Lewy body dementia). *Brain*, **110**, 1131–53.

Hansen, L., Salmon, D., Galasko, D. et al. (1990). Lewy body variant of Alzheimer's disease: a clinical and pathological entity. *Neurology*, **40**, 1–8.

Hansen, L. A., Masliah, E., Galasko, D. & Terry, R. D. (1994a). Plaque-only Alzheimer disease is usually Lewy body variant, and vice versa. *J. Neuropathol. Exp. Neurol.*, **52**, 648–54.

Hansen, L. A., Galasko, D., Samuel, W., Xia, Y., Chen, X. & Saitoh, T. (1994b). Apolipoprotein-E epsilon-4 is associated with increased neurofibrillary pathology in the Lewy body variant of Alzheimer's disease. *Neurosci. Lett.*, **182**, 63–5.

Harrington, C. R., Louwagie, J., Rossau, R. et al. (1994). Influence of apolipoprotein E genotype on senile dementia of the Alzheimer and Lewy body types. Significance for etiological theories of Alzheimer's disease. *Am. J. Pathol.*, **145**, 1472–84.

Hughes, A. J., Daniel, S. E., Blankson, S. & Lees, A. J. (1993). A clinicopathologic study of 100 cases of Parkinson's disease. *Arch. Neurol.*, **50**, 140–8.

Ince, P., Irving, D., MacArthur, F. & Perry, R. H. (1991). Quantitative neuropathological study of Alzheimer-type pathology in the hippocampus: comparison of senile dementia of Alzheimer type, senile dementia of Lewy body type, Parkinson's disease and nondemented elderly control patients. *J. Neurol. Sci.*, **106**, 142–52.

Khachaturian, Z. S. (1985). Diagnosis of Alzheimer's disease. *Arch. Neurol.*, **42**, 1097–105.

Koller, W. C., Glatt, S. L., Hubble, J. P. et al. (1995). Apolipoprotein e genotypes in Parkinson's disease with and without dementia. *Ann. Neurol.*, **37**, 242–5.

Kosaka, K., Yoshimura, M., Ikeda, K. & Budka, H. (1984). Diffuse type of Lewy body disease: progressive dementia with abundant cortical Lewy bodies and senile changes of varying degree – a new disease? *Clin. Neuropathol.*, **3**, 185–92.

Kuzuhara, S., Mori, H., Izumiyama, N., Yoshimura, M. & Ihara, Y. (1988). Lewy bodies are ubiquitinated: a light and electron microscopic immunocytochemical study. *Acta Neuropathol.*, **75**, 345–53.

Lennox, G., Lowe, J., Morrell, K., Landon, M. & Mayer, R. J. (1989). Anti-ubiquitin immunocytochemistry is more sensitive than conventional techniques in the detection of diffuse Lewy body disease. *J. Neurol. Neurosurg. Psychiatry*, **52**, 67–71.

Lippa, C., Smith, T. W., Saunders, A. et al. (1995). Apolipoprotein E genotype and Lewy body disease. *Neurology*, **45**, 97–103.

Masliah, E., Terry, R. D., Mallory, M., Alford, M. & Hansen, L. A. (1990). Diffuse plaques do not accentuate synapse loss in Alzheimer's disease. *Am. J. Pathol.*, **137**, 1293–7.

Mirra, S. S., Heyman, A., McKeel, D. et al. (1991). The Consortium to Establish a Registry for Alzheimer's Disease (CERAD). Part II.

Standardization of the neuropathologic assessment of Alzheimer's disease. *Neurology*, **41**, 479–86.

Mizutani, T., Amano, N., Sasaki, H. et al. (1990). Senile dementia of Alzheimer type characterized by laminar neuronal loss exclusively in the hippocampus, parahippocampus and medial occipitotemporal cortex. *Acta Neuropathol.*, **80**, 575–80.

Perry, R. H., Irving, D., Blessed, G., Fairbairn, A. & Perry, E. K. (1990). Senile dementia of the Lewy body type: A clinically and neuropathologically distinct form of Lewy body dementia in the elderly. *J. Neurol. Sci.*, **95**, 119–39.

Pickering-Brown, S. M., Mann, D. M. A., Bourke, J. P. et al. (1994). Apolipoprotein E4 and Alzheimer's disease pathology in Lewy body disease and in other β-amyloid-forming diseases. *Lancet*, **343**, 1155.

Pollanen, M. S., Dickson, D. W. & Bergeron, C. (1993). Pathology and biology of the Lewy body. *J. Neuropathol. Exp. Neurol.*, **52**, 183–91.

Saunders, A. M., Strittmatter, W. J., Schmechel, D. et al. (1993). Association of apolipoprotein E allele e4 with late-onset familial and sporadic Alzheimer's disease. *Neurology*, **43**, 1467–72.

Tomlinson, B. E. (1989). Second Dorothy S. Russell Memorial Lecture: The neuropathology of Alzheimer's disease – issues in need of resolution. *Neuropathol. Appl. Neurobiol.*, **15**, 491–512.

Vermersch, P., Delacourte, A., Javoy-Agid, F., Hauw, J.-J. & Agid, Y. (1993). Dementia in Parkinson's disease: biochemical evidence for cortical involvement using the immunodetection of abnormal tau proteins. *Ann. Neurol.*, **33**, 445–50.

19

Diffuse Lewy body disease within the spectrum of Lewy body disease

K . K O S A K A and E . I S E K I

Summary

In 1980 we proposed Lewy body disease (LBD) as a disease entity and classified it into three types: brainstem, transitional, and diffuse. The brainstem type is identical to Parkinson's disease, and the diffuse type is now called diffuse LBD (DLBD).

DLBD has become the subject of much attention since the publication of our studies on DLBD. It has recently been reported that DLBD is the second most common cause of dementia among the elderly. Our recent study of 79 consecutive autopsied dementia cases suggests that also in Japan DLBD is the second most common degenerative dementia, following Alzheimer-type dementia (ATD). In 1990, we divided DLBD into two forms: a pure form and a common form. Then, it was noted that in 30% of the common form DLBD cases no parkinsonism was detected, although Parkinson pathology was present. Very recently, we proposed cerebral type of LBD as yet another type of LBD, in which cortical dementia without parkinsonism is the predominant symptom and there are as many cortical Lewy bodies as in DLBD, but Parkinson pathology is absent. This feature suggests that the development of cortical Lewy bodies can precede Parkinson pathology. Therefore, this might explain why cortical dementia precedes Parkinson symptoms in many DLBD cases. Thus, LBD is now classified into four types, and DLBD is understood within the spectrum of LBD. The frequency of cortical Lewy bodies is important. More than five or ten cortical Lewy bodies per ×100 visual field in the predilection sites are necessary for the diagnosis of DLBD or cerebral type LBD in HE or ubiquitin-immunostained sections, respectively.

19.1 Introduction

James Parkinson first described the detailed clinical features of Parkinson's disease (PD) in 1817. It was not until 1912, however, that the most important pathological marker of this disease was reported by Lewy (1912). One and a half centuries after Parkinson's report, the neuropathological basis of this disease was established by Greenfield and Bosanquet (1953) and Bethlem and Den Haltog Jager (1960).

The neuropathological features of PD are: marked depigmentation in the substantia nigra and locus ceruleus, and abiotrophic degeneration with scattered Lewy bodies in some brainstem and diencephalon nuclei, including the substantia nigra and locus ceruleus.

The predilection sites of Lewy bodies were first reported by Den Haltog Jager et al. in 1960. Lewy bodies are predominantly found in the hypothalamic nuclei, nucleus basalis of Meynert, substantia nigra, dorsal raphé nucleus, locus ceruleus, superior central nucleus, dorsal vagal nucleus, and intermediolateral nucleus. Intraneuritic Lewy bodies also occur in the sympathetic ganglia and in the intramural autonomic ganglia of the digestive tracts. It was believed, however, that few or no Lewy bodies occur in the cerebral cortex and basal ganglia.

In the late 1970s, we demonstrated that Lewy bodies frequently occur in the cerebral cortex and basal ganglia as well (Kosaka et al., 1976; Kosaka, 1978; Kosaka & Mehraein, 1979).

In 1980 we proposed Lewy body disease as a disease entity (Kosaka et al., 1980), based on our clinicopathological research.

19.2 What is Lewy body disease?

Lewy body disease is a chronic progressive neuropsychiatric disease whose clinical features are characterized by parkinsonian symptoms with or without dementia. Patients are usually senile or presenile and the disease rarely appears in the young. In some cases, progressive dementia is the predominant symptom, followed by parkinsonian symptoms in the later stages. The main neuropathological findings are the presence of numerous Lewy bodies and abiotrophic degeneration in the central nervous system, frequently combined with senile changes of various degree.

When we first proposed Lewy body disease, we classified it into three types; a brainstem type, a transitional type and a diffuse type (Kosaka et al., 1980, 1984, 1989). In the brainstem type, many Lewy bodies are found in the brainstem and diencephalon nuclei, but very few or none at all are found in the cerebral cortex or basal ganglia. In the diffuse type, numerous Lewy bodies are distributed both in the brainstem and diencephalon as well as in the cerebral cortex and basal ganglia. In the transitional type, there are many Lewy bodies in the brainstem and diencephalon, but fewer in the cerebral cortex, compared with the diffuse type. The brainstem type of Lewy body disease is identical to PD, and the diffuse type is now called diffuse Lewy body disease (DLBD). This recent nomenclature was proposed by Yoshimura (1983) who confirmed our findings.

19.3 Diffuse Lewy body disease

DLBD has become the subject of much attention among Japanese neuropathologists following the publication of our studies on DLBD cases. Since then, many similar cases have been reported in Japan (Kosaka, 1990). In our paper of 1984 (Kosaka et al., 1984) we pointed out that DLBD had been overlooked in European and North American countries, since only one case had been reported in the US by Forno et al. (1978) and a number of DLBD cases had been found in Germany and Austria by our group (Kosaka & Mehraein, 1979; Ikeda et al., 1980; Yoshimura, 1983). Since 1985, there have been many studies published on DLBD, including those from European and North American countries. It has recently been reported by certain British and American research groups (Dickson et al., 1989; Lennox et al., 1989; Perry et al., 1990) that DLBD is the second most common cause of dementia among the elderly, following Alzheimer-type dementia (ATD).

Our recent study of 79 autopsied dementia cases in a district geriatric hospital determined that in 34 cases (43.6%), the pathological diagnosis was ATD, in 18 (23.1%), it was vascular dementia, and in 12 (15.4%), it was DLBD. This suggests that in Japan DLBD is the second most common degenerative dementia, following ATD. However, all DLBD cases were clinically misdiagnosed.

In 1990 and 1993, we reviewed all DLBD cases reported in Japan (Kosaka, 1990, 1993) and divided DLBD into two forms: a pure form and a common form. With the pure form, only a few senile changes or none at all can be observed, while with the common form, numerous senile plaques can be found in the cerebral cortex and, to a greater or lesser extent, also can neurofibrillary tangles in the parahippocampal and hippocampal regions.

In about 80% of the pure form cases, the initial symptoms were parkinsonian symptoms. On the other hand, with the common form cases, the initial symptom was memory disturbance in about 60% and parkinsonian symptoms in about 15%. Most cases with the pure form showed parkinsonian symptoms with eventual progressive cortical dementia. All cases with the common form, however, had cortical dementia, but in about 30%, no parkinsonian symptoms were detected, even in the terminal stage.

Our first case with the common form of DLBD was reported in 1976 (Kosaka et al., 1976). The patient began developing memory disturbances at the age of 56. Cortical dementia progressed, followed by muscular rigidity of all extremities. In addition to the pathological features of PD, numerous cortical Lewy bodies were noted in the cerebral cortex and amygdala. In addition, numerous senile plaques and neurofibrillary tangles were observed in the cerebral cortex.

The neuropathological features of ATD are known to be: (1) diffuse brain atrophy; (2) numerous senile plaques in the cerebral cortex; (3) many neurofibrillary tangles in the parahippocampal cortex and hippocampus, although those in the neocortex are not always necessary for the diagnosis of senile dementia of the Alzheimer type (SDAT); and (4) laminar neuronal loss in the entorhinal cortex. Thus, our first case also exhibited ATD pathology. We have also reported similar cases with the common form of DLBD, although senile changes were generally milder in degree than in our first case. Neurofibrillary tangles especially were usually mild and localized in the parahippocampus, hippocampus and amygdala.

A presenile case with the pure form of DLBD involved a 62-year-old female. She first complained of finger tremor and gait disturbance. Parkinsonian symptoms progressed and were later followed by mental deterioration with auditory hallucinations and mood depressions. She eventually died at the age of 73 years. Neuropathological examination revealed numerous Lewy bodies in the cerebral cortex and brainstem nuclei. No senile plaques were present, but some neurofibrillary tangles were observed in the hippocampal regions. Most Japanese cases with the pure form of DLBD involved younger people.

A second case with the pure form of DLBD that has been reported by us (Odawara et al., 1992) involved a 48-year-old man who had a 10-year history of parkinsonian symptoms with later progressive dementia. Neuropathological examination revealed a widespread distribution of Lewy bodies in the brainstem and diencephalon as well as in the cerebral cortex.

Some neurofibrillary tangles were also present in the hippocampus, but senile plaques were absent. In addition, a great number of small spheroids were observed in the globus pallidus, substantia nigra and hippocampus.

19.4 Distribution of Lewy bodies in DLBD

As we reported previously (Kosaka, 1978), in DLBD Lewy bodies are widely distributed not only in the brainstem and diencephalon, but also in the cerebral cortex and basal ganglia. Cortical Lewy bodies are scattered throughout the cerebral cortex, but are preferentially found in the frontal, anterior cingulate, insular and temporal cortices. Rare ones are also present in the hippocampus. They are usually localized in small nerve cells at the fifth and sixth cortical layers. Figure 19.1 shows the distribution pattern of Lewy bodies in one of our DLBD cases.

In 1978 we (Kosaka, 1978) pointed out for the first time that many Lewy bodies can be found in the amygdala. However, their detailed distribution in that portion of the brain remained unclear. Our recent examination (Iseki et al., 1995) has disclosed the characteristic distribution pattern of Lewy bodies in the amygdala. As shown in Fig. 19.2 they are present throughout the amygdala, but are preferentially found in the medial parts of the accessory basal and basal nuclei and in the cortico-amygdaloid transition area. These nuclei are known to be closely associated with the hippocampus and parahippocampus. Therefore, Lewy bodies in the amygdala might contribute to memory disturbance in DLBD.

19.5 Other specific findings in DLBD

Our recent investigation (Iseki et al., 1996) disclosed that many specific ubiquitin-positive spheroid-like structures are present in the central nucleus of the amygdala in DLBD brains as well as in some with PD, but none have been found in cases involving ATD. These structures are tau-negative. Ubiquitin-immunoelectron microscopic examination revealed that these structures are identical to spheroid bodies and have occasional synaptic structures. The central nucleus receive dense cathecolaminergic fibers from the substantia nigra and locus ceruleus. Therefore, these structures may develop as a result of the degeneration of distal or terminal axons of nerve cells in the substantia nigra and locus ceruleus.

Dickson et al. (1991) reported that ubiquitin-positive neuritic structures are specifically found in the CA2-3 areas of the hippocampus in

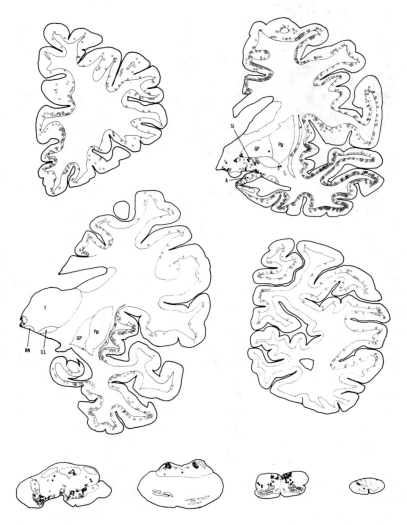

Fig. 19.1 Distribution of Lewy bodies in a DLBD case. Pu: Putamen; GP: Globus pallidus; SI: Substantia innomonata; A: Amygdala; T: Thalamus; CL: Corpus Luysi; RN: Red nucleus; An open circle means an intracytoplasmic Lewy body, and a dot indicates an intraneuritic Lewy body.

cases involving DLBD. We have been able to confirm their findings. Our recent examination (Iseki et al., 1996) disclosed that these structures were found in the CA2-3 areas in 10 of 12 DLBD cases, but none were found in ATD and PD cases. They differ from neuropil threads in that they are

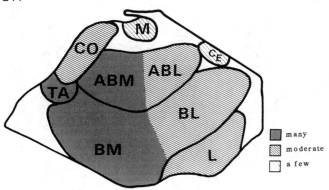

Fig. 19.2 Distribution of Lewy bodies in the amygdala. M: Median nucleus; CO: Cortical nucleus; CE: Central nucleus; TA: Cortico-amygdaloid transition area; ABM: Accessory basal nucleus, medial part; ABL: Accessory basal nucleus, lateral part; BM: Basal nucleus, medial part; LM: Basal nucleus, lateral part; L: Lateral nucleus.

tau-negative. Unlike Dickson et al. (1991), however, we could not find any correlation in frequency between these structures and cortical Lewy bodies. In addition, we found similar ubiquitin-positive structures in the transentorhinal cortex and amygdala as well as in the parafascicular nucleus of Meynert and hypothalamus. Our examination has revealed that these neuritic structures occur as two types; fibrillary and rod-like. The former type is found in the transentorhinal cortex and amygdala as well as in the CA2/CA3 areas of the hippocampus, while the latter is found in the other areas. It was suggested that the latter structures are derived from proximal axons of the brainstem type – Lewy body – containing neurons, since they are always present quite near the brainstem type of Lewy bodies. On the other hand, the former structures are suggested to be derived from distal axons of the neurons unassociated with Lewy bodies since the ubiquitin-immunoelectron microscopic examination revealed that they are filled with neurofilaments, mitochondria and synaptic vesicles or with dense lamellar bodies.

Recently, we also found tau2-positive glial cells in the basal ganglia and brainstem nuclei of DLBD brain tissue (Odawara et al., 1995). These cells were rod-like, GFAP negative, ferritin positive and predominantly observed in the putamen, subthalamic nucleus and substantia nigra. It was suggested that they were microglial cells activated by the degeneration process common to certain neurodegenerative disorders including DLBD.

19.6 Cerebral type of Lewy body disease

Very recently, we proposed a 'cerebral type of Lewy body disease' as yet another type of Lewy body disease (Kosaka et al., 1996). An example of this type involved a male patient who started becoming forgetful at the age of 77 years. From that point, cortical dementia progressed. He was admitted to a geriatric hospital because of delirious episodes. By then, the dementia was profound. No parkinsonism was detected. He died at the age of 79 years.

Macroscopical examination revealed that the substantia nigra and locus ceruleus were well pigmented. This was not observed, however, in DLBD cases. On microscopic examination, no degeneration was found in the substantia nigra or locus ceruleus, although rare occurrences of Lewy bodies were observed in some brainstem nuclei. Thus, this case had no PD pathology. It was very interesting, however, that there were as many cortical Lewy bodies in the cerebral cortex and amygdala as in cases of DLBD.

The features of this cerebral type of Lewy body disease suggest that the development of cortical Lewy bodies precedes PD pathology. Therefore, this might explain why cortical dementia precedes parkinsonian symptoms in many DLBD cases.

19.7 A classification of types of Lewy body disease

As mentioned above, Lewy body disease can be now classified as follows:

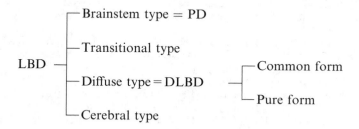

Thus, we understand DLBD within the spectrum of Lewy body disease.

19.8 Other Lewy body dementias

With respect to Alzheimer pathology and how it relates to DLBD, Hansen et al. (1990) proposed a 'Lewy body variant of Alzheimer disease'.

They looked upon it as being within the spectrum of ATD. We do not, however, agree with them.

Our recent investigation concerning senile changes in cases with the common form of DLBD (Odawara et al., 1994) revealed that 75% had combined mild or early SDAT pathology, 17% had a borderline pathology between SDAT and physiological aging, and 8% had physiological aging. Thus, all cases involving the common form of DLBD cannot be understood to come within the spectrum of ATD. Furthermore, the pure form of DLBD has no Alzheimer pathology.

On the other hand, Perry et al. (1989, 1990) proposed a type which they termed 'senile dementia of Lewy body type' (SDLT). Their view was that SDLT is consistent with our transitional type of Lewy body disease with dementia.

References

Bethlem, J. & Den Haltog Jager, W.A. (1960). The incidence and characteristics of Lewy bodies in idiopathic paralysis agitans (Parkinson's disease). *J. Neurol. Neurosurg. Psychiatry*, **23**, 74–80.

Byrne, E.J., Lennox, G. & Lowe, J. (1989). Diffuse Lewy body disease: clinical features in 15 cases. *J. Neurol. Neurosurg. Psychiatry*, **52**, 709–17.

Den Haltog Jager, W.A. & Bethlem, J. (1960). The distribution of Lewy bodies in the central and autonomic nervous system in idiopathic paralysis agitans. *J. Neurol. Neurosurg. Psychiatry*, **23**, 283–90.

Dickson, D.W., Crystal, H., Mattiace, L.A. et al. (1989). Diffuse Lewy body disease: light and electron microscopic immunocytochemistry of senile plaques. *Acta Neuropathol.*, **78**, 572–84.

Dickson, D.W., Davies, P., Mayeux, R. et al. (1987). Diffuse Lewy body disease: Neuropathological and biochemical studies of six cases. *Acta Neuropathol.*, **75**, 8–15.

Dickson, D.W., Ruan, D., Crystal, H. et al. (1991). Hippocampal degeneration differentiates diffuse Lewy body disease (DLBD) from Alzheimer's disease: Light and electron microscopic immunocytochemistry of CA2-3 neurites specific to DLBD. *Neurology*, **41**, 1402–9.

Forno, L.A., Barbour, P.J. & Norville, R.L. (1978). Presenile dementia with Lewy bodies and neurofibrillary tangles. *Arch. Neurol.*, **75**, 818–22.

Greenfield, J. D. & Bosanquet, F. D. (1953). The brainstem lesion in parkinsonism. *J. Neurol. Neurosurg. Psychiatry*, **16**, 213–26.

Hansen, L., Salmon, D., Galasco, D. et al. (1990). The Lewy body variant of Alzheimer's disease. A clinical and pathologic entity. *Neurology*, **40**, 1–8.

Ikeda, K., Hori, A. & Boda, G. (1980). Progressive dementia with 'diffuse Lewy-type inclusion' in cerebral contex. *Arch. Psychiatr. Nervenkr.*, **228**, 243–8.

Iseki, E., Odawara, T., Kosaka, K. et al. (1995). A quantitative study of Lewy bodies and senile changes in the amygdala in diffuse Lewy body disease. *Neuropathol. Appl. Neurobiol*, **15**, 112–116.

Iseki, E., Odawara, T., Kosaka, K. et al. (1996). Age-related ubiquitin-positive granular structures in non-demented subjects and neurodegenerative disorders. *J. Neurol. Sci.* (in press).

Kosaka, K. (1978). Lewy bodies in cerebral cortex. Report of three cases. *Acta Neuropathol.*, **42**, 127–34.

Kosaka, K. (1990). Diffuse Lewy body disease in Japan. *J. Neurol.*, **237**, 197–204.

Kosaka, K. (1993). Dementia and neuropathology in Lewy body disease. *Adv. Neurol.*, **60**, 456–63.

Kosaka, K. & Mehraein, P. (1979). Dementia-parkinsonism with numerous Lewy bodies and senile plaques in cerebral cortex. *Arch. Psychiatr. Nervenkr.*, **226**, 241–50.

Kosaka, K., Oyanagi, S., Matsushita, M. et al. (1976). Presenile dementia with Alzheimer-, Pick-, and Lewy body changes. *Acta Neuropathol.*, **36**, 221–33.

Kosaka, K., Matsushita, M., Oyanagi, S. et al. (1980). A clinicopathological study of 'Lewy body disease'. *Psychiat. Neurol. Japan*, **82**, 292–311.

Kosaka, K., Yoshimura, M., Ikeda, K. et al. (1984). Diffuse type of Lewy body disease: Progressive dementia with abundant cortical Lewy bodies and senile changes of various degree – a new disease? *Clin. Neuropathol.*, **3**, 185–92.

Kosaka, K., Tsuchiya, K. & Yoshimura, M. (1989). Lewy body disease with and without dementia: a clinicopathological study of 35 cases. *Clin. Neuropathol.*, **7**, 299–205.

Kosaka, K., Iseki, E., Odawara, T. et al. (1996). Cerebral type of Lewy body disease. *Neuropathology*, **16**, 32–5.

Lennox, G., Lowe, J., Byrne, E. J. et al. (1989). Diffuse Lewy body disease. *Lancet*, **1**, 323–4.

Lewy, F. H. (1912). Paralysis agitans. I. Pathologische Anatomie. In *Handbuch der Neurologie,* Vol. 3, ed. M. Lewandowsky, pp. 920–33. Berlin: Springer.

Odawara, T., Iseki, E., Yagishita, S. et al. (1992). An autopsied case of juvenile parkinsonism and dementia, with a widespread occurrence of Lewy bodies and spheroids. *Clin. Neuropathol.*, **11**, 131–4.

Odawara, T., Iseki, E., Kosaka, K. et al. (1994). Incidence and distribution of senile plaques and neurofibrillary tangles in late-onset diffuse Lewy body disease. *Neuropathology*, **14**, 7–11.

Odawara, T., Iseki, E., Kosaka, K. et al. (1995). Investigation of tau-2 positive microglia cells in the subcortical nuclei of human neurodegenerative disorders. *Neurosci. Lett.*, **192**, 145–8.

Perry, R. H., Irving, D., Blessed, G. et al. (1989). Senile dementia of Lewy body type and spectrum of Lewy body disease. *Lancet*, **1**, 1088.

Perry, R. H., Irving, D., Blessed, G. et al. (1990). Senile dementia of Lewy body type. A clinically and neuropathologically distinct form of Lewy body dementia in the elderly. *J. Neurol. Sci.*, **95**, 119–39.

Yoshimura, M. (1983). Cortical changes in the Parkinsonian brain: a contribution to the delineation of 'diffuse Lewy body disease'. *J. Neurol.*, **229**, 17–32.

20

Temporal lobe immunohistochemical pathology for tangles, plaques and Lewy bodies in diffuse Lewy body disease, Parkinson's disease, and senile dementia of Alzheimer type

S. KUZUHARA, M. YOSHIMURA,
T. MIZUTANI, H. YAMANOUCHI and
Y. IHARA

Summary

Cortical Lewy bodies (LBs), neurofibrillary tangles (NFTs) and senile plaques (SPs) in the limbic and neocortical cortices of the temporal lobe were studied with anti-ubiquitin, anti-tau and anti-β-protein immunohistochemistry in senile dementia of Alzheimer type (SDAT), diffuse Lewy body disease (DLBD), Parkinson's disease (PD) with and without dementia, and normal controls. DLBD was characterized by numerous cortical LBs together with marked senile changes similar to those of SDAT though neocortical NFTs were significantly less than in SDAT. There were rare or no cortical LBs and neocortical NFTs in most PD cases with and without dementia while there were a few cortical LBs and moderate senile changes, in some cases with dementia. These findings suggest that either of the abundant cortical LBs and senile change, or both have produced dementia in DLBD, while the neuropathological background for dementia in PD cases may be heterogeneous and vary among individual cases.

20.1 Introduction

Diffuse Lewy body disease (DLBD) is a neuropathological entity in which abundant Lewy bodies (LBs) are found throughout the cerebral cortex as well as in the brainstem nuclei in the manner identical to Parkinson's disease (Kosaka et al., 1980, 1984). Marked senile changes including abundant senile plaques (SPs) and Alzheimer neurofibrillary tangles (NFTs) are also found in this condition. Immunohistochemical

248

stains with tau and β-protein antibodies respectively demonstrate NFTs and SPs selectively and sensitively. Ubiquitin immunohistochemistry can immunostain LBs of both brainstem and cortical types sensitively (Kuzuhara et al., 1988; Lowe et al., 1988), and detect far more LBs than the conventional techniques (Lennox et al., 1989). In this paper, we report the immunohistochemial study on NFTs, SPs and LBs in the temporal lobe cortex of the autopsy case of DLBD, Parkinson's disease (PD) and senile dementia of Alzheimer type (SDAT).

20.2 Materials and methods

Submitted for the study were autopsy brains from nine cases of DLBD, 13 cases of PD including nine with dementia and four without dementia, five cases of SDAT, and five normal controls. The diagnoses were made on the bases of both clinical and neuropathological findings although a variety of clinical diagnoses including SDAT, PD with dementia, normal pressure hydrocephalus, and Shy-Drager syndrome had been made in DLBD cases. The slices of the temporal lobe of the formalin-fixed brains at the level of the lateral geniculate body, which included the hippocampus, the parahippocampal gyrus, the occipitotemporal gyrus, and the inferior, middle and superior temporal gyri (T3, T2 and T1) were cut into 8 μm sections and immunohistochemical staining was performed as previously reported; for NFT, antisera to human phosphorylated tau (anti-tau) (Ihara, 1988) was used; for SP, antisera to synthetic polypeptide (1–24) of amyloid β-protein (anti-ABP) (Yamaguchi et al., 1988; Kuzuhara et al., 1991); for LB, monoclonal or polyclonal antibody to ubiquitin (anti-UB) (Kuzuhara et al., 1988). NFTs, SPs, and LBs of the parahippocampal gyrus and the occipitotemporal gyrus were counted in a rectangular area of 1 mm^2 with an eyepiece graticule at a magnification of $\times$330.

20.3 Results

The findings are shown in Table 20.1. The most characteristic feature in the immunohistochemical pathology of DLBD was the appearance of abundant cortical LBs in the deeper layers of the temporal lobe cortex, and no other conditions showed the similar finding although a few cortical LBs were present in the parahippocampal gyrus of some of the SDAT cases. Alzheimer changes including NFTs and SPs were nearly similar to those of SDAT in the parahippocampal gyrus, but NFTs in the

Table 20.1. *Semiquantitative immunohistochemical data for NFT, SP and LB in the temporal lobe cortex of the parahippocampal and occipitotemporal gyri*

	SDAT	DLBD	PDcD	PDsD	Control
Case nos	5	9	9	4	5
Age (years)	78–96	51–91	65–86	73–91	68–86
	(86.4 ± 6.9)	(78.4 ± 11.5)	(77.8 ± 7.2)	(81.5 ± 7.8)	(79.8 ± 6.9)
Parahip Gyr (number/mm^2)					
NFT	13–65	8–64	0–53	7–33	1–20
	(35.0 ± 23.1)	(26.2 ± 24.1)	(13.1 ± 15.9)	(17.5 ± 11.7)	(7.0 ± 7.4)
SP	20–58	5–36	0–20	0–2	0–22
	(36.2 ± 18.2)	(21.4 ± 8.6)	(2.8 ± 6.7)	(0.5 ± 1.0)	(7.8 ± 10.8)
LB	0–4	4–309	0–12	0–4	0
	(1.2 ± 1.8)	(11.0 ± 7.9)	(3.7 ± 4.5)	(0.8 ± 1.8)	
Oc-Tmp Gyr (number/mm^2)					
NFT	10–62	1–54	0–4	0–1	0–3
	(36.8 ± 22.7)	(12.1 ± 19.1)	(1.1 ± 1.5)	(0.3 ± 0.5)	(0.6 ± 1.3)
SP	17–47	7–46	0–20	0–4	0–16
	(27.6 ± 12.7)	(24.3 ± 11.1)	(2.8 ± 6.7)	(0.8 ± 1.8)	(5.0 ± 7.3)
LB	0	3–30	0–4	0	0
		(9.8 ± 8.3)	(0.9 ± 1.3)		

Data are expressed as the range and (mean $\pm$ SD).
Statistical differences between the individual groups (Mann–Whitney's U-test) were as follows:

	NFT	SP	LB	
Parahip Gyr				
DLBD:SDAT	NS	NS	$p < 0.01$	
DLBD:PDcD	NS	$p < 0.005$	$p < 0.05$	
DLBD:PDsD	NS	$p < 0.05$	$p < 0.05$	
DLBD:Control	$p < 0.05$	$p < 0.05$	$p < 0.005$	
SDAT:PDcD	$p < 0.05$	NS	NS	
PDcD:PDsD	$p < 0.05$	NS	NS	
PDcD: Control	NS	NS	NS	
PDsD: Control	NS	NS	NS	
Oc-Tmp Gyr				
DLBD:SDAT	$p < 0.05^*$	NS	$p < 0.005$	*DLBD < SDAT
DLBD: PDcD	$p < 0.05$	$p < 0.005$	$p < 0.001$	
DLBD:PDsD	$p < 0.05$	$p < 0.01$	$p < 0.01$	
DLBD:Control	$p < 0.05$	$p < 0.01$	$p < 0.005$	
SDAT:PDcD	$p < 0.005$	$p < 0.01$	NS	
PDcD:PDsD	NS	NS	NS	
PDcD: Control	NS	NS	NS	
PDsD: Control	NS	NS	NS	

*DLBD = diffuse Lewy body disease; SDAT = senile dementia of Alzheimer type; PDcD = Parkinson's disease with dementia; PDsD; Parkinson's disease without dementia Parahip Gyr = parahippocampal gyrus; Oc-Temp Gyr = occipitotemporal gyrus occipitotemporal gyrus were significantly less than in SDAT and significantly more than in PD with or without dementia. Some of the PD cases with dementia showed cortical Lewy bodies in a moderate number, but senile changes were minimal and there was no significant difference in the number of NFTs, SPs and LBs between normal controls and PD with or without dementia, and between PD with dementia and PD without dementia. Abundant cortical LBs together with marked senile changes were thus the hallmark of DLBD while NFTs were far less than in SDAT.

20.4 Discussion

Rare cases of atypical dementia with parkinsonism with abundant cortical Lewy bodies was first described in the US by Okazaki et al. (1961), but little attention had been paid to the condition until Kosaka and his colleagues (1980, 1984) proposed the concept of Lewy body disease (LBD – see also introduction) which included a spectrum of neuropathological conditions that are characterized by appearance of LBs in the central nervous system. On the basis of the topographical distribution and frequency of LBs, Kosaka and his colleagues (1980, 1984) have classified LBD into three subgroups; diffuse type (DLBD or group A, clinically presenting with severe dementia), transitional type (group B, clinically presenting with PD usually followed by dementia of mild to moderate degree) and brainstem type (group C, clinically presenting with classical PD). Since the proposal by Kosaka and his colleagues (1980, 1984), many cases of LBD of diffuse and transitional types have been accumulated not only from Japan but also from Europe and North America. Since they presented with atypical dementia clinically, these cases have been designated, in addition to the term DLBD (Dickson et al., 1987; Burkhardt et al., 1988; Byrne et al., 1989; Kuzuhara & Yoshimura 1993), as 'Lewy body dementia without Alzheimer changes' (Sima et al., 1986), 'cortical Lewy body dementia' (Gibb et al., 1989), 'Lewy body variant of Alzheimer's disease' (Hansen et al., 1990) or 'senile dementia of Lewy body type' (Perry et al., 1990). Some of these names imply that LBs are responsible for the development of dementia though this has not been fully substantiated.

The present study aimed to clarify the neuropathological findings related to dementia in LBD. In our previous study on NFTs and SPs with anti-tau and anti-β-protein immunohistochemistry in more than 300 autopsy cases aged between 60 and 103 years (Kuzuhara et al., 1991), we have found that the neocortex of the temporal lobe including the occipitotemporal gyrus was affected by many NFTs in SDAT cases but was spared in nondemented cases while the limbic cortex including the hippocampus and parahippocampal gyrus was affected in both the demented and nondemented elderly cases, and that the limbic cortex and neocortex were equally affected by SPs in both the nondemented and SDAT cases although significantly more SPs were found in the latter. Thus, the immunohistochemical findings in the occipitotemporal gyrus are a better indicator of the difference in senile changes between nonde- mented and SDAT cases than those of the hippocampus and parahippo- campal gyrus. The same areas of the temporal lobe were examined in the present study.

The present study showed that abundant cortical LBs were the most characteristic feature of DLBD and that marked senile changes were another characteristic feature although the number of NFTs in the occi- pitotemporal gyrus was significantly less than in SDAT – as described previously in studies with conventional staining techniques (Kosaka et al., 1984; Sima et al., 1986; Gibb et al., 1989; Hansen et al., 1990). A recent biochemical study on the neurotransmitters in the basal ganglia and cerebral cortex of Lewy body variant of Alzheimer's disease (nearly identical to DLBD) have demonstrated that reduction in basal ganglia dopamine was similar to PD and activity of choline acetyltransferase was lower than in SDAT (Langlais et al., 1993). These findings support the idea that either, or both, cortical LBs and senile Alzheimer-type changes could be the neuropathological substrate for dementia in DLBD. In contrast, immunohistochemical neuropathology of LBs, NFTs and SPs varied among the individual PD cases with dementia; some showed cor- tical LBs and neocortical NFTs in a moderate number while others, none, or very occasional LBs. According to Jellinger and Riederer (1984), there are several subgroups in PD from morphological as well as clinical points of view. The morphological changes of PD without dementia are limited to the brainstem with little or no extranigral Alzhei- mer changes; whereas those of PD with dementia vary in severity and distribution of the nigral and cortical changes, cortial Lewy bodies, Alz- heimer changes, and other aging or degenerative changes. Yoshimura (1988) examined the brains of 37 PD cases with dementia of Japanese elderly people and has found that 24 cases (64.9%) showed Alzheimer changes, 5 cases (13.5%), combined senile-vascular changes, and the remaining 8 cases (21.6%), neither senile nor vascular changes. Dementia in PD cases may be heterogeneous in nature, and there may be some other lesions than LBs, NFTs or SPs responsible for dementia.

Acknowledgements

The present study was supported in part by a Grant-in-Aid for Scientific Research (B-03454240) from the Ministry of Education, Science and Culture of Japan. We thank Mr Aikyo N. and Ms Saishoji J. for their technical assistance.

References

Burkhardt, C. R., Filley, C. M., Kleinschmidt-DeMasters, B. K., de la Monte, S. et al. (1988). Diffuse Lewy body disease and progressive dementia. *Neurology*, **38**, 1520–8.

Byrne, E. J., Lennox, G., Lower, J. & Godwin-Austen, R. B. (1989). Diffuse Lewy body disease: clinical features in 15 cases. *J. Neurol. Neurosurg. Psychiatry*, **52**, 709–17.

Dickson, D. W., Davies, P., Mayeux, R., Crystal, H. et al. (1987). Diffuse Lewy body disease. Neuropathological and biochemical studies of six patients. *Acta Neuropathol. (Berl.)*, **75**, 8–15.

Gibb, W. R. G., Luthert, P. J., Janota, I. & Lantos, P. L. (1989). Cortical Lewy body dementia: clinical features and classification. *J. Neurol. Neurosurg. Psychiatry*, **52**, 185–92.

Hansen, L., Salmon, D., Galasko, D., Masliah, E. et al. (1990). The Lewy body variant of Alzheimer's disease: a clinical and pathologic entity. *Neurology*, **40**, 1–8.

Ihara, Y (1988). Massive somatodendritic sprouting of cortical neurons in Alzheimer's disease. *Brain Res.*, **459**, 138–44.

Jellinger, K. & Riederer, P. (1984). Dementia in Parkinson's disease and (pre) senile dementia of Alzheimer type: morphological aspects and changes in the intracerebral MAO activity. In *Advances in Neurology*, Vol. 40, ed. R. G. Hassler & J. F. Christ, pp. 199–210. New York: Raven Press.

Kosaka, K., Matsushita, M., Oyanagi, S. & Mehraein, P. (1980). A clinicopathological study of the 'Lewy body disease'. *Psychiat. Neurol. Jpn*, **82**, 292–311.

Kosaka, K., Yoshimura, M., Ikeda, K. and Budka, H. (1984). Diffuse type of Lewy body disease: progressive dementia with abundant cortical Lewy bodies and senile changes of varying degree – A new disease? *Clin. Neuropathol.*, **3**, 185–92.

Kuzuhara, S. & Yoshimura, M. (1993). Clinical and neuropathological aspects of diffuse Lewy body disease in the elderly. In *Advances in Neurology* Vol. 60, ed. H. Narabayashi, T. Nagatsu, N. Yanagisawa and Y. Mizuno, pp. 464–69. New York: Raven Press.

Kuzuhara, S., Mori, H., Izumiyama, N., Yoshimura, M. et al. (1988). Lewy bodies are ubiquitinated: a light and electron microscopic immunocytochemical study. *Acta Neuropathol. (Berl.)*, **75**, 345–53.

Kuzuhara, S., Ihara, Y., Shimada, H. & Toyokura Y. (1991). β-Protein and tau immunohistochemistry on brains of normal aging and dementia. In *Frontiers of Alzheimer Research* (Excerpta Medica International Congress Series 946), ed. T. Ishii, D. Allsop and D. J. Selkoe, pp. 87–97. Amsterdam: Elsevier.

Langlais, P. J., Thal, L., Hansen, L., Galasko, D. et al. (1993). Neurotransmitters in basal ganglia and cortex of Alzheimer's disease with and without Lewy bodies. *Neurology*, **43**, 1927–34.

Lennox, G., Lowe, J., Morrel, K., Landon, M. et al. (1989). Anti-ubiquitin immunocytochemistry is more sensitive than conventional techniques in the detection of diffuse Lewy body disease. *J. Neurol. Neurosurg. Psychiatry*, **52**, 67–71.

Lowe, J., Blanchard, A., Morrell, K., Lennox, G. et al. (1988). Ubiquitin is a common factor in intermediate filament inclusion bodies of diverse type in man, including those of Parkinson's disease, Pick's disease, and Alzheimer's disease, as well as Rosenthal fibers in cerebellar astrocytomas, cytoplasmic bodies in muscle, and Mallory bodies in alcoholic liver disease. *J. Pathol.*, **155**, 9–15.

Okazaki, H., Lipkin, L. E. & Aronson, S. M. (1961). Diffuse intracytoplasmic ganglionic inclusions (Lewy type) associated with progressive dementia and quadriparesis in flexion. *J. Neuropathol. Exp. Neurol.*, **20**, 237–44.

Perry, R. H., Irving, D., Blessed, G., Fairbairn, A. & Perry, E. K. (1990). Senile dementia of Lewy body type. A clinically and neuropathologically distinct form of Lewy body dementia in the elderly. *J. Neurol. Sci.*, **95**, 119–39.

Sima, A. A. F., Clark, N. A., Sternberger, N. A. & Sternberger, L. A. (1986). Lewy body dementia without Alzheimer changes. *Can. J. Neurol. Sci.*, **13**, 490–7.

Yamaguchi, H., Hirai, S., Morimatsu, M., Shoji, M. et al. (1988). A variety of cerebral amyloid deposits in the brains of the Alzheimer-type dementia demonstrated by β protein immunostaining. *Acta Neuropathol. (Berl.)*, **76**, 541–9.

Yoshimura, M. (1988). Pathologic basis for dementia in elderly patients with idiopathic Parkinson's disease. *Eur. Neurol.*, **28**, suppl. 1, 29–35.

21

Pathological and clinical features of Parkinson's disease with and without dementia

R. A. I. de VOS, E. N. H. JANSEN,
D. YILMAZER, H. BRAAK and E. BRAAK

Summary

The pathology of Parkinson's disease (PD) is characterized by the presence of neuronal loss, Lewy bodies (LBs), and Lewy neurites (LNs) at predilection sites in the nervous system. During the course of PD a characteristic pattern of lesions develops in both the central and peripheral nervous system, with a predominant involvement of 'efferent' subcortical structures such as the substantia nigra and amygdala. 'Afferent' cortical structures such as the entorhinal region are frequently involved in Alzheimer-type pathology. In this chapter the clinical features and post-mortem findings of 33 patients with PD are reviewed and compared, with special attention being paid to the frequent but not exclusive association of LBs/LNs with Alzheimer-type pathology. Although a clear relationship between the neuropathological findings and the clinical features of psychopathology and/or dementia could not be observed, one could speculate that the Parkinson-specific lesions in cortical and subcortical structures and the Alzheimer-type pathology, which is seen most often in the entorhinal region, reinforce each other and thus are responsible for the development of dementia in PD. CA2 ubiquitin-immunoreactive neurites were found in almost all patients with PD and should be considered a normal finding in PD, irrespective of whether or not the patient is demented.

21.1 Introduction

Thirty-three patients with a clinical history of Parkinson's disease (PD), with or without concomitant affective, behavioral, and/or cognitive changes were assessed. They were referred to the Department of Neurology of the Medisch Spectrum Twente, The Netherlands, to determine the relationship, if any, between clinical PD with or without dementia and neuropathological changes.

21.2 Clinical data

Thirty-three patients with a clinical diagnosis of PD, who had been reviewed for many years in the outpatient clinic of the Department of Neurology, died in hospital and a postmortem examination and neuro-pathological diagnosis was made. All patients had undergone comprehensive psychogeriatric and neurologic assessment, and detailed case notes covering the period from first presentation until death were available. Generally, the patients with a diagnosis of idiopathic PD had had the disease for many years and therefore had had a long exposure to dopamimetic medication. All patients who had symptoms of PD and subsequent dementia were responsive to levodopa. Special attention was given to assessing the presence of visual or auditory hallucinations, episodes of confusion, lucid intervals (as in delirium) and to the cognitive status. Dementia was defined as a Mini-Mental State examination score of less than 20 in a patient fulfilling DSM-IIIR criteria for dementia (Folstein et al., 1975; American Psychiatric Association, 1987). The clinical data are summarized in Table 21.1.

21.3 Neuropathology

Samples of 33 brains were taken from the superior and medial frontal gyri, superior and inferior parietal lobules, superior and middle temporal gyri, occipitotemporal gyrus and striate area, nucleus basalis of Meynert, and the anterior part of the cingulate gyrus (at the level of the midpoint of the anterior commissure), basal ganglia, hippocampal formation and entorhinal cortex, cerebellum, midbrain, pons and medulla oblongata. Sections (8–10 μm thick) were stained with hematoxylin and eosin and modified Bielschowsky silver impregnation. Sections from patients 23 to 33 were stained with the Gallyas silver technique. Immunocytochemical studies were performed with a polyclonal antibody to ubiquitin (1:80, DAKO), and monoclonal antibodies to TAU-2 (1:1000, SIGMA), beta A4 (1:50, DAKO), and ALZ-50 (kindly supplied by Abbott Laboratories, Chicago, Illinois, USA). A semiquantitative analysis of Lewy bodies (LBs) was done as described previously (de Vos et al., 1995). When counting the LBs in the anterior cingulate gyrus, we distinguished

Table 21.1. *Frequency of key clinical symptoms in 33 consecutive patients with Parkinson's disease*

Symptoms	No dementia $n = 9$	Dementia $n = 24$
Rest tremor	7 (78%)	18 (75%)
Delirium	3 (33%)	15 (62%)
Hallucinations	4 (44%)	12 (50%)
Delusions	2 (22%)	6 (25%)
Disturbed Consciousness	2 (11%)	9 (37%)
Dopa response	8 (89%)	21 (87%)
Autonomic Features	6 (67%)	17 (71%)
H and Y stage (mean)[a]	3.6	4.1

[a]H and Y = Hoehn and Yahr disability rating scale

between patients with more than five cortical LBs (CLBs) per field (CLBs + +) and patients with fewer than five CLBS (CLBs +). The neuropathological diagnosis of Alzheimer's disease (AD) was based on the CERAD criteria (Mirra et al., 1991). For staging of the neurofibrillary changes according to the criteria of Braak and Braak (1991), a block of the temporal lobe containing the hippocampal formation and entorhinal region was embedded in polyethylene glycol (PEG 1000, Merck), sectioned into 100-μm slices, and stained with aldehydefuchsin-darrow red for lipofuchsin pigment and Nissl material, Gallyas for Alzheimer-related neurofibrillary changes and the Campbell-Switzer silver technique for demonstration of A4-amyloid deposits and LBs and Lewy neurites (LNs). This staging could be performed for 28 patients. There was insufficient material available from the other five patients to enable this staging to be performed. In six patients the entire hemisphere was sectioned as described by Braak et al. (1994).

21.4 Morphological features specific to Parkinson's disease

A key feature of Parkinson's disease (or Lewy body disease) is the occurrence of LBs and LNs at predilection sites in both the central (nigral and extranigral) and peripheral (autonomic) nervous system. Although the distribution of LBs and LNs was quite irregular in our patients, a characteristic pattern of PD-related lesions was detected.

21.4.1 Nigral lesions

Extraneural melanin, gliosis, and LBs were present in the substantia nigra in all subjects. This was associated with a moderate-to-severe loss of large pigmented neurons. Pale bodies were often present.

21.4.2 Extranigral lesions

Neo/allocortex. CLBs were present, although in varying density, in all our patients. The CLBs were most easily seen in the anterior proneocortex (cingulate gyrus, predominantly in the multiform layer), and in the insular and entorhinal cortices. More than five CLBs per field were detected in six patients, all of whom had overt dementia.

Amygdala. In all patients LBs and LNs were distributed in a specific manner throughout the nuclear complex. The most prominent changes occurred in the corticomedial region (especially the accessory cortical nucleus) and in the central nucleus. In general, there were no LBs or LNs in the basal and lateral nuclei.

Hippocampus CA 2. Ubiquitin-immunoreactive neurites were seen in preparations from 30 patients. In only three cases did we fail to find these structures. This may be a sampling error, as only one hippocampal section was available for each of these patients.

Basal forebrain nuclei, nucleus of stria terminalis, thalamic (midline) nuclei, hypothalamic nuclei (tuberomamillary and posterior hypothalamic nuclei), reticular formation (periaqueductal gray, locus coeruleus, peripeduncular nuclei, raphe nuclei, medial and lateral reticular formation), and dorsal vagal complex. PD-related lesions were seen in these locations in all patients.

Autonomic nervous system. PD-related lesions were seen in all patients, and especially in the sympathetic and enteric (esophagus, distal part) division (Figs 21.1 and 21.2).

21.5 Morphological features additional to Parkinson's disease

21.5.1 Alzheimer-type lesions

Table 21.2 summarizes the neuropathological diagnoses of AD, based on the CERAD criteria (Mirra et al., 1991). Of the nine patients who were not demented, one was diagnosed as possible AD and the other eight were diagnosed as being normal. Seven out of 24 demented patients were classified as normal, two as possible AD, ten as probable AD, and five as

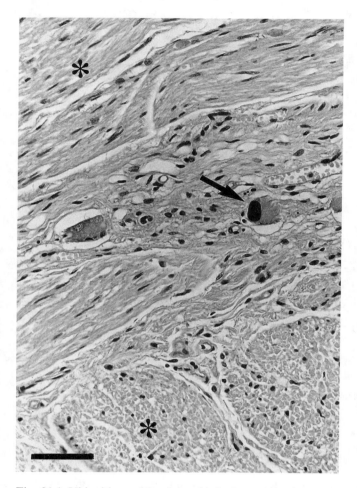

Fig. 21.1 Ubiquitin-positive Lewy body (arrow) in the myenteric (Auerbach's) plexus of the esophagus. * = external muscular layer. Ubiquitin, ×300. Bar is 50 μm.

definite AD. It was possible to stage AD according to the Braak and Braak criteria in 28 patients (Table 21.3). The three patients with the isocortical stage all had clinically defined dementia (Folstein et al., 1975; American Psychiatric Association 1987). Nine of 19 patients with dementia had already reached a limbic stage (mostly stage III). Seven demented patients were in transentorhinal stages I and II. Amyloid deposits, which occurred most often as diffuse plaques, were seen in 24 patients, with and without dementia. Amyloid angiopathy in combina-

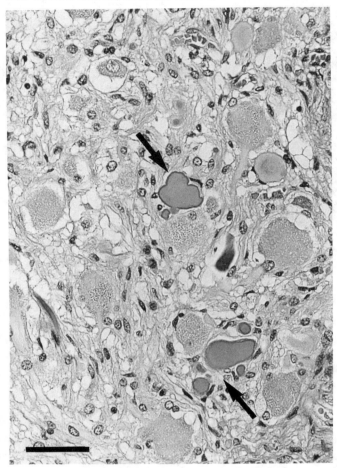

Fig. 21.2 Lewy neurites (arrow) in a ganglion of the sympathetic trunk. Hematoxylin-eosin, ×300. Bar is 50 μm.

tion with a moderate-to-severe amount of amyloid was seen in nine of these patients.

21.5.2 Argyrophilic grains

One of our patients (no. 28) had argyrophilic grains and coiled bodies in the hippocampal formation (especially CA1), entorhinal/transentorhinal cortex, and adjoining temporal isocortex and amygdala. Only slight neurofibrillary changes were present in the transentorhinal/entorhinal region

Table 21.2. *Clinicopathological diagnosis in 33 consecutive patients with Parkinson's disease*

Patient no.	Dementia	CLB[a]	ARP score[b]	CERAD classification
10, 11, 16, 17, 20, 21, 27	No	+	0	Normal
14	No	+	±	Normal
9	No	+	+	AD[c] possible
4, 28, 29, 30, 32, 33	Yes	+	0	Normal
3	Yes	+ +	0	Normal
18	Yes	+	±	AD possible
25	Yes	+ +	±	AD possible
1, 2, 6, 19, 26	Yes	+	±	AD probable
5, 12, 23	Yes	+	+	AD probable
24, 31	Yes	+ +	+	AD probable
7, 13, 15	Yes	+	+ +	AD definite
8, 22	Yes	+ +	+ +	AD definite

[a]CLB = Cortical Lewy bodies/Gyrus cinguli (+ = < 5/field, + + = ⩾ 5/field)
[b]ARP = Age-related plaque score (0 = absent, ± = sparse, + = moderate, + + = frequent)
[c]AD = Alzheimer's disease

of this patient (stage II Braak and Braak). Sparse to moderate amyloid deposits were present in the occipital region.

21.5.3 Vascular lesions

Moderate atherosclerosis of the large vessels of the circle of Willis was present in 11 patients. In none of these patients were macroscopically visible infarcts larger than 1 cm seen. In nine patients (two of whom were not demented) small, less than 1 cm, mostly lacunar infarcts were found, accompanied by arteriosclerotic changes of the vessel wall. These infarcts were most commonly found in the basal ganglia. In five (demented) patients there was a slight loss of myelin in the deep periventricular white matter, due to (hyaline) arteriosclerosis of the small penetrating vessels. In three patients the globus pallidus showed calcification in and around the blood vessels. No vascular abnormalities were seen in the remaining 13 patients.

Table 21.3. *Clinicopathological diagnosis in 28 out of 33 consecutive patients with Parkinson's disease*

No dementia	Dementia	Braak and Braak[a]
10, 11, 21		0
20, 27	3, 4, 29	I
16, 17	26, 28, 30, 32	II
9	15, 18, 19, 23, 24, 25, 31, 33	III
14	22	IV
	7, 18, 13	V
		VI

[a]I/II transentorhinal stage; III/IV limbic stage; V/VI isocortical stage

21.6 Possible causes of dementia

21.6.1 *Lewy bodies/Lewy neurites*

Cortex

Although the patients without dementia seemed to have a lower density of CLBs, we could not find a significant correlation between the cognitive status and the number of CLBs. However, all six patients with many CLBs (five or more at 100×) were demented. One of the predilection sites for CLBs was the entorhinal cortex. Many LBs were found in one of the deep cellular layers, a layer which is responsible for the feedback projection of hippocampal data to the neocortex. It is possible that these cellular changes interfere with cognitive function. One of our patients was particularly interesting because he had severe dementia and a high density of CLBs, but minimal Alzheimer-type pathology (sparse neurofibrillary tangles in the transentorhinal region, no amyloid). This patient fulfills Kosaka's criteria for 'pure type' diffuse Lewy body disease. Kosaka (1990) uses five or more CLBs per field in the preferred sites (anterior frontal, cingulate, temporal and insular cortices) as criterion for diffuse Lewy body disease. On the basis of our findings, we consider it inappropriate to diagnose this disease solely on the basis of the presence of five CLBs per field (de Vos et al., 1995).

Amygdala

The severity of PD-related lesions was not related to the presence or absence of cognitive impairment. Amygdala involvement (in a specific pattern) may well contribute to the behavioral changes and autonomic dysfunctions seen in patients with PD. The amygdala is the origin of major projections to the neocortex, in particular the cingulate area, limbic system, and centers regulating endocrine and autonomic functions. We cannot exclude that it influences cognitive functions as well, but these amygdaloid lesions did not correlate with the occurrence of dementia. Interestingly, in a recent report the central nucleus was said to be a preferred site for LBs in diffuse Lewy body disease (Odawara et al., 1994), as it was in our patients with PD.

Hippocampus CA 2

The CA 2–3 ubiquitin-positive neurites described as a characteristic marker for diffuse Lewy body disease (Dickson et al., 1994) bear a close resemblance to the LNs within the amygdala and basal forebrain nuclei. In our patients these neurites did not extend into the CA 3 sector and are, therefore, referred to as CA 2 LNs. These neurites were present in most of our patients (30 out of 33), and we consequently consider the presence of these positive neurites to be a normal finding in PD and not related to the cognitive status. It is worthwhile mentioning that this region probably receives a projection from the tuberomamillary nucleus, a nucleus which also showed PD-related lesions.

Cholinergic, noradrenergic, and serotonergic nuclei

All patients had severe lesions in the basal forebrain nuclei, the dorsal raphe nuclei, and the locus coeruleus. Considering that there are projections to the cortex (either direct or indirect via the mediodorsal nuclei of the thalamus), the loss of cholinergic neurons may contribute to the cognitive impairment. A lesion in the locus coeruleus and the dorsal raphe seems to be related to a loss of vigilance (bradyphrenia) and to the development of depression (Saper, 1987).

21.6.2 Alzheimer-type pathology

Patients with dementia had a substantially higher degree of cortical Alzheimer-type pathology (neurofibrillary changes), in many cases corresponding to stage III of the Braak and Braak criteria. Amyloid deposits were present in both demented and nondemented subjects. Five patients had coexisting PD and AD (according to the CERAD system). The

Alzheimer-type pathology was restricted to the entorhinal region in many patients, which stresses the need for careful examination of this region in patients with PD. Seven demented patients showed minor Alzheimer-type pathology (stage I-II of the Braak and Braak criteria). We consider the presence of Alzheimer-type pathology in combination with specific lesions in cortical and subcortical structures to be critical to the development of cognitive decline in patients with PD.

21.6.3 Argyrophilic grains

Argyrophilic grains, which were first described by Braak and Braak (1989), and which were detected in one of our patients, almost certainly contribute to the cognitive impairment. This patient had only slight neurofibrillary changes in the transentorhinal region (stage I-II, Braak and Braak). To our knowledge, there are only two reports of a patient with PD and argyrophilic grains in the literature (Braak & Braak, 1989).

21.6.4 Vascular lesions

We cannot exclude that the white matter lesions have a role in the decline in cognitive function of patients with PD. However, these lesions are also seen in asymptomatic (especially older) subjects, so their exact role cannot be elucidated.

Conclusion

Parkinson's disease is characterized neuropathologically by a specific distribution of lesions. Apart from the destruction of the substantia nigra, an impressive pattern of extranigral lesions is seen in PD. The specific lesions in limbic structures, which are so abundant in PD, are probably the morphological substrates for the behavioral and psychiatric features of the disease and for the autonomic dysfunction seen in patients with PD. The frequency of dementia in our 33 patients was very high, 73%. This frequency may be biased by the referral of patients with severe PD to our Department of Neurology. Referral would increase the likelihood that an autopsy would be performed on these patients with 'end stages' of PD. The same bias is probably also present with respect to the psychopathological features of these patients. Confusional states, delirious episodes, and visual hallucinations are often seen in severely disabled PD patients who have had the disease for a long time and who have thus had a long exposure to therapy with dopamine precursors, dopamine agonists, anticholinergics, and MAO-B inhibitors. None of our patients were referred from a psychogeriatric ward, and consequently no patients in this series had slight 'parkinsonism' and severe dementia. This makes our patient population quite distinct from that of McKeith et al. (1994). The cause of the cognitive decline and the psychiatric features of PD is still obscure, especially in patients with PD but without concomitant AD. A common cholinergic correlate of the cognitive impairment in PD and AD has been proposed (Perry et al., 1985). We were unable to establish a clear relationship between the neuropathological and the clinical presence of psychopathology or dementia in the patients we studied. Although CLBs and especially Alzheimer-type pathology are both important, especially in combination, they are not likely to be the only factors in the development of dementia. The correlation of the neuropathological staging of the neurofibrillary changes with the cognitive status was not so high in our study as in the recent study of Bancher (Bancher et al., 1993). This is an argument for a nosological distinction between the entities of AD and PD/dementia, and provides support for the hypothesis that entorhinal Alzheimer-type pathological changes are not the only components underlying the cognitive decline seen in PD. However, many of our demented patients showed full-blown PD-related lesions in combination with Alzheimer-type pathology corresponding to the limbic stage III. It is remarkable that the Alzheimer-type pathology was restricted to the entorhinal region in most patients. In our experience Alzheimer-type pathology remains nonprogressive for many years, as evidenced by the presence of 'burned out' neurofibrillary tangles. The pathological changes did not extend to the hippocampus and neocortex, as they do in AD. We hypothesize that PD-specific lesions in combination with Alzheimer-type pathology increase the likelihood that a patient with PD will develop dementia. This does not rule out that there are other causes of dementia, such as vascular pathology or argyrophilic grains (as in one of our patients). We consider CA2 hippocampal LNs to be a normal finding in PD and not related to cognitive decline. The dementia and psychopathological features of PD cover a broad spectrum of pathological features. We found a high frequency of hallucinations and episodes of delirium in our patients. The role of dopamimetic therapy in provoking these symptoms is well understood in general neurological practice. These hallucinations are possibly comparable to the hallucinations and delusions described in senile dementia of Lewy body type by McKeith et al. (1992). Hallucinations are also seen in many patients with Alzheimer's disease (Lerner et al., 1994). Dementia is part of the clinical spectrum of PD, but neither the clinical nor the morphological criteria for the dementia are strictly defined or characterized and do not fit in a diagnostic framework such as 'Lewy body dementia'. Current data suggest that 'Lewy body disease' covers a broad spectrum of clinical and pathological features. The pathological basis for the dementia of PD thus remains controversial, and there is still much debate about the nosological state of Lewy body dementia and especially about the role of cortical LBs. Yet the fact remains that LBs and LNs are found throughout the brain. The task is now to determine their biological significance and to develop a unifying concept to explain their presence in combination with Alzheimer-type lesions and vascular lesions.

Acknowledgements

The authors wish to thank Wies vom Bruch for secretarial assistance, Liane Stokkink and Harry Begthel for technical assistance, Richard Rieksen for photographic work and Jane Bär-Sykes, MD, for linguistic advice. This work was supported by grants from the Stichting Wetenschappelijk Onderzoek Medische Staf Streeklaboratorium (SWOMSS), Enschede, The Netherlands, and Upjohn Nederland BV, and Stichting Neurologisch Onderzoek Twente (SNOT) of the Medisch Spectrum Twente in Enschede.

References

American Psychiatric Association (1987). *Diagnostic and Statistical Manual of Mental Disorders*, 3rd revised edn. (DSM-IIIR). Washington, DC: American Psychiatric Association.

Bancher, C., Braak, H., Fischer, P. & Jellinger, K. A. (1993). Neuropathological staging of Alzheimer lesions and intellectual status in Alzheimer's and Parkinson's disease patients. *Neurosci. Lett.*, **162**, 179–82.

Braak, H. & Braak, E. (1989). Cortical and subcortical argyrophilic grains characterize a disease associated with adult onset dementia. *Neuropathol. Appl. Neurobiol.*, **15**, 13–26.

Braak, H. & Braak, E. (1991). Neuropathological stageing of Alzheimer-related changes. *Acta Neuropathol.*, **82**, 239–59.

Braak, H., Braak, E., Yilmazer, D. et al. (1994). Amygdala pathology in Parkinson's disease. *Acta Neuropathol.*, **88**, 493–500.

de Vos, R. A. I., Jansen, E. N. H., Stam, F. C., Ravid, R. & Swaab, D. F. (1995). 'Lewy body disease': clinico-pathological correlations in 18 consecutive cases of Parkinson's disease with and without dementia. *Clin. Neurol. Neurosurg.*, **97**, 13–22.

Dickson, D. W., Schmidt, M. L., Lee, V. M.-Y., Zhao Meng-Liang Yen, S. -H. & Trojanowski, J. Q. (1994). Immunoreactivity profile of hippocampal CA2/3 neurites in diffuse Lewy body disease. *Acta Neuropathol.*, **87**, 269–76.

Folstein, M. F., Folstein, S. E. & McHugh, P. R. (1975). 'Mini-Mental State'. A practical method for grading the cognitive state of patients for the clinician. *J. Psychiat. Res.*, **23**, 56–62.

Kosaka, K. (1990). Diffuse Lewy body disease in Japan. *J. Neurol.*, **237**, 197–204.

Lerner, A. J., Koss, E., Patterson, M B. et al. (1994). Concomitants of visual hallucinations in Alzheimer's disease. *Neurology*, **44**, 523–7.

McKeith, I. G., Fairbairn, A., Perry, R., Thompson, P. & Perry, E. (1992). Neuroleptic sensitivity in patients with senile dementia of Lewy body type. *BMJ*, **305**, 673–8.

McKeith, I. G., Fairbairn, A. F., Bothwell, R. A. et al. (1994). An evaluation of the predictive validity and inter-rater reliability of clinical diagnostic criteria for senile dementia of Lewy body type. *Neurology*, **44**, 872–7.

Mirra, S. S., Heyman, A., McKeel, D. et al. (1991). The Consortium to Establish a Registry for Alzheimer's Disease. Part II. *Neurology*, **41**, 479–86.

Odawara, T., Iseki, E., Akiyama, H. & Ikeda, K. (1994). Incidence and distribution of Lewy bodies and senile changes in the amygdala of diffuse Lewy body disease (DLBD) brains. *Brain Pathol.*, **4**, 533.

Perry, E. K., Curtis, M., Dick, D. J. et al. (1985). Cholinergic correlates of cognitive impairment in Parkinson's disease: comparisons with Alzheimer's disease. *J. Neurol. Neurosurg. Psychiatry*, **48**, 413–21.

Saper, C. B. (1987). Function of the locus coeruleus. *Trends Neurosci.*, **10**, 343–4.

22

Dementia with Lewy bodies: relationships to Parkinson's and Alzheimer's diseases

K. A. JELLINGER and C. BANCHER

Summary

Among 290 demented subjects in a consecutive autopsy series of elderly individuals with or without parkinsonian signs, 41 cases or 14.1% showed abundant subcortical and cortical Lewy bodies satisfying the diagnosis of Lewy body dementia (LBD); they represented 35.7% of demented patients with parkinsonism (54% of those with idiopathic Parkinson's disease) (IPD) and 26.1% of confirmed cases of Alzheimer's disease (AD) with parkinsonism. Both elderly subjects without clinical parkinsonism ($n = 83$) and IPD patients ($n = 39$) showed significant negative correlations between Mini-Mental State and neuritic Alzheimer stages, while 10 of 18 LBD cases clinically presenting with IPD and dementia did not satisfy the CERAD criteria for AD but represented 'plaque-only' type of AD. The 41 cases of autopsy-proven LBD showed a female preponderance (31/10), mean age at death of 76 ± 10.8 years and mean duration of 5.2 ± 4.1 years. Among 31 clinically well documented LBD cases, all except 4 were severely demented, with initial cognitive impairment in 58%, parkinsonian symptoms in 26%, and later combination of both in 84%. Neuropathology revealed LBD without AD pathology in one, LBD with 'plaque-predominant' AD and CERAD-definite AD in 15 cases each. Morphometric analyses showed about 70% neuronal loss in the cholinergic nucleus basalis of Meynert in LBD, demented IPD, and AD cases. While these data suggest the importance of both cortical AD pathology and dysfunction of the ascending cholinergic system for mental decline in these disorders, both the significance of cortical Lewy bodies and the pathogenic relationships between IPD, LBD and LBD + AD await further elucidation.

268

22.1 Introduction

A group of dementing disorders morphologically characterized by the presence of abundant cortical Lewy bodies (cLB) has been referred to as (diffuse) Lewy body disease (LBD) (Kosaka et al., 1984; Burkhardt et al., 1988; Lippa et al., 1994), senile dementia of Lewy body type (SDLT) (Perry et al., 1990) or Lewy body variant of AD (LBV-AD) (Hansen et al., 1990). Since cLB are seen in almost all cases of idiopathic Parkinson's disease (IPD) (Perry et al., 1991; Hughes et al., 1992) and in many cases of AD (Kazee & Han, 1995), the diagnostic criteria of LBD and the question whether IPD with concurrent AD, LBD without neuritic AD pathology, combined LBD and AD or LBV-AD, and AD with nigral lesions and occasional cLB represent separate disorders that can sometimes coexist, particularly in the very old, or whether they provide a spectrum of diseases with 'pure' AD, LBD and IPD with or without AD as poles and cases of 'mixed pathology' are still under discussion (Lippa et al., 1994; Dababo et al., 1995). While the recent demonstration of biochemical differences between cLB in IPD and LBD (Smith & Perry 1994), the different distribution and quantity of neuritic Alzheimer pathology (Lippa et al., 1994), of paired helical filaments and pathological tau proteins (Harrington et al., 1994), and differences in cholinergic biochemistry (Perry et al., 1993) argue for a separation of LBD, IPD and AD, concurrence of these disorders with motor neuron disease (Hedera et al., 1995) and similar other neurodegenerative 'overlap' syndromes have been reported (Uitti et al., 1995). Although neither the frequency of cLB nor the intensity of cortical AD pathology have been shown to relate directly to the severity of dementia in many LBD patients (Jansen et al., 1994), the contribution of both types of lesions to cognitive impairment are under discussion. The purpose of the present study was to determinate the relationships between LBD, IPD and AD based on the clinical and neuropathological findings in 31 well documented cases of LBD observed in a large consecutive autopsy series of demented aged subjects with or without parkinsonian symptoms.

22.2 Clinical materials and methods

Between 1989 and 1994, 120 subjects with the clinical diagnosis of IPD or parkinsonism and 290 demented elderly came to autopsy. Clinical data were assessed retrospectively from the hospital records using DSM-IIIR (1987) and WHO-ICD-9 criteria. The majority of the patients had been examined at least once by a skilled neurologist/psychiatrist. Diagnosis of IPD was mainly based on the UK Parkinson Disease Society Brain Bank criteria (Gibb & Lees, 1988), that of 'probable' AD on the NINCDS–ADRDA criteria (McKhann et al., 1984). Neuropathological examination was performed on paraffin blocks of superior frontal, cingulate, superior parietal, and temporal gyri including hippocampus and para-hippocampal regions, basal ganglia, brainstem, and cerebellum using conventional, silver (methenamine, modified Bielschowsky and Reusche), and immunohistochemical methods (for tau, AT-8, ubiquitin, and paired helical filaments using monoclonal antibody 3.39). Neuropathological diagnosis was performed using current criteria: AD was diagnosed according to the NIA (Khachaturian, 1985) and CERAD criteria (Mirra et al., 1991) and the staging of neuritic Alzheimer lesions (Braak & Braak 1991); LBD from the presence of abundant LB in both subcortical and cortical areas (Kosaka et al., 1984) with densities in cingulate and/or hippocampal regions of or exceeding one cLB/sqmm. Comparative studies of psychometrically assessed mental status using the Mini-Mental State (Folstein et al., 1975) not longer than six months prior to death were performed prospectively in a cohort of 39 patients with IPD (mean age 79.4 years), all Hoehn and Yahr stages IV or V, with a mean duration of illness of 10 years, and in 83 age-matched elderly subjects from the Vienna Prospective Dementia study using the same methods (for details see Bancher et al., 1993). Quantitative assessment of neuronal numbers and densities in the magnocellular part of the nucleus basalis of Meynert (NBM) was performed in 50 cases of IPD (32 demented, 18 nondemented), 43 cases of AD, 10 cases of LBD (8 LBD + neuritic AD stages V or VI, 2 LBD + 'plaque only' type AD), and 29 age-matched controls (for methods see Jellinger, 1987).

22.2.1 Incidence of Lewy body forms of dementia

Among 120 consecutive autopsy cases of clinically diagnosed IPD/parkinsonism, 104 showed the morphological features of brainstem LB type of IPD with or without additional pathologies, while 16 brains (13.3%) revealed other pathological entities, such as AD with or without nigral lesions or other brainstem disorders. The prevalence of moderate to severe dementia in the total group was 38.8% but only 30.8% for the IPD group, mainly related to AD lesions and, rarely, to other pathologies (degeneration of the NBM, internal hydrocephalus, post-traumatic lesions). LB dementia accounted for 35.7% of all demented parkinsonian

Table 22.1. *Pathology of 120 consecutive autopsy cases of parkinsonism (1989–1994)*

Neuropathology	Total	With dementia	
		n	%
Parkinson dis. LB type (IPD)	54	1	1.8
IPD + lacunar state	10	0	0
IPD + cerebrovascular lesions	7	0	0
IPD + AD/DAT	15	15	100.0
LB variant AD	13	13	100.0
IPD + MIX (AD/MIE)	1	1	100.0
IPD + other pathology	4	2	50.0
Primary IPD	104	32	30.8
AD/DAT°	8	8	100.0
Prog. supranucl. palsy	3	2[*]	66.7
Multisystem atrophy	3	2[*]	66.7
Corticobasal degen.	1	1	100.0
SAE Binswanger	1	1	100.0
Second. Park. Syndromes	16	14	87.5
TOTAL	120	46	38.3

°with nigral lesion 4; [*]with AD

patients and for 54% of those with IPD which was more frequent than IPD associated with AD (IPD + AD) or AD with or without nigral lesions (Tables 22.1 and 22.2). There was no significant difference in sex distribution, age at death, and duration of illness between demented and nondemented IPD patients except for a significant female preponderance in the LBD group and much shorter illness in AD subjects with parkinsonian symptoms (Table 22.3). Among the 290 elderly demented patients, most diagnosed clinically with 'probable' AD, 23 with additional IPD features, almost all fulfilled the neuropathological NIA criteria for AD, but CERAD criteria for probable or definite AD were satisfied in only 235 cases (81%). Almost all showed Braak stages V and VI, occasionally stages IV to V (with only few isocortical neurofibrillary tangles). Among 211 confirmed AD cases without clinical parkinsonian signs, 15 (7.1%) revealed more than single occasional cLB satisfying the diagnosis of LBD or LBV-AD, while six of 23 (26.1%) AD cases with clinical parkinsonism showed abundant cLB in the limbic areas. Thus the incidence of LBD in the total autopsy series of demented elderly subjects was 14.1% (Table 22.2). The mean age at death in the

Table 22.2. *Lewy body forms of dementias (autopsies 1989–1994)*

Clinical diagnosis	n	LB-dementias	%
Alzheimer's disease (AD)[*]	211	15	7.1
AD + parkinsonism	23	6	26.1
Parkinson's disease + dementia[**]	56	20	35.7
Dementias, total	290	41	14.1

[*]CERAD confirmed
[**]19 AD or other non-IPD disorders

LBV-AD group (78.7 years) was slightly lower than that in the other AD patients with parkinsonian signs (81 years), but duration of illness in the latter group (mean 3 years) was much shorter than in the LBV-AD group (mean 9.7 years) (Table 22.3).

22.2.2 *Morphological substrates of dementia in Parkinson's disease*

In 100 consecutive autopsy cases of IPD, there was no significant difference in the mean age at death between demented (78.8 years) and nondemented subjects (78.5 years), the latter, however, showing a longer duration of illness (10.1 vs. 8.0 years). In addition to classical histological features of IPD (focal loss of pigmented neurons, particularly in the ventral tier, and gliosis in substantia nigra zona compacta and other brainstem nuclei), with typical subcortical LB, occasional cLB were observed in 91% (58 out of 64) of the nondemented IPD cases but in all demented IPD patients. The majority of the nondemented IPD cases revealed no or only mild Alzheimer lesions, mainly diffuse amyloid deposits without neuritic changes; 78% had negative NIA neuropathological AD criteria and only 6.2% satisfied the CERAD criteria for possible AD. Neurofibrillary tangles (NFT) were either absent or were restricted to the limbic areas. In contrast, the majority of the demented IPD subjects fulfilled the NIA criteria for AD, and 73% satisfied the CERAD criteria for probable or definite AD, with isocortical neuritic AD changes present in 61% (Table 22.4). Comparison between the mental status (severely demented versus nondemented), neuritic AD stages, and age at death in this cohort gave similar results (Fig. 22.1). The majority of nondemented IPD patients, irrespective of their age at death, showed negative CERAD criteria for AD and neuritic pathology either absent or restricted to the entorhinal region without involvement of both the hippocampus and isocortex (corresponding to Braak stages 0

Table 22.3. *Parkinson's disease with and without dementia*

Pathology	Nondemented				Demented			
	n	(M/F)	age yrs (mean ± S.D.)	Duration	n	(M/F)	age yrs (mean ± S.D.)	Duration
IPD (Lewy)	54	(21/27)	78.4 ± 4.7	10.7 ± 5.8	1	(1/0)	79	2.0
IPD + CVD	17	(7/10)	80.4 ± 3.1	7.1 ± 3.0		–		–
IPD + AD	–				15	(8/7)	75.8 ± 7.0	7.8 ± 5.2
LBV-AD	–				13	(3/10)	77.5 ± 7.1	7.0 ± 5.6
AD					8	(4/4)	81.0 ± 5.6	2.9 ± 1.2

CVD = Cerebrovascular disease; LBV = Lewy body variant, AD = Alzheimer's disease.

Table 22.4. *Clinico-pathological features of 100 consecutive autopsy cases with the clinical diagnosis of Parkinson's disease (1989–1994)*

N pat.	Mean age	Dementia	cLB	CERAD	Khachat.	Braak/Braak
50	75.0	0	45/50	0	0	0–II
2	82.5	0	2/2	0	+	I–II
3	77.7	0	3/3	0	+	III
5	81.8	0	5/5	0/A	+	IV
4	81.0	0	4/4	possible AD	+	IV
64	78.5	nondemented	59/64			
3	80.0	+	3/3	0/A	0/+	III
4	79.0	+	4/4	0	+	II–III
3	78.7	+	3/3	0/A	0	III–IV,IV
4	77.5	+	4/4	probable AD	+	IV
8	78.2	+	8/8	probable AD	+	IV,IV–V
2	80.0	+	2/2	probable AD	+	V
12	77.4	+	12/12	definite AD	+	V–VI
36	78.8	demented	36/36			
100	78.6	Total	94/100			

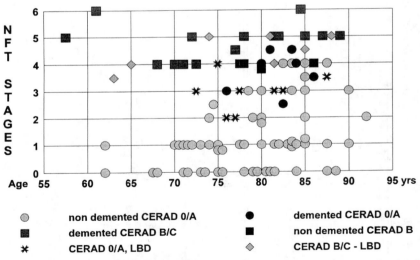

Fig. 22.1 Relations between mental state, Alzheimer stages, and age at death of 100 consecutive autopsy cases with clinical diagnosis of Parkinson's disease.

to II). Only a small number of nondemented IPD subjects showed extension of NFT to the hippocampus (Braak stages III and IV); only three such brains met the CERAD criteria for probable AD, while isocortical NFT were not seen. The demented IPD cases showed variable brain pathology: while the majority met the NIA criteria for AD, almost 30% were CERAD negative or 'possible' AD, with neuritic lesions restricted to the hippocampus (Braak stages III and IV). Only 61% of the demented IPD subjects showed considerable isocortical neuritic AD pathology (Braak stages IV–V to VI). Whereas in the nondemented IPD subjects, the intensity of neuritic AD lesions showed some relationship with age, no such relations were seen in the demented ones (Fig. 22.1). It should be emphasized that 10 of the 18 demented IPD cases without isocortical NFT showed abundant cLB and, therefore, were diagnosed as LBD, while only three of them met the CERAD criteria for probable or definite AD, corresponding to Braak stage V, all of them fulfilled the morphological NIA criteria suggesting that most of them represented the 'plaque predominant' type of AD (Hansen et al., 1993), corresponding to Braak stages II and III or to the 'limbic' type of AD, with Braak stages III and IV (Fig. 22.1).

The relationship between mental status and neuritic Alzheimer staging in 39 consecutive autopsy cases of IPD (including five LBD) and 83 age-matched elderly subjects without clinical IPD signs (including eight cases of LBD) is shown in Fig. 22.2a and b. In both series, there was a highly significant negative correlation between Mini-Mental State scores and neuritic AD staging, the majority of severely demented subjects showing extensive isocortical NFT (Braak stages V and VI) although these were less frequent in severely demented IPD cases. While in the non-IPD group all except one of the severely demented LBD cases showed Braak stages V and VI, in the IPD group with severe dementia, 2 of 5 LBD cases and two IPD cases with few cLB were free of isocortical NFT corresponding to hippocampal stage IV (Fig. 22.2b).

22.2.3 Clinical and morphological features of LBD

In our consecutive series of 290 elderly subjects and 120 parkinsonian patients, there were 41 brains showing abundant cLB allowing the morphological diagnosis of LBD. There were 31 females and 10 males, ranging in age at death from 44 to 91 (mean 76.1 ± 10.8) years, with a duration of illness ranging from one to 20 (mean 5.2 ± 4.1) years. In 31 well documented cases, the major clinical features at presentation were

Consecutive autopsies of aged (mean age 79.0 yrs)

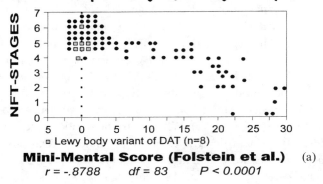

Mini-Mental Score (Folstein et al.)   (a)

r = -.8788   *df = 83*   *P < 0.0001*

Consecutive autopsy cases of LB-PD (mean age 79.4 yrs)

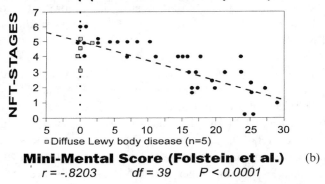

Mini-Mental Score (Folstein et al.)   (b)

r = -.8203   *df = 39*   *P < 0.0001*

Fig. 22.2 (a) Correlation between neuropsychologically assessed psychostatus (Mini-Mental-State score) and neuropathological stages of neuritic Alzheimer lesions in 83 consecutive elderly subjects without parkinsonian features; (b) correlation between psychostatus and neuritic Alzheimer stages in 39 consecutive cases of Parkinson's disease.

cognitive impairment in 58%, PD features in 26%, cognitive impairment with PD signs in one, and other presenting symptoms in four patients: two with schizophrenia, one with affective psychosis and another one with falls and fluctuating cognition (Table 22.5). Clinical diagnosis was IPD with or without dementia in eight patients, AD in 19 (10 with IPD features), and others in four (schizophrenia with ensuing neuroleptic-induced rigid-akinetic parkinsonism in two), affective (manic-depressive) psychosis terminating in akinetic state, and possible Creutzfeldt–Jakob disease in one each). Most of the patients fulfilled the operational criteria

Table 22.5. *Clinical features in 31 cases of Lewy body dementia*

Main clinical features	At presentation (in %)	Late stage (in %)
Cognitive impairment	58	9.7
PD features only	25.8	0
Cognitive impairment and PD features	3.2	83.9
Other presentations	12.8	
Schizophrenic psychosis	6.4	
Manic-depressive psychosis	3.2	
Dizziness and falls	3.2	
Fluctuating cognition		

7 males, 24 females; age 44–91 (mean 76.1 ± 10.8) years; duration of illness: 1–20 (mean 5.2 ± 4.1) years

for SDLT (McKeith et al., 1992), although visual hallucinations were reported only in 22 of 31 patients (71%). The duration of illness was longest in LBD patients presenting with IPD symptoms; the age at death was highest in the group presenting with primary dementia (Table 22.6). Morphologically, all brains showed numerous LB in cortical, mainly limbic, less frequently in insular and other isocortical and subcortical regions; 25 or 81% had ubiquitin-positive neurites in the CA2/CA3 region of the hippocampus and showed subcortical lesions with focal neuronal loss in the ventral tier of substantia nigra zona compacta, in the locus coeruleus and dorsal vagal nucleus indistinguishable from IPD. The remaining nine brains displayed only mild nigral lesions, either diffuse or in the posterolateral portion with few LB; subcortical NFT were seen in 12 brains. All except for one (female aged 44 years with schizophrenia-parkinsonism and only mild cognitive deficits) fulfilled the NIA criteria for AD, but only 19 satisfied the CERAD criteria for probable or definite AD. While 15 brains represented AD of 'plaque-only' type with no isocortical NFT, the other 15 cases revealed extensive isocortical NFT pathology (Braak stages V or VI) or represented a combination of LBD with 'true' AD (Table 22.7). The correlation between mental status (severe vs no dementia), neuritic AD stages, and age (Fig. 22.3) shows that in all four nondemented, but also in 11 severely demented subjects the neuritic AD lesions were restricted to the allocortex, only three of them satisfying the CERAD criteria for probable AD, while the other half of the severely demented cases showed isocortical neuritic pathology fulfilling the CERAD criteria

Table 22.6. *Lewy body dementia (LBD): clinical features*

Clinical diagnosis	PD ($n=8$)	AD+PD ($n=10$)	AD ($n=9$)	Others ($n=4$)
Age/death (mean, yr)	74.4	78.5	80.1	67.8
Duration (mean, yr)	7.5	5.3	5.2	4.3
PD symptoms	8/8	10/10	4/9	4/4
Fluctuating cognition	6/8	10/10	7/9	4/4
Visual hallucinations	6/8	8/10	5/9	3/4
Repeated falls	8/8	7/10	6/9	3/4
Disturbed consciousness	6/8	9/10	7/9	4/4
Delusions	6/8	10/10	8/9	4/4
Dementia, severe	7/8	10/10	9/9	1/4

for probable or definite AD. The mean Braak stage value for all cases was 3.7. In general, there was no definite relationship between the age at death and the severity of neuritic AD pathology.

Morphometric analysis of the neuronal numbers and density in the cholinergic magnocellular part of the nucleus basalis of Meynert revealed severe cell depletion in IPD, more severe in demented than in nondemented cases, in AD and in LBD, all ranging about 70% of age matched controls, while neuronal density was most severely reduced in LBD and

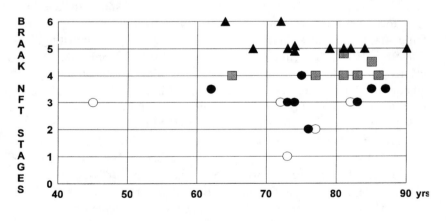

not severely demented CERAD 0/A   severely demented CERAD 0/A
severely demented CERAD B   severely demented CERAD C

Fig. 22.3 Correlation between neuritic Alzheimer stages and age: 31 autopsy cases of Lewy body disease.

Table 22.7. *Lewy body dementia (LBD): neuropathological features*

Clin. DX	PD + Dem (n = 8)	AD + PD (n = 10)		AD (n = 9)		Other (n = 4)
SN lesion	3 +	3 +	1 +	3 +	1 +	3 +
Cort. LB (> 1/mm²)						
Cingulate gyrus	8	6	4	4	5	4
Parahippocampus	8	6	4	4	5	4
Lewy neurites. CA2-3	8	5	2	3	4	3
LB L. coeruleus	8	6	4	4	4	4
Dors. X nucleus	7	6	4	4	4	4
AD pathology						
Khachaturian +	8	6	4	4	5	3
CERAD/Braak	−	−	−	−	−	
stages 0/1	−	−	−	−	−	1 A
0/2,3	4			−	−	3
A/3	−	3	−	1	−	− B
B/4	2	1	−	−	1	−
B/5	2	1	−	1	−	−
C/5,6	−	2	3	2	4	− C
Subcort. NFT	−	2	4	2	3	1
Brain weight (mean)	1153	1090		1146		1185

Type of LBD: DLBD/no AD (n = 1);
DLBD + AD/plaque type (n = 15), 'LB variant of AD;
DLBD + true AD (n = 15) of AD'

AD (Fig. 22.4a and b). There were no major differences in NBM cell loss between LBD with 'plaque-only' AD (two cases) and with 'true' AD (eight cases with Braak stages V or VI). LB and NFT in the NBM neurons were seen in eight brains of LBD each.

22.3 Discussion

The presence of cLB in a substantial proportion of elderly demented subjects meeting the clinical and morphological criteria of IPD, AD or other neurodegenerative disorders is now being recognized (Hughes et al., 1992; Pollanen et al., 1993; Kazee & Han, 1995). However, the nosological relevance and the contribution of cLB to the dementing process has not been fully explained. cLB that are frequently associated with LB in the brainstem and/or other subcortical regions, may occur with or without amyloid deposits (plaques) and neuritic Alzheimer or tau pathology (neuritic plaques, NFT, neuropil threads) in the cerebral cortex. Therefore, when numerous cLB are found, a variety of diagnoses may

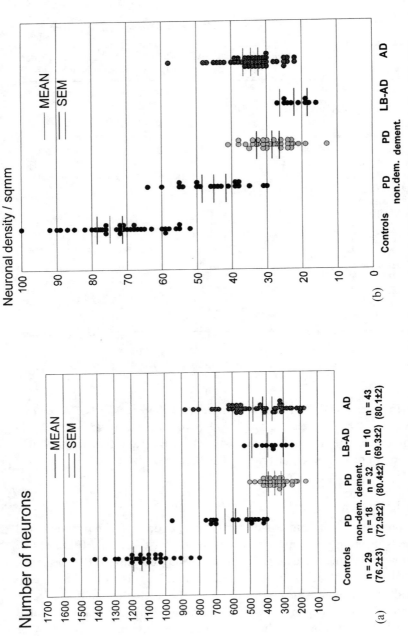

Fig. 22.4 Total number (a) and mean density of neurons (b) in the magnocellular (Ch4) part of the nucleus basalis of Meynert in **IPD** with/without dementia, AD, LBV-AD, and age-matched controls.

be considered, including LBD, LBD with amyloid plaques in the absence of neuritic lesions ('plaque only' type of AD), or 'pathological aging' (Dickson et al., 1992), LBV-AD, AD with cLB, or brainstem LBD with variable numbers of cLB. Major problems may arise due to frequent overlap conditions and coincidental association between AD, IPD and other conditions with cLB.

LBD featured by the presence of abundant cLB has been considered a frequent cause of dementia in the elderly, second only to AD, comprising seven up to 30% of all dementias (Perry et al., 1993; Harrington et al., 1994). Among 290 demented elderly subjects in our 5-year autopsy series of, 235 or 81% meeting the CERAD criteria for AD, and 120 parkinsonian patients (104 with confirmed IPD), LBD accounted for 14.1% representing 26.1% of the AD cases with, and 7.1% without parkinsonism, 35.7% of demented parkinsonians and 54% of demented IPD cases. While the majority of nondemented IPD patients, 75% showing occasional cLB, did not meet the morphological CERAD criteria for AD, cortical Alzheimer pathology with or without abundant cLB was the most frequent organic substrate of dementia in IPD, although only 70% satisfied the CERAD criteria for probable or definite AD. The majority of these CERAD-negative cases were LBD with plaque-predominant AD lacking isocortical neuritic lesions which otherwise have been referred to as pathological aging of the brain and have been distinguished from AD (Dickson et al., 1992, 1995). Whereas in the majority of elderly subjects with or without IPD there was a strict correlation between the clinical severity of dementia and NFT formation, which is consistent with findings of other studies (McKee et al., 1992; Bancher et al., 1993; Bierer et al., 1995a, Nagy et al., 1995) some of the severely demented LBD cases were free of isocortical neuritic Alzheimer pathology, suggesting that in these patients neurodegeneration indicated by NFT formation was not a critical determinant of mental decline. A comparison of neuritic Alzheimer changes using the Braak staging (Braak & Braak, 1991) in six diagnostic groups of our consecutive autopsy series showed considerable morphological overlap between nondemented aged controls, nondemented IPD, and pure LBD cases on one hand, and between demented IPD, LBV-AD, and AD patients on the other (Fig. 22.5). Brains of aged nondemented elderly subjects mainly were Braak stages 0 to III, and only very rarely stage IV; the same stages occupied by about 85% of the nondemented and by pure LBD patients (demented and nondemented). While almost 60% of the demented IPD and about half of the LBV-AD brains were limbic stages III and IV, corresponding to plaque-predominant AD

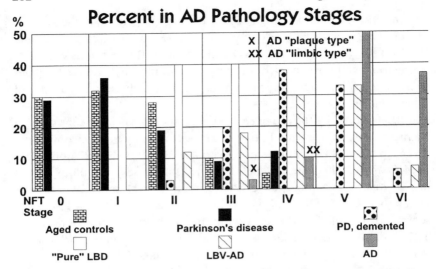

Fig. 22.5 Extent of neuritic Alzheimer changes using Braak stages in six diagnostic groups of our autopsy series: aged controls ($n = 50$), Parkinson's disease without/with dementia ($n = 66/34$), 'pure' Lewy body disease (LBD) ($n = 5$), Lewy body variant of Alzheimer's disease (LBV/AD) ($n = 26$), and Alzheimer's disease (AD) ($n = 225$). Incidence of neuritic AD pathology stages is expressed as percentage of cases in each diagnostic category.

or CERAD probable AD (see also Fig. 22.3), about 40% each of the demented IPD and LBV-AD brains as well as the majority of typical AD cases were isocortical stages V and VI, meeting the CERAD criteria of definite AD.

The group of 41 patients with autopsy-proven LBD showed a similar age at death as IPD and AD cases, but a striking female preponderance (31 vs 10) and much shorter duration of illness than both demented and nondemented IPD patients (mean 5.2 vs 7.8 and 10.7 years, respectively). Since cognitive impairment was the most frequent presenting clinical feature often followed by parkinsonian symptoms, AD with or without IPD was diagnosed in 60%; IPD with dementia in 25%, while the remaining four patients showed other (psychotic) presentations. Retrospectively, most patients met the diagnostic criteria for SDLT (McKeith et al., 1992) although visual hallucinations were not reported in 30%. Morphologically, in addition to abundant cLB, mainly in limbic and, less frequent, in isocortical regions, 71% of the brains showed subcortical lesions including severe nigral damage with predilection to the ventral tier indistinguishable from IPD, while in the others there was only mild rather diffuse nigral damage as often seen in AD (Kazee & Han, 1995; Kazee et al., 1995). While all except one mildly demented young female met the NIA anatomical criteria for AD, only 61% satisfied the CERAD criteria for probable or definite AD and one half of the brains each were either plaque-only or true plaque and tangle type of AD. These data also suggest that NFT formation in a considerable proportion of LBD cases may not be an essential structural basis of cognitive decline and other mental disorders. On the other hand, LBD, like AD and IPD with dementia, show severe neuronal loss in the cholinergic NBM ranging between 50% and 75% of controls (Jellinger, 1987; Perry et al., 1993), the accompanying decrease in cortical cholinergic markers being highly correlated with severity of dementia in both LBD and AD (Bierer et al., 1995b; Dickson et al., 1995). While in AD, secondary degeneration of the cholinergic basal forebrain system suggested by significant correlations between NBM neuron depletion and neuritic AD lesions in their cortical target areas has been confirmed by defective retrograde transport of nerve growth factor to the NBM (Mufson et al., 1995), the variability of NBM depletion and loss of cholinergic markers in neocortex and hippocampus, irrespective of cortical neuritic pathology in both IPD and LBD, suggest a primary degeneration of the cholinergic basal forebrain system causing a major cholinergic derangement as a major component of dementia in these disorders (Jellinger, 1987; Perry et al., 1993, 1995).

Based on the anatomical findings in our and other case series, we propose to distinguish at least six subsets of disorders with cLB:

1. Predominant brainstem LBD with subcortical lesions characteristic of IPD and small numbers of cLB without Alzheimer pathology = IPD, often without dementia;
2. LBD with and/or rarely without subcortical IPD type lesions with no cortical amyloid or neuritic Alzheimer lesions = pure LBD with or without dementia, or IPD, or transitional LBD (Kosaka et al., 1984);
3. LBD with/rarely without subcortical IPD type lesions associated with diffuse plaques or limbic AD lacking isocortical neuritic AD/tau pathology (CERAD negative) = LBV-AD (frequently demented, with/without IPD);
4. LBD, brainstem and cortical, with isocortical neuritic AD pathology (CERAD positive, Braak V and VI), with or without subcortical IPD type lesions = LBD-AD or LBD + true AD (usually severely demented), or IPD + AD;

5. AD of plaque-only or plaque and tangle type with small numbers of cLB and subcortical IPD type lesions (nigral damage with LB) = IPD + AD or AD + IPD; LBV-AD;
6. AD of both types with small numbers of cLB with mild subcortical (nigral damage = AD with cLB.

This proposed subgrouping of LBD is in general accordance with, but goes beyond, the morphological classification suggested by the *Consortium on Dementia with Lewy Bodies* on October 6, 1995. Despite variable overlaps, these data do not confirm the notion that LBV-AD usually represents coexistence of AD and IPD (Dababo et al., 1995), but the final classification and pathogenetic relations between these disorders and their clinical relevance await further elucidation.

References

Bancher, C., Braak, H., Fischer, P. & Jellinger, K. (1993). Neuropathological staging of Alzheimer lesions and intellectual status in Alzheimer's and Parkinson's disease. *Neurosci. Lett.*, **162**, 179–82.

Bierer, L. M., Hof, P. R., Purohit, D. P. et al. (1995a). Neocortical neurofibrillary tangles correlate with dementia severity in Alzheimer's disease. *Arch. Neurol.*, **52**, 81–8.

Bierer, L. M., Haroutunian, V., Gabriel, S. et al. (1995b). Neurochemical correlates of dementia severity in Alzheimer's disease: relative importance of the cholinergic deficits. *J. Neurochem.*, **64**, 749–60.

Braak, H. & Braak, E. (1991). Neuropathological staging of Alzheimer-related changes. *Acta Neuropathol.*, **82**, 239–59.

Burkhardt, C. R., Filley, C. M., Kleinschmidt-DeMasters, B. K., de la Monte, S., Norenberg, M. D. & Schneck, S. A. (1988). Diffuse Lewy body disease and progressive dementia. *Neurology*, **38**, 1520–8.

Dababo, M. A., Bigio, E. H., Hladik, C. L. & White, C. L. III. (1995). Neuropathological evidence that the Lewy body variant of Alzheimer disease represents coexistence of Alzheimer disease and idiopathic Parkinson disease (abstr). *J. Neuropathol. Exp. Neurol.*, **54**, 429.

Dickson, D. W., Crystal, H. A., Mattiace, L. A. et al. (1992). Identification of normal and pathological aging in prospectively studied nondemented elderly humans. *Neurobiol. Aging*, **13**, 179–89.

Dickson, D. W., Crystal, H. A., Bevona, C., Honer, W., Vincent, I. & Davies, P. (1995). Correlations of synaptic markers with cognitive status in prospectively studied elderly humans. *Neurobiol. Aging*, **16**, 285–98.

DSM-IIIR. (1987). *Diagnostic and Statistical Manual of Mental Disorders*. 3rd edn, revised. Washington: American Psychiatric Association.

Folstein, M. F., Folstein, S. E. & McHugh, P. R. (1975). 'Mini-Mental State': a practical method grading the cognitive state of patients for the clinician. *J. Psychiat. Res.*, **12**, 189–98.

Gibb, W. R. G. & Lees, A. J. (1988). The relevance of Lewy bodies to the pathogenesis of idiopathic Parkinson's disease. *J. Neurol. Neurosurg. Psychiatry*, **51**, 745–52.

Hansen, L., Salmon, D., Galasko, D. et al. (1990). The Lewy body variant of Alzheimer's disease: a clinical and pathologic entity. *Neurology*, **40**, 1–8.

Hansen, L. A., Masliah, E., Galasko, D. & Terry, R. D. (1993). Plaque-only Alzheimer disease is usually the Lewy body variant and vice versa. *J. Neuropathol. Exp. Neurol.*, **52**, 648–54.

Harrington, C. R., Perry, R. H., Perry, E. K. et al. (1994). Senile dementia of Lewy body type and Alzheimer type and biochemically distinct in terms of paired helical filaments and hyperphosphorylated tau protein. *Dementia*, **5**, 215–28.

Hedera, P., Lerner, A. J., Castellani, R. & Friedland, R. P. (1995). Concurrence of Alzheimer's disease, Parkinson's disease, diffuse Lewy body disease, and amyotrophic lateral sclerosis. *J. Neurol. Sci.*, **128**, 219–24.

Hughes, A. J., Daniel, S. E., Kilford, L. & Lees, A. J. (1992). Accuracy of clinical diagnosis of idiopathic Parkinson's disease. A clinico-pathological study of 100 cases. *J. Neurol. Neurosurg. Psychiatry*, **55**, 181–4.

Jansen, F. N. H., De Vos, R. A. I., Stam, F. C., Ravid, R. & Swaab, D. F. (1994). Lewy bodies, with and without dementia: clinico-pathological correlations in 22 consecutive cases of Parkinson's disease. In: *Dementia in Parkinson's disease*. ed. A. D. Korczyn, pp. 207–9. Bologna: Monduzzi Ed.

Jellinger, K. (1987). Neuropathological substrates of Alzheimer's and Parkinson's disease. *J. Neural Transm.* (suppl), **24**, 109–29.

Kazee, A. M. & Han, L. Y. (1995). Cortical Lewy bodies in Alzheimer's disease. *Arch. Pathol. Lab. Med.*, **199**, 448–53.

Kazee, A. M., Cox, C. & Richfield, E. K. (1995). Substantia nigra lesions in Alzheimer disease and normal aging. *Alzheimer Dis. Assoc. Disord.*, **9.**, 61–7.

Khachaturian, Z. S. (1985). Diagnosis of Alzheimer's disease. *Arch. Neurol.*, **42**, 1097–105.

Kosaka, K., Yoshimura, M., Ikeda, K. & Budka, H. (1984). Diffuse type of Lewy body disease: progressive dementia with abundant cortical Lewy bodies and senile changes of various degree – a new disease? *Clin. Neuropathol.*, **3**, 185–92.

Lippa, C. F., Smith, T. W. & Swearer, J. M. (1994). Alzheimer's disease and Lewy body disease: a comparative clinicopathological study. *Ann. Neurol.*, **35**, 81–8.

McKee, A. C., Kosik, K. S. & Kowall, N. W. (1992). Neuritic pathology and dementia in Alzheimer's disease. *Ann. Neurol.*, **30**, 156–65.

McKeith, I. G., Perry, R. H., Fairbairn, A. F., Jabeen, S. & Perry, E. K. (1992). Operational criteria for senile dementia of Lewy body type (SDLT). *Psychol. Med.*, **22**, 911–22.

McKhann, G., Drachman, D., Folstein, M., Katzman, R., Price, D. & Stadlan, E. M. (1984). Clinical diagnosis of Alzheimer's disease: Report of the NINCDS-ADRDA work group under the auspices of the Department of Health and Human Services Task Force of Alzheimer's Disease. *Neurology*, **34**, 939–44.

Mirra, S. S., Heyman, A., McKheel, D. et al. (1991). The Consortium to establish a registry for Alzheimer's disease (CERAD). II. Standardization of the neuropathologic assessment of Alzheimer's disease. *Neurology*, **41**, 479–86.

Mufson, E. J., Conner, J. M. & Kordower, J. H. (1995). Nerve growth factor in Alzheimer's disease. Defective retrograde transport to nucleus basalis. *Neuroreport*, **6**, 1063–6.

Nagy, Z., Esiri, M. M., Jobst, K. A. et al. (1995). Relative roles of plaques and tangles in the dementia of Alzheimer's disease: correlations using three sets of neuropathological criteria. *Dementia*, **6**, 21–31.

Perry, R. H., Irving, I., Blessed, G., Fairbairn, A. & Perry, E. K. (1990). Senile dementia of Lewy body type. A clinically and neuropathologically distinct form of Lewy body dementia in the elderly. *J. Neurol. Sci.*, **95**, 119–39.

Perry, E. K., Irving, D., Kerwin, J. M. et al. (1993). Cholinergic transmitter and neurotrophic activities in Lewy body dementia. Similarity to Parkinson's and distinction from Alzheimer disease. *Alzheimer Dis. Assoc. Disord.*, **7**, 69–79.

Perry, E. K., Morris, C. M., Court, J. A. et al. (1995). Alterations in nicotine binding sites in Parkinson's disease, Lewy body dementia and Alzheimer's disease: possible index of early neuropathology. *Neuroscience*, **64**, 385–95.

Perry, E. K., McKeith, I. G., Thompson, P. et al. (1991). Topography, extent, and clinical relevance of neurochemical deficits in dementia of Lewy body type, Parkinson's disease and Alzheimer's disease. *Ann. NY Acad. Sci.*, **640**, 197–202.

Pollanen, M. S., Dickson, D. W. & Bergeron, C. (1993). Pathology and biology of the Lewy body. *J. Neuropathol. Exp. Neurol.*, **52**, 183–91.

Smith, M. A. & Perry, G. (1994). Is a Lewy body always a Lewy body? In *Dementia in Parkinson's Disease*, ed. A. D. Korczyn, pp. 187–93. Bologna: Monduzzi Ed.

Uitti, R. J., Berry, K., Yasuhara, O. et al. (1995). Neurodegenerative 'overlap' syndrome: clinical and pathological features of Parkinson's disease, motor neuron disease, and Alzheimer's disease. *Park. Rel. Dis.*, **1**, 21–34.

23

What do Lewy bodies tell us about dementia and parkinsonism?

R. DE LA FUENTE-FERNÁNDEZ
and D. B. CALNE

Summary

Lewy bodies remain an enigma. Their presence in the substantia nigra is often taken as a diagnostic criterion for idiopathic parkinsonism (IP, Parkinson's disease). Yet the first report of Lewy bodies in IP is an account of their appearance in the dorsal motor nucleus of the vagus, and the nucleus basalis of Meynert. More serious problems have arisen in recent years, partly as a result of improved techniques for detecting Lewy bodies. The more they have been looked for, the more they have been found. A further complicating factor is that they have different appearances in different regions of the brain. We know that Lewy bodies are made up from cytoskeletal products and they are associated with the death of neurons. They may contribute to the mechanism driving cell death. Alternatively, their formation may represent a compensatory adjustment in an attempt to ameliorate the demise of neurons. They have not helped us in an attempt to find the aetiology of IP, because they occur in such widely diverse settings as hereditary neurodegeneration (e.g. Hallervorden–Spatz disease) and viral infection (e.g. subacute sclerosing panencephalitis). Thus our knowledge, and our ignorance, concerning Lewy bodies leaves us in a tantalizing situation. Surely they are important clues to neurodegeneration, but as yet we have not been able to reveal the secrets that they should provide to help us unravel the pathogenesis of IP.

23.1 Introduction

James Parkinson described the clinical features of the disorder that bears his name in 1817 (Parkinson, 1817). In 1912, Lewy demonstrated the existence of neuronal inclusion bodies in the dorsal motor nucleus of the vagus and nucleus basalis of Meynert in Parkinson's disease. Seven years later Trétiakoff established the basic pathologic substrate of Parkinson's disease: severe neuronal loss in the substantia nigra and the presence of the neuronal inclusions previously reported by Lewy (and since then called Lewy bodies) in surviving neurons. This is, in short, the history that links Parkinson's disease and Lewy bodies. The term Incidental Lewy body disease appeared later, when Forno demonstrated the presence of Lewy bodies in subjects who had died without parkinsonism (Forno, 1969; Forno & Alvord, 1971; see also Introduction).

Lewy bodies have been found in a diversity of locations, including monoaminergic and cholinergic neurons of the brainstem, diencephalon, basal forebrain, cerebral cortex, and autonomic ganglia (Gibb, 1989; Fearnley & Lees, 1994). Besides, it is known that their ultrastructural appearance can differ according to their specific topographic location. Thus, for example, while the classic Lewy body (brainstem type Lewy body) appears as an eosinophilic, intracytoplasmic inclusion with a hyaline core and a pale-staining peripheral halo, cortical Lewy bodies generally do not have a distinct peripheral halo (Lowe, 1994). These differences could be due to different aetiologic or pathogenetic factors, but it is more likely that they represent only topographically distinct aspects of the same structure.

The meaning of Lewy bodies remains unclear but, in the absence of any linkage to disordered function, the concept of Lewy body disease remains popular. Its clinical spectrum is enlarging, and now includes parkinsonism (Parkinson's disease), dementia (diffuse Lewy body disease) (Gibb et al., 1987), autonomic failure (Gibb, 1988), dystonia (Meige syndrome) (Mark et al., 1994), pure akinesia (Quinn et al., 1989), supranuclear gaze palsy (Fearnley et al., 1991), and lower motor neuron disease (Kato et al., 1988). This clinical spectrum will probably continue to expand, complicating further the concept of Lewy body disease. If it is already difficult to arrive at an accurate clinical diagnosis of Lewy body disease in patients with parkinsonism (Hughes et al., 1992), it will be much more difficult for the clinician to recognize this entity in the absence of parkinsonism. At present, there is a series of clinical criteria to help one to recognize Lewy body disease in cases of parkinsonism, with and without dementia (Crystal et al., 1990; Calne et al., 1992), but there are no clinical clues to identify Lewy body disease in other settings.

Despite the existence of this wide variety of clinical manifestations, two presentations dominate the spectrum of Lewy body disease: a classical form, characterized by parkinsonian signs (bradykinesia, rigidity and tremor at rest), and a second form where dementia of Alzheimer-type or symptoms of organic psychosis combined with parkinsonian deficits are the most relevant clinical features. While in the former the pathology (Lewy bodies and neuronal loss) is largely confined to the brainstem (Parkinson's disease), in the latter the pathologic changes are widely distributed throughout the brain, not only in the brainstem but also in the neocortex (diffuse Lewy body disease) (Gibb et al., 1987; Kosaka, 1993). It is important to note, however, that a careful examination, particularly if ubiquitin immunocytochemistry is used, can reveal the presence of a few cortical Lewy bodies in a substantial number of patients with Parkinson's disease, and that, on the other hand, most, if not all, patients with diffuse Lewy body disease have pathological features of Parkinson's disease (Lennox et al., 1989b,c). These findings reinforce the concept of Lewy body disease as a clinico-pathological spectrum.

As we mentioned before, Lewy bodies are quite common in brains of neurologically normal persons aged 60 or older ('incidental' Lewy bodies). Although the meaning of this finding remains elusive, it is possible that these cases represent presymptomatic Parkinson's disease (Forno, 1969; Forno & Alvord, 1971; Gibb & Lees, 1988; Fearnley & Lees, 1991; Fearnley & Lees, 1994). The preferential distribution of 'incidental' Lewy bodies in the ventrolateral region of the substantia nigra, similar to that occurring in Parkinson's disease, supports this contention (Gibb & Lees, 1991).

Finally, there are other neurodegenerative disorders, such as Hallervorden–Spatz disease, neuroaxonal dystrophy, ataxia-telangiectasia, subacute sclerosing panencephalitis, spinocerebellar degeneration, progressive supranuclear palsy, multiple system atrophy, cortical-basal ganglionic degeneration, and Alzheimer's disease, where Lewy bodies can be present in addition to the pathologic features characteristic of each one of these entities (Gibb & Lees, 1988; Alvord & Forno, 1992).

It is clear, therefore, that (1) Lewy bodies are neither a selective marker of dopaminergic degeneration nor a selective marker of Parkinson's disease, and (2) the clinical presentation of Lewy body disease depends only on which structures are predominantly damaged. We do not know whether Parkinson's disease has a single aetiology and pathogenesis (Calne, 1989), and, therefore, we do not know whether the term 'Parkinson's disease' is appropriate. We think that 'idiopathic parkinsonism' is a more prudent term, and so we shall use it instead of 'Parkinson's disease' (Calne, 1994).

23.2 Lewy bodies and neuronal death

The aim of this review is to answer the question 'What do Lewy bodies tell us about dementia and parkinsonism?'. Hence, the first question that we should pose would be 'Do Lewy bodies play a pathogenetic role in Lewy body disease?' or 'Are they only a mere histological marker?'. In other words, 'Are Lewy bodies responsible for neuronal dysfunction or neuronal death?'. This is a very important issue, because if the answer is affirmative one should look into the structure and composition of Lewy bodies in an attempt to understand how to prevent their formation, and so prevent the development of idiopathic parkinsonism. On the other hand, Lewy bodies may also represent an epiphenomenon in some types of neurodegenerative processes, either without any implication in the pathogenesis of the disease (marker) or with only a secondary participation in the death of the nerve cell. Finally, it is also possible, hypothetically, that they may represent compensatory mechanisms directed to preserve the survival of the neurons (Gibb et al., 1990). We do not know if the formation of the Lewy bodies is linked to specific environmental causes or is related to the existence of a genetically determined susceptibility of the individual.

If Lewy bodies were primarily involved in neuronal death one would expect to find a substantial number of Lewy bodies and little or no neuronal loss during the presymptomatic stage of the disorder (incidental Lewy bodies?). Equally, if, as it appears, pale bodies are an early form of Lewy bodies (Lowe, 1994), the highest pale bodies/Lewy bodies ratio should occur during the presymptomatic period. Meticulous studies comparing this 'relative' number of Lewy bodies in presymptomatic and symptomatic idiopathic parkinsonism have not been carried out, but it is known that: (1) individuals with 'incidental' Lewy bodies can have either a substantial loss of neurons in the ventrolateral region of the substantia nigra (Gibb & Lees, 1988; Fearnley & Lees, 1991; Gibb & Lees, 1991) or no cell loss (Hansen et al., 1990; Perry et al., 1990b); (2) cases of 'incidental' Lewy bodies can have greater numbers of Lewy bodies than patients with idiopathic parkinsonism of long duration (Forno, 1986); and (3) the degree of dementia in patients with diffuse Lewy body disease seems to be directly related to the number of Lewy bodies in the neocortex (Lennox et al., 1989a,c; Kosaka, 1993). Overall, these findings suggest that although the formation of Lewy bodies is an early feature, it might not be a prerequisite for neuronal death.

Another possibility is that, without being directly related to the process of neuronal death, Lewy bodies could cause a functional compromise of the cell. However, the fact that cases of incidental Lewy bodies can present with a very high number of Lewy bodies argues against this possibility. Up to now there is no evidence that Lewy bodies are toxic *per se* for the cell. Normal cell constituents, such as lipids, enzymes, and neurofilaments, are involved in their composition (Forno, 1986; Pollanen et al., 1993).

The most widely accepted theory suggests that Lewy bodies are the consequence of cellular stress. Supporting this contention is the fact that ubiquitin, a known cell stress-associated protein thought to play a role in the degradation of abnormal proteins, has been found within the Lewy bodies (Lowe, 1994). We do not know, however, if the formation of Lewy bodies depends on the presence of pathologic mechanisms responsible for stress, or if it is secondary to compensatory mechanisms working in response to stress. In addition, the existence of a higher prevalence of incidental Lewy bodies in the elderly (Gibb & Lees, 1988) suggests that ageing could play a role in their pathogenesis. In the MPTP experimental model of parkinsonism in monkeys, Lewy body-like inclusions appear almost exclusively in elderly animals (Forno et al., 1993).

Both specific external causes (environmental factors) and individual predisposition (genetic factors) seem to be involved in the formation of Lewy bodies. In this context, MPTP-induced human parkinsonism (Langston & Ballard, 1984) and autosomal dominant parkinsonism (Golbe et al., 1990) represent extreme examples of environmental and genetic factors, respectively.

Because of the uncertainty of the role played by the Lewy bodies in the processes of neuronal dysfunction or neuronal death, we will analyse the relationship between Lewy bodies and dementia, and Lewy bodies and parkinsonism, considering the Lewy bodies only as a marker of neuronal pathology.

23.3 Lewy bodies and dementia

The relationship between Lewy bodies and dementia is complex because both cortical and subcortical pathological changes, affecting different neuronal systems, may be additive or potentiate one another (Gaspar & Gray, 1984; Yoshimura, 1988).

23.3.1 Subcortical involvement

In some cases the dementia may have a predominantly subcortical pathological substrate. Thus, some of the memory disturbances that can be found in patients with idiopathic parkinsonism might be due to neuronal loss in the nucleus basalis of Meynert. Indeed, the dysfunction of this ascending cholinergic system has been correlated with dementia in patients with idiopathic parkinsonism without concomitant cortical pathological changes (Whitehouse et al., 1983; Gaspar & Gray, 1984; Nakano & Hirano, 1984). Nevertheless, this finding is difficult to reconcile with the fact that patients with olivopontocerebellar degeneration sometimes show a severe neuronal depopulation in this nucleus but do not develop any cognitive deterioration (Berciano, 1993). Equally, there are several reports that some patients with idiopathic parkinsonism of long duration can show normal cognitive function despite severe pathology in the nucleus of Meynert (Quinn et al., 1989).

Dysfunction of the noradrenergic system has been implicated in the pathogenesis of dementia in Lewy body disease because the degree of neuronal loss in the locus coeruleus is greater in demented patients with Lewy body disease (Zweig et al., 1993). However, there are cases of parkinsonism of prolonged duration presenting with severe neuronal loss and Lewy bodies or neurofibrillary tangles in the locus coeruleus, but no dementia (Rajput et al., 1989; Paulus & Jellinger, 1991).

A dopaminergic dysfunction may also be implicated in the development of dementia in Lewy body disease (Eggerston & Sima, 1986). It is known that the neurons of the medial portion of the substantia nigra project mainly to the caudate nucleus, and to limbic and cortical areas (mesolimbic and mesocortical dopaminergic systems) (De Keyser et al., 1990), and a correlation has been recently demonstrated between dementia and neuronal loss in the medial substantia nigra (Rinne et al., 1989; Paulus & Jellinger, 1991). In addition, although more related to depression and bradyphrenia, damage of the ventral tegmental area (the other major origin of the mesolimbocortical dopaminergic system) could also play a role in the pathogenesis of dementia (Torack & Morris, 1988; Zweig et al., 1993).

23.3.2 Cortical involvement

The role of the cerebral cortex in the dementia associated with Lewy body disease is supported by the fact that the great majority of the patients with Lewy body disease who develop frank dementia have substantial pathological changes at the level of the cerebral cortex, showing a large number of cortical Lewy bodies (diffuse Lewy body disease) (Kosaka, 1993). In fact, diffuse Lewy body disease may be the second most common form of degenerative dementia after Alzheimer's disease (Byrne et al., 1989; Lennox et al., 1989a,b,c). Diverse denominations, such as 'cortical Lewy body dementia' (Gibb et al., 1989a), 'senile dementia of Lewy body type' (Perry et al., 1990a) and 'Lewy-body variant of Alzheimer's disease' (Hansen et al., 1990) are alternative names for this same entity, representing one end of the spectrum of Lewy body disease (Kosaka, 1993).

Two forms of diffuse Lewy body disease have been recognized: a common form associated with Alzheimer-type changes (senile plaques and neurofibrillary tangles), and a pure form without these changes (Kosaka, 1993). Although some authors have suggested that the association of Lewy bodies and Alzheimer-type changes might be due to chance alone (Gibb et al., 1989b), more brains with Alzheimer's disease have Lewy bodies within the substantia nigra than could be expected by the effect of the ageing alone, or chance association (Joachim et al., 1988; Pollanen et al., 1993). This supports the idea of a close relationship between these two entities (diffuse Lewy body disease and Alzheimer's disease) (Bergeron & Pollanen, 1989; Calne & Eisen, 1989). Furthermore, it is known that Lewy bodies contain neurofilaments that share epitopes with Alzheimer's neurofibrillary tangles, and may also contain beta-amyloid precursor proteins (Galloway et al., 1988; Arai et al., 1992). Biochemically there is an overlap between diffuse Lewy body disease and Alzheimer's disease (Whitehouse, 1989); for example, the cortical levels of somatostatin are reduced in both conditions (Dickson et al., 1987). Therefore, in the same way that Lewy body disease can display a spectrum of clinical dementia, there seems to be a spectrum of pathologic findings linking Lewy body disease, and Alzheimer's disease. Several possibilities could explain this association. For instance, Lewy body disease and Alzheimer's disease could be: (1) two different entities that share the same aetiology; or (2) two different manifestations of the same pathogenic process. These possibilities are illustrated in Fig 23.1.

It remains unclear whether the formation of Lewy bodies in both substantia nigra and cerebral cortex (and other areas of the nervous system) occurs simultaneously (Hughes et al., 1992). Curiously, the distribution of cortical Lewy bodies may coincide with the distribution of dopamine terminals or with the distribution of cortical neurons containing mRNA for tyrosine hydroxylase (Kuljis et al., 1989). So the dementia associated with Lewy body disease could be a predominantly dopaminergic dementia.

23.4 Lewy bodies and parkinsonism

In the absence of a definite biological marker, the presence of Lewy bodies in the substantia nigra remains a good diagnostic indicator for idiopathic parkinsonism. Thus, the diagnosis of idiopathic parkinsonism depends on the presence of Lewy bodies, the existence of depletion of dopaminergic neurons in the substantia nigra (over 50%), and the exclusion of other causes of parkinsonism. It has been suggested that idio-

A)

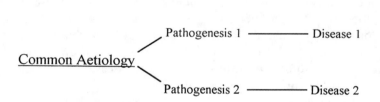

B)

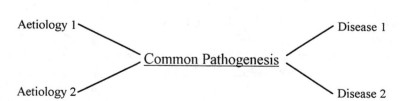

Fig. 23.1 Possible relationship between Lewy body disease and Alzheimer's disease. These putative mechanisms are predicated upon the disease resulting from an interaction between environmental and genetic factors.

pathic parkinsonism can be excluded if no Lewy bodies are found in two 7 μm-thick nigral sections, 330 pigmented nigral nerve cells, or 150 pigmented nerve cells in the locus coeruleus (Gibb, 1989). This proportion is built upon the premise that idiopathic parkinsonism *must* have nigral Lewy bodies; not all neurologists agree with these criteria (Duvoisin & Golbe, 1989).

A striking pathological finding in idiopathic parkinsonism is the characteristic distribution of the lesion in the substantia nigra, with severe loss of neurons in the ventrolateral region of the zona compacta (Hassler, 1938; Fearnley & Lees, 1991; Gibb & Lees, 1991; Fearnely & Lees, 1994). Why this region is more vulnerable to the pathologic process remains unclear; the answer to this question could provide important clues for understanding the pathogenesis and aetiology of idiopathic parkinsonism. Unfortunately, this topographic distribution of lesions in the substantia nigra is not specific for idiopathic parkinsonism, but can also be found in multiple system atrophy (Fearnley & Lees, 1991).

The significance of incidental Lewy bodies remains unclear, although many believe that these cases represent presymptomatic idiopathic parkinsonism. Supporting this contention is the fact that the distribution of nigral and extranigral lesions in these incidental Lewy body cases overlaps with symptomatic cases. Thus, there are Lewy bodies in the substantia nigra, and cell depletion, when present, occurs with preferential involvement of the ventrolateral region (Gibb & Lees, 1988; Fearnley & Lees, 1991; Gibb & Lees, 1991; Fearnley & Lees, 1994). Furthermore, in these cases the degree of neuronal loss in the substantia nigra is intermediate between normal and idiopathic parkinsonism, which agrees with the hypothesis of a clinically latent stage leading to a loss up to 80% of striatal dopamine and 50% of nigral neurons (Bernheimer et al., 1973; Kish et al., 1988; Fearnley & Lees, 1991). However, it is unclear whether the age-specific prevalence of 'incidental' Lewy bodies correlates with the age-specific prevalence of idiopathic parkinsonism (Gibb & Lees, 1988; Marttila, 1992 and Perry et al., 1990b).

There are other forms of neurodegenerative parkinsonism not associated with the presence of Lewy bodies. Most of them, however, have other histological markers, such as neurofibrillary tangles (progressive supranuclear palsy, Lytico-Bodig of Guam), oligodendroglial argyrophilic inclusions (multiple system atrophy), Pick bodies (Pick's disease), and achromatic neurons with basophilic inclusions (cortical-basal ganglionic degeneration). Although the topographic distribution of the lesions in these diseases tends to be more widespread than in idiopathic parkinsonism, there are cases (clinically indistinguishable from idiopathic parkinsonism) associated with neurofibrillary tangles in the substantia nigra and locus coeruleus alone (Forno & Alvord, 1971; Rajput et al., 1989). Why these patients react to the nigral insult with the formation of neurofibrillary tangles instead of Lewy bodies remains uncertain. One possibility is that these patients have been exposed to different environmental factors or different doses of the same factor. Four recently reported patients had an early onset parkinsonism (mean age, 40 years), suggesting that a different individual response (perhaps age-related) may be the cause of the appearance of different histological markers (Rajput et al., 1989).

Finally, 2% of the brains from parkinsonian patients show no histological marker, and there is only a severe neuronal loss in the substantia nigra (Hughes et al., 1992). If this subgroup represents a different pathological entity, it is possible that some of the cases labelled as Lewy body disease have in reality another kind of idiopathic neuronal degeneration of the substantia nigra *plus* incidental Lewy bodies.

23.5 Conclusions

Currently, very little is known about the structure and composition of Lewy bodies, and much less about their origin or the role that they might play in the pathogenesis of the disease(s) they define (Lewy body disease). However, despite the fact that they are not pathognomonic for any particular disease, in the absence of any more specific biological marker, Lewy bodies continue to be a useful tool to classify cases of idiopathic parkinsonism and/or dementia (and, less frequently, other clinical pictures).

The concept of Lewy body disease entails an enlarging spectrum of clinical and pathological manifestations. It constitutes the most common form of parkinsonism (idiopathic parkinsonism) and may be the second most common form of degenerative dementia (diffuse Lewy body disease) after Alzheimer's disease. As more is known about Lewy body disease, it begins to lose its clinical and pathological independence as a separate and individual entity. By analogy, we are using Lewy bodies to define disease as previous physicians might have used leukocytes before the discovery of infective microorganisms. We should not be lulled into the expectation that the study of Lewy bodies will reveal the aetiology of neurodegeneration, but we can anticipate that further understanding of their nature will unravel pathogenetic mechanisms. More than one histologic marker of pathology (e.g. Lewy bodies and neurofibrillary tangles) can be present within the same neuron. Occasionally we know the cause of neuronal death associated with these markers, as in the patient reported by Gibb et al. (1990) with subacute sclerosing panencephalitis. When we know how these intracellular structures are formed we may be able to draw some more insightful conclusions concerning the nature of so-called Lewy body disease.

Acknowledgements

Dr R. de la Fuente-Fernández is supported in part by a grant from the Xunta de Galicia, Spain. The collaboration of Susan Calne is gratefully appreciated. We also thank the Medical Research Council of Canada, The National Parkinson Foundation, the Parkinson Foundation of Canada, and the Movement Disorder Institute.

References

Alvord, E. C. Jr & Forno, L. S. (1992). Pathology. In *Handbook of Parkinson's disease*, 2nd edn. revised and expanded, ed. W. C. Koller, pp. 255–84. New York: Marcel Dekker.

Arai, H., Lee, V.M.-Y., Hill, W. D., Greenberg, B. D. & Trojanowski, J. Q. (1992). Lewy bodies contain beta-amyloid precursor proteins of Alzheimer's disease. *Brain Res., **585**, 386–90.

Berciano, J. (1993). Olivopontocerebellar atrophy. In *Parkinson's Disease and Movement Disorders*, 2nd edn. ed. J. Jankovic & E. Tolosa, pp. 163–89. Baltimore: Williams & Wilkins.

Bergeron, C. & Pollanen, M. (1989). Lewy bodies in Alzheimer disease: One or two diseases? *Alzheimer Dis. Assoc. Disord.*, **3**, 197–204.

Bernheimer, H., Birkmayer, W., Hornykiewicz, O., Jellinger, K. & Seitelberger, F. (1973). Brain dopamine and the syndromes of Parkinson and Huntington: Clinical, morphological and neurochemical correlations. *J. Neurol. Sci.*, **20**, 415–55.

Byrne, E. J., Lennox, G., Lowe, J. & Godwin-Austen, R. B. (1989). Diffuse Lewy body disease: Clinical features in 15 cases. *J. Neurol., Neurosurg. Psychiatry*, **52**, 709–17.

Calne, D. B. (1989). Is 'Parkinson's disease' one disease? *J. Neurol., Neurosurgery and Psychiatry*, Special Supplement, 18–21.

Calne, D. B. (1994). Is idiopathic parkinsonism the consequence of an event or a process? *Neurology*, **44**, 5–10.

Calne, D. B. & Eisen, A. (1989). The relationship between Alzheimer's disease, Parkinson's disease and motor neuron disease. *Can. J. Neurol. Sci.*, **16**, 547–50.

Calne, D. B., Snow, B. J. & Lee, C. (1992). Criteria for diagnosing Parkinson's disease. *Ann. Neurol.*, **32**, S125–7.

Crystal, H. A., Dickson, D. W., Lizardi, J. E., Davies, P. & Wolfson, L. I. (1990). Antemortem diagnosis of diffuse Lewy body disease. *Neurology*, **40**, 1523–8.

De Keyser, J., Herregodts, P. & Ebinger, G. (1990). The mesoneocortical dopamine neuron system. *Neurology*, **40**, 1660–2.

Dickson, D. W., Davies, P., Mayeux, R. et al. (1987). Diffuse Lewy body disease: Neuropathological and biochemical studies of six patients. *Acta Neuropathologica*, **75**, 8–15.

Duvoisin, R. C. & Golbe, L. I. (1989). Toward a definition of Parkinson's disease. *Neurology*, **39**, 746.

Eggerston, D. E. & Sima, A. A. F. (1986). Dementia with cerebral Lewy bodies. A mesocortical dopaminergic defect? *Arch. Neurol.*, **43**, 524–7.

Fearnley, J. M. & Lees, A. J. (1991). Ageing and Parkinson's disease: Substantia nigra regional selectivity. *Brain*, **114**, 2283–301.

Fearnley, J. & Lees, A. (1994). Pathology of Parkinson's disease. In *Neurodegenerative Diseases*, ed. D. B. Cane, pp. 545–54. Philadelphia: W. B. Saunders Company.

Fearnley, J. M., Revesz, T., Brooks, D. J., Frackowiak, R. S. & Lees, A. J. (1991). Diffuse Lewy body disease presenting with a supranuclear gaze palsy. *J. Neurol., Neurosurg. Psychiatry*, **54**, 159–61.

Forno, L. S. (1969). Concentric hyalin intraneuronal inclusions of Lewy type in the brains of elderly persons (50 incidental cases): Relationship to parkinsonism. *J. Am. Geriatr. Soc.*, **17**, 557–75.

Forno, L. S. (1986). The Lewy body in Parkinson's disease. In *Parkinson's disease. Advances in Neurology*, vol. 45, ed. M. D. Yahr & K. J. Bergmann, pp. 35–43. New York: Raven Press.

Forno, L. S. & Alvord, E. C. (1971). The pathology of parkinsonism. In *Recent Advances in Parkinson's Disease*, ed. F. H. McDowell & C. H. Markham, pp. 120–61. Oxford: Blackwell.

Forno, L. S., DeLanney, L. E., Irwin, I. & Langston, J. W. (1993). Similarities and differences between MPTP-induced parkinsonism and Parkinson's disease: Neuropathologic considerations. In *Parkinson's disease: From Basic Research to Treatment. Advances in Neurology*, vol. 60, ed. H. Narabayashi, T. Nagatsu, N. Yanagisawa & Y. Mizuno, pp. 600–8. New York: Raven Press.

Galloway, P. G., Grundke-Iqbal, I., Iqbal, K. & Perry, G. (1988). Lewy bodies contain epitopes both shared and distinct from Alzheimer neurofibrillary tangles. *J. Neuropathol. Exp. Neurol.*, **47**, 654–63.

Gaspar, P. & Gray, F. (1984). Dementia in idiopathic Parkinson's disease: A neuropathological study of 32 cases. *Acta Neuropathol.*, **64**, 43–52.

Gibb, W. R. G. (1988). The Lewy body and autonomic failure. In *Autonomic Failure*, 2nd edn. ed. R. Bannister, pp. 484–97. Oxford: Oxford University Press.

Gibb, W. R. G. (1989). Neuropathology in movement disorders. *J. Neurol., Neurosurg. Psychiatry*, Special Supplement, 55–67.

Gibb, W. R. G. & Lees, A. J. (1988). The relevance of the Lewy body to the pathogenesis of idiopathic Parkinson's disease. *J. Neurol., Neurosurg. Psychiatry*, **51**, 745–52.

Gibb, W. R. G. & Lees, A. J. (1989). The significance of the Lewy body in the diagnosis of idiopathic Parkinson's disease. *Neuropathol. Appl. Neurobiol.*, **15**, 27–44.

Gibb, W. R. G. & Lees, A. J. (1991). Anatomy, pigmentation, ventral and dorsal subpopulations of the substantia nigra, and differential cell death in Parkinson's disease. *J. Neurol. Neurosurg. Psychiatry*, **54**, 388–96.

Gibb, W. R. G., Esiri, M. M. & Lees, A. J. (1987). Clinical and pathological features of diffuse cortical Lewy body disease (Lewy body dementia). *Brain*, **110**, 1131–53.

Gibb, W. R. G., Luthert, P. J., Janota, I. & Lantos, P. L. (1989a). Cortical Lewy body dementia: Clinical features and classification. *J. Neurol., Neurosurg. Psychiatry*, **52**, 185–92.

Gibb, W. R. G., Mountjoy, C. Q., Mann, D. M. A. & Lees, A. J. (1989b). A pathological study of the association between Lewy body disease and Alzheimer's disease. *J. Neurol., Neurosurg. Psychiatry*, **52**, 701–8.

Gibb, W. R. G., Scaravilli, F. & Michaud, J. (1990). Lewy bodies and subacute sclerosing panencephalitis. *J. Neurol. Neurosurg. Psychiatry*, **53**, 710–11.

Golbe, L. I., Di Iorio, G., Bonavita, V., Miller, D. C. & Duvoisin, R. C. (1990). A large kindred with autosomal dominant Parkinson's disease. *Ann. Neurol.*, **27**, 276–82.

Hansen, L., Salmon, D., Galasko, D. et al. (1990). The Lewy body variant of Alzheimer's disease: A clinical and pathologic entity. *Neurology*, **40**, 1–8.

Hassler, R. (1938). Zur Pathologie der Paralysis agitans und des postenzephalitischen Parkinsonismus. *J. Psychologie Neurologie*, **48**, 387–476.

Hughes, A. J., Daniel, S. E., Kilford, L. & Lees, A. J. (1992). Accuracy of clinical diagnosis of idiopathic Parkinson's disease: A clinico-pathological study of 100 cases. *J. Neurol. Neurosurg. Psychiatry*, **55**, 181–4.

Joachim, C. L., Morris, J. H. & Selkoe, D. J. (1988). Clinically diagnosed Alzheimer's disease. Autopsy results in 150 cases. *Ann. Neurol.*, **24**, 50–6.

Kato, T., Katagiri, T., Hirano, A., Sasaki, H. & Arai, S. (1988). Sporadic lower motor neuron disease with Lewy body-like inclusions: A new subgroup? *Acta Neuropathol.*, **76**, 208–11.

Kish, S. J., Shannak, K. & Hornykiewicz, O. (1988). Uneven pattern of dopamine loss in the striatum of patients with idiopathic Parkinson's disease: Pathophysiologic and clinical implications. *New Engl. J. Med.*, **318**, 876–80.

Kosaka, K. (1993). Dementia and neuropathology in Lewy body disease. In *Parkinson's disease: From Basic Research to Treatment. Advances of Neurology*, vol. 60. ed. H. Narabayashi, T. Nagatsu, N. Yanagisawa & Y. Mizuno, pp. 456–463. New York: Raven Press.

Kuljis, R. O., Martin-Vasallo, P. & Peress, N. S. (1989). Lewy bodies in tyrosine hydroxylase-synthesizing neurons of the human cerebral cortex. *Neurosci. Lett.*, **106**, 49–54.

Langston, J. W. & Ballard, P. (1984). Parkinsonism induced by 1-methyl-r-phenyl-1,2,3,6-tetrahydropropyridine (MPTP): Implications for the treatment and pathogenesis of Parkinson's disease. *Can. J. Neurol. Sci.*, **11**, 160–5.

Lennox, G., Lowe, J. S., Godwin-Austen, R. B., Landon, M. & Mayer, R. J. (1989a). Diffuse Lewy body disease: An important differential diagnosis in dementia with extrapyramidal features. *Prog. Clin. Bio. Res.*, **317**, 121–30.

Lennox, G., Lowe, J., Landon, M., Byrne, E. J., Mayer, R. J. & Godwin-Austen, R. B. (1989b). Diffuse Lewy body disease: Correlative neuropathology using anti-ubiquitin immunocytochemistry. *J. Neurol. Neurosurg. Psychiatry*, **52**, 1236–47.

Lennox, G., Lowe, J., Morrell, K., Landon, M. & Mayer, R. J. (1989c). Anti-ubiquitin immunocytochemistry is more sensitive than conventional techniques in the detection of diffuse Lewy body disease. *J. Neurol. Neurosurg. Psychiatry*, **52**, 67–71.

Lewy, F. H. (1912). Paralysis agitans I. Pathologische anatomie. In *Handbuch der Neurologie*, vol. 3, ed. M. Lewandowsky, pp. 920–33. Berlin: Springer.

Lowe, J. (1994). Lewy bodies. In *Neurodegenerative Diseases*, ed. D. B. Calne, pp. 51–69. Philadelphia: W.B. Saunders.

Mark, M. H., Sage, J. I., Dickson, D. W. et al. (1994). Meige syndrome in the spectrum of Lewy body disease. *Neurology*, **44**, 1432–6.

Marttila, R. J. (1992). Epidemiology. In *Handbook of Parkinson's Disease*, 2nd edn. revised and expanded, ed. W. C. Koller, pp. 35–57. New York: Marcel Dekker.

Nakano, I. & Hirano, A. (1984). Parkinson's disease: Neuron loss in the nucleus basalis without concomitant Alzheimer's disease. *Annals of Neurology*, **15**, 415–18.

Parkinson, J. (1817). *An Essay on the Shaking Palsy*. London: Whittingham and Rowland, for Sherwood, Neely, and Jones.

Paulus, W. & Jellinger, K. (1991). The neuropathologic basis of different clinical subgroups of Parkinson's disease. *J. Neuropathol. Exp. Neurol.*, **50**, 743–55.

Perry, R. H., Irving, D., Blessed, G., Fairbairn, A. & Perry, E. K. (1990a). Senile dementia of Lewy body type: A clinically and neuropathologically distinct form of Lewy body dementia in the elderly. *J. Neurol. Sci.*, **95**, 119–39.

Perry, R. H., Irving, D. & Tomlinson, B. E. (1990b). Lewy body prevalence in the aging brain: Relationship to neuropsychiatric disorders, Alzheimer-type pathology and catecholaminergic nuclei. *J. Neurol. Sci.*, **100**, 223–33.

Pollanen, M. S., Dickson, D. W. & Bergeron, C. (1993). Pathology and biology of the Lewy body. *J. Neuropathol. Exp. Neurol.*, **52**, 183–91.

Quinn, N. P., Luthert, P., Honavar, M. & Marsden, C. D. (1989). Pure akinesia due to Lewy body Parkinson's disease: A case with pathology. *Mov. Disord.*, **4**, 85–9.

Rajput, A. H., Uitti, R. J., Sudhakar, S. & Rozdilsky, B. (1989). Parkinsonism and neurofibrillary tangle pathology in pigmented nuclei. *Ann. Neurol.*, **25**, 602–6.

Rinne, J. O., Rummukainen, J., Paljärvi, L. & Rinne, U. K. (1989). Dementia in Parkinson's disease is related to neuronal loss in the medial substantia nigra. *Ann. Neurol.*, **26**, 47–50.

Torack, R. M. & Morris, J. C. (1988). The association of ventral tegmental area histopathology with adult dementia. *Arch. Neurol.*, **45**, 4097–501.

Trétiakoff, C. (1919). Contribution à l'étude de l'anatomie pathologique du locus niger de Soemmering avec quelques déductions relatives à la pathogénie des troubles du tonus musculaire et de la maladie de Parkinson. (Thesis). Paris, University of Paris.

Whitehouse, P. J. (1989). Parkinson's disease and Alzheimer's disease: New neurochemical parallels. *Mov. Disord.*, **4** (Suppl 1), 57–62.

Whitehouse, P. J., Hedreen, J. C., White, C. L. & Price, D. L. (1983). Basal forebrain neurons in the dementia of Parkinson's disease. *Ann. Neurol.*, **13**, 243–8.

Yoshimura, M. (1988). Pathological basis for dementia in elderly patients with idiopathic Parkinson's disease. *Euro. Neurol.*, **28**, 29–35.

Zweig, R. M., Cardillo, J. E., Cohen, M., Giere, S. & Hedreen, J. C. (1993). The locus ceruleus and dementia in Parkinson's disease. *Neurology*, **43**, 986–91.

24

Pathogenesis of the Lewy body

C. BERGERON and M. S. POLLANEN

Summary

The constitutive fibrils of the Lewy body contain all three neurofilament subunits in an altered form. Our recent in situ hybridization studies of the low molecular weight subunit of the neurofilament suggest that altered neurofilament expression is not implicated in the formation of the Lewy body. Using the Mallory body of the liver as a dynamic model of intermediate filament inclusion formation, we also demonstrated that the filaments are first normally assembled and modified in a subsequent step. We propose a speculative model of Lewy body pathogenesis in which neurofilaments are assembled normally and subsequently undergo phosphorylation, proteolysis and crosslinking at a post-translational/post-assembly stage.

24.1 Introduction

The Lewy body (LB) is a major pathological feature of Lewy body disorders including idiopathic Parkinson's disease (PD) and diffuse Lewy body disease (DLB). As we discussed in our recent review (Pollanen et al., 1993), direct and indirect analysis of the LB has shown that its constitutive fibrils contain all three neurofilament (NF) subunits of molecular weights 68 kD (NF-L), 150 kD (NF-M) and 200 kD (NF-H) in both phosphorylated and nonphosphorylated forms. The NF epitopes are spatially distributed with a predominance of NF-L or amino-termini of NF subunits in the central portion of the inclusion, a phenomenon which suggests a possible segregation of proteolytic fragments. The presence of ubiquitin, ubiquitin-C-terminal hydrolase and ingestin (multicatalytic proteinase or proteasome) in the LB also suggests that proteolysis is implicated in its pathogenesis. Finally, the detergent-insolubility of these fibrils indicates that the NF proteins which form the LB are further altered and probably crosslinked. Taken together, these studies suggest that altered phosphorylation/dephosphorylation and proteolysis of NF are key post-translational events in LB pathogenesis. We have so far been unable to define the sequence of events which underlie LB formation because of the lack of a suitable tissue culture or animal model. We also have limited knowledge of neurofilament expression in LB disorders. In this communication we discuss the contribution of NF expression to LB pathogenesis as well as the use of the Mallory body as a dynamic model of LB formation.

24.2 Neurofilament expression in Lewy body disorders

We recently performed in situ hybridization (ISH) using a tritiated riboprobe to measure the mRNA levels of the low molecular weight neurofilament subunit (NF-L) in the nigral dopaminergic neurons of Lewy body disorders (Bergeron et al., 1996). We found a small but significant decrease in the NF-L mRNA levels of the LB group when compared with age matched controls. When we compared the NF-L mRNA levels in LB bearing neurons with that observed in non-Lewy body bearing neurons in a direct paired study, however, we were unable to demonstrate a significant difference in NF-L mRNA levels between these two neuronal populations. These results suggest that NF expression is unlikely to represent an important step in the development of LB.

The difference observed between the LB and control groups in the overall nigral dopaminergic neuronal population, which consists mostly of non-LB bearing neurons, probably reflects a non-specific response to neuronal injury and is independent of LB formation. Such a decrease in NF mRNA levels is seen in several other pathological conditions including Alzheimer's disease (Somerville et al., 1991) and amyotrophic lateral sclerosis (ALS) (Bergeron et al., 1994).

24.2.1 *The Mallory body as a model*

Both the LB and the Mallory body (MB) of the liver (found in alcoholic liver disease) are composed of aggregates of intermediate filaments which are native to the cell type in which the inclusion is found. Although biochemical studies of the LB are limited to material extracted from postmortem human brain, MBs can be produced in murine models by chemical induction (Denk et al., 1976). The remarkable biochemical similarities of LBs and MBs indicate that studies of induced MBs may provide basic information relevant to both LB and MB pathogenesis.

Previous biochemical studies on murine MBs indicate that MB filaments are composed of cytokeratin isoforms which are constitutively expressed in the hepatocyte (Denk et al., 1979, 1982; Franke et al., 1979). Similarly, studies of filaments derived from LBs extracted from diffuse LB diseased brain indicate that all three of the constitutively expressed neurofilament gene products are present in the LB. This finding suggests that LB filaments are NFs which have been appropriately assembled from the intermediate filament subunits. To model the assembly process of LB filaments we have used the experimentally induced MB filament and studied the assembly of these filaments in vitro (Pollanen et al., 1994).

This experimental approach was based on the previously well-studied mechanism of intermediate filament assembly. Intermediate filaments assemble via a hierarchy of filamentous precursors by a process that can be reproduced in vitro (van de Klundert et al., 1993). Studies using this approach have revealed that intermediate filaments assemble from polymers which spontaneously organize into protofilaments, subsequently form protofibrils and then intermediate filaments (Aebi et al., 1983). The precursors 'subfilaments' have a highly conserved 21 nm axial periodicity which is a structural feature indicative of appropriate filament assembly (Milam & Erickson, 1982).

The in vitro reassembled normal liver cytokeratin and MB-derived cytokeratin filaments had a similar ultrastructural appearance. In both cases, aggregates of electron-dense filaments ranging in diameter from 2 to 11 nm which corresponded to the previously reported structural precursor 'subfilaments' which associate and intertwine to produce cytokeratin intermediate filaments were observed. Many protofilaments showed direct transition to higher order structures indicating the later stages of intermediate filament assembly.

The fine-structure of the reassembled filaments was also assessed with atomic force microscopy. No structural differences were observed in the morphologic appearance of the protofilaments ($\sim$1.2 nm), protofibrils ($\sim$2.4 nm) and intermediate filaments (9–11 nm) in preparations of reassembled normal liver or MB-derived cytokeratin. The axial periodicities for the protofilaments and protofibrils of both the reassembled normal liver cytokeratin and MB filaments were similar and measured approximately 21 nm.

The similarity in the fine structure and axial periodicities of reassembled protofilaments derived from normal and pathological filaments indicates that the assembly process of MB-derived subunits is not impaired or otherwise different from the situation of normal filament assembly. The most important implication of the normal in vitro reassembly of MB filaments is the implication for the ordering of the molecular events of MB pathogenesis. These data indicate that cytokeratin proteins may either be directly incorporated into pre-existing MB filaments or first assembled into intermediate filaments prior to incorporation into the MB.

If MBs are a legitimate model for LBs, it is likely that LB pathogenesis is characterized by normal neurofilament assembly, and a post-translation/post-assembly event(s) renders the filaments insoluble and pathological.

24.2.2 Pathogenesis of the Lewy body

On the basis of these and other studies we would like to propose the following speculative model of LB formation (Fig. 24.1). Based on our

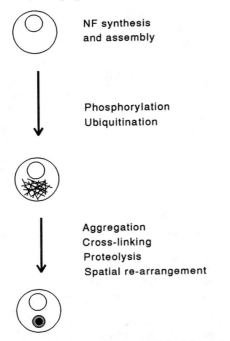

NF synthesis
and assembly

Phosphorylation
Ubiquitination

Aggregation
Cross-linking
Proteolysis
Spatial re-arrangement

Fig. 24.1 A speculative model of Lewy body pathogenesis.

ISH and Mallory body studies, it is likely that the neurofilament subunits are assembled normally and subsequently modified at the post-translational level. An early step in LB pathogenesis is probably the accumulation of aberrantly phosphorylated NF aggregates in the neuronal cytoplasm as a pre-Lewy body or pale body; the presence of ubiquitin in a subset of pale bodies (Dale et al., 1992) suggests that ubiquitination occurs as a second step, followed by partial proteolysis. The latter transformation is accompanied by a spatial reorganization of the accumulated neurofilaments with the segregation of NF proteolytic fragments in the central part of the LB and the appearance of the typical LB core (Hill et al., 1991). Additional modifications, as yet unknown, are necessary to crosslink the filaments and render them insoluble. In the Mallory body model this occurs in the latest stage of development and it is associated with the formation of covalent crosslinks by γ-glutamyl-ϵ-lysine. In contrast, the LB can be solubilized in formic acid, suggesting a different noncovalent interaction. Glycation, which was recently observed in Alzheimer neurofibrillary tangles in the context of oxidative stress (Smith et al., 1994), could account for such a crosslink. Recent studies demonstrating extensive NF modifications after their exposure to oxidative stress in vitro (Montine et al., 1995; Troncoso et al., 1995) and the presence of increased SOD-1 immunoreactivity in the periphery of the LB also support this hypothesis (Nishikawa et al., 1995).

Further studies of the Mallory body model, continuing analysis of the LB, and further in vitro manipulation of NFs will likely provide new insights in the pathogenesis of the LB and of other events implicated in neuronal degeneration and death in LB disorders.

References

Aebi, U., Fowler, W., Rew, P. & Sun, T.-T. (1983). The fibrillar substructure of keratin filaments unraveled. *J. Cell Biol.*, **97**, 1131–43.

Bergeron, C., Beric-Maskarel, K., Muntasser, S., Weyer, L., Somerville, M. J. & Percy, M. E. (1994). Neurofilament light and polyadenylated mRNA levels are decreased in amyotrophic lateral sclerosis motor neurons. *J. Neuropathol. Exp. Neurol.*, **53**, 221–30.

Bergeron, C., Petrunka, C., Weyer, L., Pollanen, M.S. (1996). Altered neurofilament expression does not contribute to Lewy body formation. *Am J. Pathol.*, **148**, 267–72.

Dale, G., Probst, A., Luthert, P., Martin, J., Anderton, B. & Leigh, P. (1992). Relationship between Lewy bodies and pale bodies in Parkinson's disease. *Acta Neuropathol.*, **83**, 525–9.

Denk, H., Eckerstorfer, R., Gschnait, F., Konrad, K. & Wolff, K. (1976). Experimental induction of hepatocellular hyaline (Mallory bodies) in mice by griseofulvin treatment: 1. Light microscopic observations. *Lab. Invest.*, **35**, 377–82.

Denk, H., Franke, W., Kerjaschki, D. & Eckerstorfer, R. (1979). Mallory bodies in experimental animals and man. *Int. Rev. Exp. Pathol.*, **20**, 77–121.

Denk, H., Krepler, R., Lackinger, E., Artlieb, U. & Franke, W. (1982). Immunological and biochemical characterization of the keratin-related component of Mallory bodies: a pathological pattern of hepatocytic cytokeratins. *Liver*, **2**, 165–75.

Franke, W., Denk, H., Schmid, E., Osborn, M. & Weber, K. (1979). Ultrastructural, biochemical and immunological characterization of Mallory bodies in livers of griseofulvin-treated mice. Fimbriated rods of filaments containing prekeratin-like polypeptides. *Lab. Invest.*, **40.**, 207–20.

Hill, W. D., Lee, V. M.-Y., Hurtig, H. I., Murray, J. M. & Trojanowski, J. Q. (1991). Epitopes located in spatially separate domains of each neurofilament subunit are present in Parkinson's disease Lewy bodies. *J. Comp. Neurol.*, **309**, 150–60.

Milam, L. & Erickson, H. (1982). Visualization of a 21-nm axial periodicity in shadowed keratin filaments and neurofilaments. *J. Cell Biol.*, **94**, 592–6.

Montine, T. J., Farris, D. B. & Graham, D. G. (1995). Covalent crosslinking of neurofilament proteins by oxidized catechols as a potential mechanism of Lewy body formation. *J. Neuropathol. Exp. Neurol.*, **54**, 311–19.

Nishikawa, K., Murayama, S., Shimizu, J. et al. (1995). Cu/Zn superoxide dismutase-like immunoreactivity is present in Lewy bodies from Parkinson's disease: a light and electron microscopic immunocytochemical study. *Acta Neuropathol.*, **89**, 471–4.

Pollanen, M. S., Dickson, D. W. & Bergeron, C. (1993). Pathology and biology of the Lewy body. *J. Neuropathol. Exp. Neurol.*, **52**, 183–91.

Pollanen, M. S., Markiewicz, P., Weyer, L., Goh, M. C. & Bergeron, C. (1994). Mallory body filaments become insoluble after normal assembly into intermediate filaments. *Am. J. Pathol.*, **145**, 140–7.

Smith, M. A., Taneda, S., Richey, P. L. et al. (1994). Advanced Maillard reaction end products are associated with Alzheimer disease pathology. *Proc. Natl. Acad. Sci. USA*, **91**, 5710–14.

Somerville, M. J., Percy, M. E., Bergeron, C., Yoong, L. K. K., Grima, E. A. & McLachlan, D. R. C. (1991). Localization and quantitation of 68 kDA neurofilament and superoxide dismutase-1 mRNA in Alzheimer brain. *Mol. Brain Res.*, **9**, 1–8.

Troncoso, J. C., Costello, A. C., Kim, J. H. & Johnson, G. V. W. (1995). Metal-catalyzed oxidation of bovine neurofilaments in vitro. *Free Radical Biol. Med.*, **18**, 891–9.

van de Klundert, F., Raats, J. & Bleomendal, H. (1993). Intermediate filaments; regulation, gene expression and assembly. *Eur. J. Biochem.*, **214**, 351–66.

25

Altered tau processing: its role in development of dementia in Alzheimer's disease and Lewy body disease

C. R. HARRINGTON, M. ROTH and
C. M. WISCHIK

Summary

Altered processing of tau protein is a characteristic feature of Alzheimer's disease (AD) that, unlike the accumulation of amyloid β-protein, is strongly correlated with clinical dementia. In AD, tau is substantially redistributed from its soluble, predominantly axonal form into insoluble PHF-tau that accumulates in the somatodendritic compartment. Although hyperphosphorylated tau also accumulates, this accounts for no more than 5% of the total PHF-tau during any stage of the development of AD. In contrast, cortical Lewy body dementia in the elderly is not associated with these changes in tau processing and such patients have less than one-tenth of the levels of both PHF-tau and neurofibrillary pathology as those found in AD. These findings support the notion that the pathobiology of these two disorders is distinct and provide the opportunity to compare non-PHF- with PHF-type dementias. Both these late-onset dementias are associated with comparable increases in the frequency of the apolipoprotein E (APO E) type $\epsilon4$ allele (in excess of 30%, as compared with 14% in controls and 10% in Parkinson's disease). The extent of abnormal PHF-tau levels in AD is unaffected by the presence of an $\epsilon4$ allele, suggesting that APO E polymorphisms do not directly influence the pathological processing of tau. These findings suggest that cortical Lewy body dementia has an aetiopathogenesis that is distinct from AD. Furthermore, APO E polymorphisms influence the development of dementia in both AD and cortical, but not subcortical Lewy body disease by mechanisms(s) that remain to be identified.

25.1 Introduction

The discovery of cortical Lewy body dementia as a new form of primary dementia with a clinical picture distinct from Alzheimer's disease (AD) provides a new avenue with which to investigate the molecular basis of dementia in the elderly. A detailed comparison between structural, biochemical and molecular changes in AD and Lewy body dementia should assist in deciding which molecular lesions are both specific and essential for dementia and, therefore, of central importance to the particular phenotype. It was this possibility that prompted us to investigate the biochemical changes in Lewy body dementia, studies which in turn led us to a number of new observations that have relevance for the pathogenesis of not only Lewy body dementia, but also AD.

The pathology of Alzheimer's disease is characterized by the presence of neurofibrillary tangles and neuritic plaques in medial temporal cortex and other neocortical regions of the brain. Several studies have demonstrated that the neurofibrillary lesions are stronger indicators of clinical dementia than the extracellular deposits of amyloid β-protein (Aβ) within plaques. Neurofibrillary tangles, neuritic plaques and dystrophic neurites throughout the neuropil share the presence of paired helical filaments (PHFs) that constitute the neurofibrillary lesions. The molecular biology that surrounds the deposition of Aβ in AD and the processing of its precursor protein has been the subject of extensive investigations. In contrast to Aβ, it is only recently that the biology of neurofibrillary pathology has been addressed by a growing number of investigators. This has meant that a Schmitt Symposium, held in May 1994, was the first meeting virtually dedicated to discussions on the neurofibrillary alterations in AD. For more detailed references, the reader is directed to a special issue that was prepared in conjunction with the latter meeting and which reviews in detail much of our current understanding of tau pathology in AD (Coleman et al., 1995), and to a recent review (Wischik et al., 1995a).

25.2 Structure and composition of PHFs

Neurofibrillary tangles are found within the somatodendritic compartment of large pyramidal cells. Their formation is closely linked with the death of these cells, leaving the residue of a 'ghost' extracellular tangle. The main structural constituent of these tangles is the PHF. Tau protein is the only protein representing an integral constituent of the core struc-

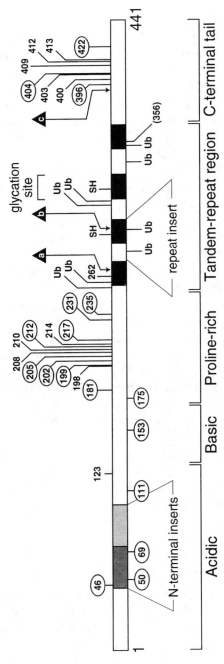

Fig. 25.1 Tau protein – its domains and post-translational modifications. The largest tau isoform in the human brain is 441 amino acid residues in length, including two N-terminal inserts and tandem repeat insert. Residue numbers above and below the sequence correspond to Ser or Thr phosphorylation sites. The residues above are those which have been identified in tau and/or PHF-tau by mass spectrometry or by the use of site-specific, phosphorylation-dependent antibodies. Most phosphorylation sites flank the tandem-repeat region and only Ser-262 is within the repeats, although it remains outwith the PHF-core tau fragment. The latter truncated fragment corresponds to the region, indicated by the arrows, between Leu-266 (a), or Ile-297 (b), through to Glu-391 [recognized by mAb 423] (c). The latter fragment also contains the mab 7.51 epitope (residues 350–368). Putative phosphorylation sites that have not been identified in vivo are indicated below. SH denotes the two Cys residues in the repeat region that can potentially form either intra- or inter-chain disulfide bonds. At least four lysine residues in PHF-tau serve as ubiquitin acceptors and these are all within the microtubule-binding region (U; indicated above the sequence) (Morishima-Kawashima et al., 1993). Evidence of four other possible ubiquitination sites (U; below the sequence) has yet to be confirmed. A prominent site of glycation in PHF-tau has been identified within residues 317–335, a sequence containing three Lys residues (Ledesma, Bonay & Avila, 1995).

ture of the PHF (Wischik et al., 1988). In the adult human brain, tau protein exists in six isoforms, ranging from 352 to 441 amino acids in length, and derived by alternative splicing of mRNA encoded by a single gene located on chromosome 17q21 (Goedert, 1993). No mutations or polymorphisms in this gene have been identified. Tau exists as a family of phosphoproteins and the expression of the different tau isoforms and the extent to which they are phosphorylated are both developmentally regulated (Goedert, 1993). The isoforms contain either three- or four-tandem repeat domains of 31 or 32 amino acids, each containing an 18-residue tubulin-binding domain (Fig. 25.1).

Tau extracted from PHF-core preparations is derived from both the three- and four-repeat isoforms, but is restricted to the length of three repeats (Jakes et al., 1991). Thus it is 93/95 residues in length but shifted with respect to the tandem repeats, such that it starts within the first repeat of the three-repeat isoform, or within the second repeat of the four-repeat isoform, and terminates C-terminal to the repeat domains at Glu-391. Truncation at Glu-391 creates an epitope that is specifically recognized by the monoclonal antibody (mAb) 423 (Novak et al., 1993; see Fig. 25.1). Thus the limits for proteolytic susceptibility differ between normal tau and PHF-core tau, indicating that the method of incorporation of tau into PHFs is distinct from its involvement in microtubule assembly. PHFs are surrounded by a protease-sensitive fuzzy coat that contains epitopes to those domains that are N- and C-terminal to the core PHF-tau. These include all of the sites of phosphorylation that have been identified (see Fig. 25.1). The binding of full-length tau to the core PHF makes no structural contribution to the regular paracrystalline structure of the core indicating that the structural integrity of the PHF is dependent neither on the presence of the full length of the molecule nor on the phosphorylation of tau protein at sites not present in the core PHF-tau. Based upon molecular mass measurements, it is considered that only one in six molecules of the PHF extends to the N-terminus (Wischik et al., 1995a).

25.3 Post-translational modifications of tau protein

Tau proteins are susceptible to a number of post-translational modifications that may be important in the assembly of PHFs in AD. These include phosphorylation, ubiquitination, glycation, oxidation and proteolysis, and sites at which such changes have been identified are summarized in Fig. 25.1.

Despite a wealth of experimental data (predominantly in vitro) on these modifications, the temporal sequence with which these changes occur and the relative importance of specific changes is uncertain. This does not infer that only the early events need be important. For example, a modification that occurs after the formation of PHFs could lead to inadequate clearance of PHFs or induce an abnormal cellular response in the brain. Both of these circumstances, despite occurring late on in the process, would still be pathologically important in disease development.

Phosphorylation of tau protein suppresses its competence in the assembly of microtubules in vitro. There are many sites of phosphorylation in tau and all, with the exception of Ser-262, are outwith the tandem repeat region (Fig. 25.1). With the discovery that normal adult tau from epileptic brain tissue is subjected to rapid dephosphorylation over time after re-section (Matsuo et al., 1994), it is now the extent of tau phosphorylation rather than the *abnormal* phosphorylation of disease-specific sites that is distinctive in AD. Although exact levels remain to be quantified, the extent of tau phosphorylation is greatest in PHF-tau, then fetal tau and, finally, normal adult tau. Thus one might best use the term *hyperphosphorylated* tau to describe the type of tau found in AD brains.

A molecular study of early stage AD found that no more than 5% of PHF-tau is phosphorylated, an amount that is inadequate to account for the substantial accumulation of PHFs found in AD (Wischik et al., 1995b). Likewise, a proportion of neurofibrillary tangles can develop in neurons in the absence of hyperphosphorylation (Bondareff et al., 1995). These studies indicate that phosphorylation of tau may be a secondary event. Furthermore hyperphosphorylation is found in neurodegenerative disorders other than AD, such as Lewy body disease (see below), progressive supranuclear palsy and amyotrophic lateral sclerosis–parkinsonism dementia complex of Guam. This suggests that the presence of hyperphosphorylated tau may be a phenomenon that is more general than in just AD.

Tau proteins can be glycated in vitro and advanced glycation endproducts (AGEs) colocalize with both neurofibrillary tangles and PHFs. PHF-tau isolated from the brains of AD patients is glycated in the tubulin-binding region present in tau (Ledesma et al., 1995; see Fig. 25.1). AGE formation can result in production of free radicals which can cause oxidative damage to proteins and other macromolecules. Glycated tau, introduced into cultivated cells, can generate oxygen-free radicals capable of disturbing neuronal function (Yan et al., 1995). The two Cys residues in the tubulin-binding domain are particularly prone to oxidative damage and such alterations could lead to protein cross-linking. This would accelerate polymer aggregation and the oxidized protein would also serve as a substrate for ubiquitin. Aggregation of tau might also result from the action of transglutaminase.

The accumulation of truncated tau protein in a particular conformational state in the PHF core has been considered as an important feature in AD, that does not necessarily rely upon post-translational modifications of tau protein (Wischik et al., 1995a).

25.4 Tau processing in vivo

The antigenic features of pathological tau protein present in core PHFs can be defined by two independent immunochemical procedures (Harrington et al., 1991); first, C-terminal truncation at Glu-391 which is detected by mAb 423 and second, acid-reversible occlusion of a generic tau epitope located in the tandem repeat region of tau detected by mAb 7.51 (see Fig. 25.1). That is, while mAb 7.51 can recognize normal tau protein, its epitope in PHF-bound tau is revealed only after acid exposure. The mAb 7.51 recognizes an epitope contained within the final tubulin-binding domain of four-repeat tau that is present in all six isoforms of tau. Taken together, the data suggest that the epitope for mAb 7.51 in the tubulin-binding domain is conformationally altered when incorporated into PHFs, making it inaccessible to antibody in the absence of prior formic acid treatment.

Occlusion of the mAb 7.51 epitope appears to be closely associated with the addition of a coating of full-length tau molecules as the core tau units assemble into PHFs. In addition to the labelling of tangles, mAb 423 immunoreactivity is seen in the form of diffuse cytoplasmic staining in the somatodendritic compartment of pyramidal cells lacking PHFs. These deposits are labelled also with mAb 7.51, but only after formic acid treatment of the section (Mena et al., 1996). Ultrastructurally, these deposits appear as amorphous clumps either free in the cytoplasm, or associated with membranous organelles, including mitochondria. Occasionally these deposits are associated with the cytoplasmic surface of the endoplasmic reticulum. The presence of the same protease-resistant core element at the earliest detectable stages of neurofibrillary pathology indicates that this may be a critical feature in the initiation and propagation of PHF assembly (Wischik et al., 1995a).

Immunoassays to investigate tau protein in brain tissue were developed using the properties of mAbs 423 and 7.51 (Harrington et al., 1991).

Using PHF core preparations from advanced cases of AD, it has been possible to demonstrate biochemically that there is a substantial redistribution of tau in AD as compared with age-matched controls (Mukaetova-Ladinska et al., 1993). Similarly, there is a substantial accumulation of hyperphosphorylated tau, i.e. tau phosphorylated in the vicinity of Ser-202/Thr-205 and recognized by mAb AT8 (Harrington et al., 1994a). There is no evidence that phosphorylated tau species behave as PHF precursors (Lai et al., 1995; Wischik et al., 1995b). In fact, the only species for which a clear case could be made as a PHF precursor was normal soluble tau. Since depletion of normal tau is also a feature of other neurodegenerative diseases (Harrington et al., 1994a), features that distinguish AD need to be found; namely, the conversion of tau into PHFs. The rate of PHF assembly was found to increase geometrically as the level of PHF-tau increased (Lai et al., 1995). This relationship is consistent with PHF assembly being a self-propagating process, that need not necessarily be dependent upon post-translational modifications of tau (Wischik et al., 1995).

25.5 Tau protein in Lewy body diseases

Perry and his colleagues (1990) described a group of patients as having senile dementia of the Lewy body type (SDLT), a form of dementia that is characterized by the presence of a moderate number of neocortical Lewy bodies yet with sparse or absent neurofibrillary lesions (tangles or neuritic plaques). What determines the clinical symptoms in these patients in whom the global severity of dementia is comparable with that found in AD?

We looked in detail to see if these SDLT patients had a PHF burden that might have gone undetected by classical histological staining methods undertaken by Perry et al. (1990). Infrequent PHFs and low levels of PHF-tau were observed in a minority of the SDLT cases, in parallel to the demonstration of occasional neurofibrillary tangles in tissue sections. In these cases, the extent and pattern of phosphorylation of tau could not be distinguished from that found in AD. This was ascertained using a panel of mAbs (SMI-31, SMI-33, SMI-34, AT8, AT180, AT270 and Tau-1) that are dependent on the phosphorylation status of various epitopes (Harrington et al., 1994a; C.R.H., unpublished data). We found no evidence, however, that the accumulation of either protease-resistant PHFs or hyperphosphorylated tau could distinguish SDLT patients from either age-matched controls or patients with idiopathic Parkinson's disease

(Harrington et al., 1994a) (see Fig. 25.2). The mean level of either PHFs and tangles was no greater than 5% of that found in AD. Moreover, those SDLT patients who had detectable, but low, levels of PHFs corresponded to those cases who had infrequent tangles. Thus, abundant PHFs in neurites does not appear to provide an explanation for the dementia found in these SDLT patients. In contrast, the levels of PHFs were increased in AD by more than twenty-fold when compared with controls (Harrington et al., 1994a).

Aβ accumulation did not show the same discrimination between age-matched controls and patients with neurodegenerative disorders (Fig. 25.2). There was less than a twofold increase in Aβ in AD compared with controls and substantial levels of Aβ were found in the latter (Harrington et al., 1994a). This observation is consistent with a number of reports that have demonstrated extensive numbers of Aβ deposits in non-demented elderly patients. Whereas the slight overlap between AD and controls, in terms of PHF content, might be accounted for by the existence of 'preclinical AD' cases in the elderly control group, the same could not be the case for Aβ accumulation. More than two-thirds of the AD cases had Aβ levels overlapping those found in control patients. The mean level of Aβ in SDLT was intermediate between that observed in controls and AD (Harrington et al., 1994a). Thus, although SDLT might be considered as a cerebral amyloidosis, the extent of Aβ deposition is insufficient to discriminate these patients from the non-demented elderly. Furthermore, the plaques in SDLT tend to be predominantly of the non-neuritic, tau-immunonegative type (Dickson et al., 1989), a finding corroborated by the absence of PHF-type pathology in these patients (Harrington et al., 1994a). One further conclusion from these findings with SDLT is that altered processing of APP, leading to Aβ deposition, need not necessarily trigger neurofibrillary pathology. Whether Aβ deposition triggers neurofibrillary pathology in AD, remains unproven.

The depletion of normal tau protein was not a discriminatory marker between the different neurodegenerative disorders (Fig. 25.2). Levels of normal tau are decreased with normal aging and these are depleted even further in AD (Mukaetova-Ladinska et al., 1993). Tau is depleted to a similar extent in AD, SDLT and Parkinson's disease (with or without dementia) patients. Thus the biochemical data indicate that it is the accumulation of PHFs, rather than the deposition of Aβ or depletion of normal tau, that serves as a better molecular discriminant for the clinical symptoms of AD from both normal aging and the Lewy body diseases, including both idiopathic Parkinson's disease and cortical Lewy

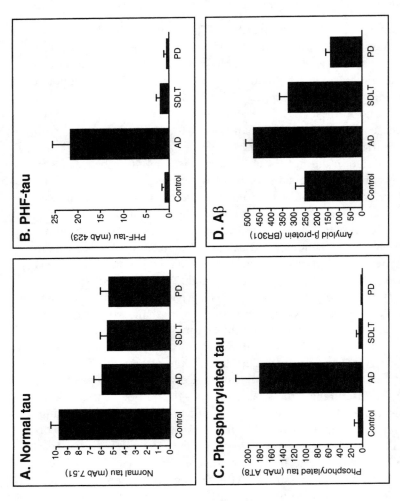

Fig. 25.2 Biochemical comparison of elderly patients with AD, SDLT, or Parkinson's disease (PD) or controls without neurological disorders (C). Normal tau was depleted in all three neurodegenerative disorders, whereas there was more than a twenty-fold accumulation of PHF-tau and hyperphosphorylated tau that was specific for AD. There was substantial deposition of Aβ in the control group and considerable overlap with that found in AD cases (1.8-fold greater in AD than C). Aβ levels in SDLT were intermediate between controls and AD. Both cingulate and occipital cortex was examined from 11–13 patients for each category; error bars represent SE about the mean values.

body dementia (Fig. 25.2). The absence of PHF-type pathology in SDLT suggests the existence of an alternative pathological mechanism from that seen in AD, and strengthens the notion that pure SDLT is a distinct disease entity from both AD and PD.

25.6 Apolipoprotein E genotype in Lewy body diseases

Polymorphisms of the APO E gene act as a susceptibility factor in the development of AD. The APO E type $\epsilon 4$ allele is a risk factor for late-onset sporadic and familial AD, whereas the rarer $\epsilon 2$ allele confers protection (Roses, 1995). From an autopsy series, the age of onset for AD is decreased by 15 years on average, for patients who are homozygous for the $\epsilon 4$ allele as compared with $\epsilon 2/\epsilon 3$ patients. Identification of the $\epsilon 4$ allele as a risk factor for AD has now been confirmed in many laboratories throughout the world. The APO E type $\epsilon 4$ allele frequency in SDLT patients is increased to a similar level to that found in age-matched, elderly sporadic AD patients (Harrington et al., 1994b). The $\epsilon 4$ allele frequencies in SDLT (36.5%) and AD (32.8%) were both significantly greater than in controls (14.7%). In contrast, neither Parkinson's disease (9.8%) nor Huntington's chorea (17%) had APO E polymorphisms that differed from controls (see also Chapters 18 and 30). There is evidence also that vascular disease (both coronary and cerebral) is associated with slight, though non-significant, increases in the $\epsilon 4$ allele (Harrington et al., 1994b). The increased $\epsilon 4$ allele frequency (25%) in the latter group was comparable with those observed in extensive studies of atherosclerosis.

25.7 Influence of APO E on development of AD and Lewy body diseases

In light of the proposal that APO E polymorphisms might exert their effect by affecting tau metabolism (Roses, 1995), we examined whether or not the $\epsilon 4$ allele exerted an influence on the depletion of normal tau and its redistribution into PHFs that has been observed in AD (Mukaetova-Ladinska et al., 1993). Those AD patients who possessed an $\epsilon 4$ allele were not associated with significantly greater accumulation of RHF-tau, when compared with those with an $\epsilon 4$ allele (Harrington et al., 1994b) (see Fig. 25.3). Galasko et al. (1994), in contrast, reported that an increased $\epsilon 4$ allele frequency was associated only with those cortical Lewy body dementia patients with Alzheimer-type pathology and not with 'pure' Lewy body disease. In our study, we observed no difference in the low level of PHFs (or tangles) between SDLT patients possessing or lacking

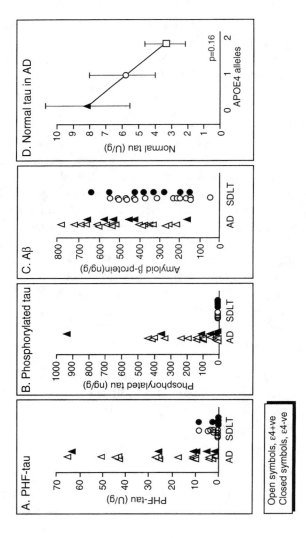

Fig. 25.3 Influence of APOE genotype on tau and Aβ pathology. There were no significant differences in PHF-tau, phosphorylated tau and Aβ accumulation in AD or SDLT when cases were separated according to the presence or absence of an $\epsilon 4$ allele (A–C). Although normal tau protein was depleted with increasing APOE $\epsilon 4$ gene dosage, this failed to reach statistical significance (D).

an $\epsilon 4$ allele (see Fig. 25.3). In fact, the only biochemical parameter that showed an association with the $\epsilon 4$ allele was an increased deposition of $A\beta$ in patients with Parkinson's disease possessing an $\epsilon 4$ allele (Harrington et al., 1994b). This provides evidence of a non-specific APO E effect since Parkinson's disease patients (with or without dementia), like controls are not associated with an increased $\epsilon 4$ allele frequency. Our findings indicate that PHF-type pathology is not an inevitable consequence of possession of the $\epsilon 4$ allele. SDLT patients who lack PHF pathology, have $\epsilon 4$ allele frequencies that are increased to the same extent as found in AD (Harrington et al., 1994b). It is worth emphasizing that for both AD and SDLT, presence of the $\epsilon 4$ allele is neither necessary nor sufficient to account for either disease. Approximately half of the patients in the two groups lacked any $\epsilon 4$ allele, and 27% of the elderly control patients having no neurological disorder possessed one $\epsilon 4$ allele. Thus, while PHF-tau is always present in AD, association with the APO E $\epsilon 4$ allele is neither specific nor essential, and therefore unlikely to be of central importance in the development of dementia in AD.

It has been mentioned above that the age of onset for AD is, on average, decreased by 15 years when one compares patients with an $\epsilon 4/\epsilon 4$ genotype with $\epsilon 2/\epsilon 3$. The comparable decrease is 10 years in the case of $\epsilon 3/\epsilon 4$ patients. We have examined the relationship between age and the association of the $\epsilon 4$ allele with SDLT and AD. In order to counter any possible protective effect that the $\epsilon 2$ allele might have, we have excluded the much rarer $\epsilon 2/\epsilon 4$ patients from our analysis. Groups have been split into two groups aged between 60 and 90 years at death using a cut-off point of 78 years (Table 25.1). In the younger group of non-demented controls, almost twice the number of patients possessing an $\epsilon 4$ allele were found, when compared with the older group. The same decrease was observed in the cortical Lewy body dementia group in which there were substantially greater numbers of $\epsilon 4$ carriers. The $\epsilon 4$ allele, however, was only marginally depleted in the older group of AD patients. We had previously noted that the apparent protective effect of the $\epsilon 2$ allele for AD was not found in SDLT (Harrington et al., 1994b); an observation that may have pathological significance in discriminating between the two disorders. The $\epsilon 2$ allele frequency was decreased in younger patients with SDLT, but increased in younger patients with AD. Whether this difference has biological significance will need to be addressed in more detail.

Thus the association with particular APO E genotypes is not identical for AD and Lewy body disease. This would be consistent with the bio-

Table 25.1. *APOE allele frequency distribution by age at death*

Category (age, yr)	Cases (n)	Mean age, yr (SD)	APO E allele frequency			E3/E4 plus E4/E4 patients as a proportion of total (%)	
			$\epsilon 2$	$\epsilon 3$	$\epsilon 4$		
Control (<78 yr)	39	71.1 (5.1)	0.077	0.744	0.179	35.9	
Control (78+yr)	67	84.3 (3.4)	0.075	0.806	0.119	17.9	$(p = 0.047)^*$
SDLT (<78 yr)	18	71.9 (4.8)	0.028	0.528	0.444	77.7	
SDLT (78+yr)	19	84.4 (4.0)	0.079	0.684	0.237	47.4	$p = (0.057)$
AD (<78 yr)	39	70.9 (2.6)	0.051	0.603	0.346	52.8	
AD (78+yr)	67	82.4 (3.6)	0.015	0.694	0.291	50.0	$(p = 0.789)$

*Pearson's chi-square test was used to compare the proportion of genotypes in the two age groups for each category. E2/E4 cases were excluded from these analyses only. Age range for each category was 60–90 yr.

Table 25.2. *Pathological, biochemical and APO E genotype profiles that distinguish clinical phenotypes*[*]

	Clinical phenotype			
	Normal aging	AD	SDLT	PD
Aβ pathology	+ +	+ + + +	+ + +	+ +
Neurofibrillary pathology	+/−	+ + + +	+/−	+/−
Neocortical Lewy bodies	+/−	+/−	+ +	+
Brainstem Lewy bodies	+/−	+	+ + +	+ + + +
Aβ accumulation	+ +	+ + + +	+ + +	+ + †
Normal tau depletion	+	+ + ‡	+ +	+ +
Abnormal tau accumulation	+/−	+ + + +	+/−	−
APOE allele distribution	normal	ϵ4↑ϵ2,ϵ3.↓	ϵ4↑; ϵ3↓	normal

[*] +/−, spare or absent; + to + + + +, increasing quantity of pathological or biochemical parameter, as compared with the level in the normal, young individual.

†Aβ is increased in those Parkinson's disease cases with an ϵ4 allele.

‡There is a tendency for normal tau to be depleted to a greater extent in AD cases associated with increasing gene dosage of the ϵ4 allele.

chemical and neuropathological differences between the two disorders, and would argue against the contention that SDLT is merely an early version of AD. The latter view would have to be reconciled also with the observation that clinical dementia in these patients is observed in the absence of PHF pathology.

The molecular features of AD and SDLT are summarized in Table 25.2. AD is a neurodegenerative disease characterized by the accumulation of abundant neocortical PHFs that is strongly correlated with cognitive decline, whereas SDLT is associated with the presence of neocortical Lewy bodies in the relative absence of PHFs. In both diseases, the burden of Aβ is greater than in the non-demented elderly. Since both SDLT and AD are associated with elevated $\epsilon 4$ allele frequencies, it seems unlikely that APO E polymorphism on its own can account for the pathological changes that are most closely correlated with the clinical signs of dementia in AD, that is, neurofibrillary lesions. Similarly it emerges that changes in the abnormal processing of tau protein, rather than of Aβ deposition, are more specifically associated with the clinical, pathological, and immunochemical factors that distinguish AD from SDLT, normal aging and other neurodegenerative disorders such as Parkinson's disease. The pathological substrate for dementia in the Lewy body diseases remains to be determined.

References

Bondareff, W., Harrington, C. R., Wischik, C. M., Hauser, D. L. & Roth, M. (1995). Absence of abnormal hyperphosphorylation in intracellular tangles in Alzheimer's disease. *J. Neuropathol. Exp. Neurol.*, **54**, 657–63.

Coleman, P.D., Goedert, M., Lee, V.M.-Y., Phelps, C. & Trojanowski, J. (eds) (1995). The Schmitt Symposium: The cytoskeleton and Alzheimer's disease. *Neurobiol. Aging*, **16**, 227–499.

Dickson, D. W., Crystal, H., Mattiace, L. A. et al. (1989). Diffuse Lewy body disease: light and electron microscopic immunohistochemistry of senile plaques. *Acta Neuropathol.*, **78**, 572–84.

Galasko, D., Hansen, L. A., Katzman, R. et al. (1994). Clinical-neuropathological correlations in Alzheimer's disease and related dementias. *Arch. Neurol.*, **51**, 888–95.

Goedert, M. (1993). Tau protein and the neurofibrillary pathology of Alzheimer's disease. *Trends Neurosci.*, **16**, 460–5.

Harrington, C. R., Mukaetova-Ladinska, E. B., Hills, R. et al. (1991). Measurement of distinct immunochemical presentations of tau protein in Alzheimer disease. *Proc. Natl. Acad. Sci. USA*, **88**, 5842–6.

Harrington, C. R., Perry, R. H., Perry, E. K. et al. (1994a). Senile dementia of Lewy body type and Alzheimer type are biochemially distinct in terms of paired helical filaments and hyperphosphorylated tau protein. *Dementia*, **5**, 215–28.

Harrington, C. R., Louwagie, J., Rossau, R. et al. (1994b). Influence of apolipoprotein E genotype on senile dementia of the Alzheimer and Lewy body types. Significance for etiological theories of Alzheimer's disease. *Am. J. Pathol.*, **145**, 1472–84.

Jakes, R., Novak, M., Davison, M. & Wischik, C. M. (1991). Identification of 3- and 4-repeat tau isoforms within the PHF in Alzheimer's disease. *EMBO J.*, **10**, 2725–9.

Lai, R. Y. K., Gertz, H.-J., Wischik, D. J. et al. (1995). Examination of phosphorylated tau protein as a PHF-precursor at early stage Alzheimer's disease. *Neurobiol. Aging*, **16**, 433–45.

Ledesma, M. D., Bonay, P. & Avila, J. (1995). Protein from Alzheimer's disease patients is glycated at its tubulin-binding domain. *J. Neurochem.*, **65**, 1658–64.

Matsuo, E. S., Shin, R.-W., Billingsley, M. L. et al. (1994). Biopsy-derived adult human brain tau is phosphorylated at many of the same sites as Alzheimer's disease paired helical filament tau. *Neuron*, **13**, 989–1002.

Mena, R., Edwards, P.C., Harrington, C.R., Mukaetova-Ladinska, E.B. & Wischik, C. M. (1996). Staging the pathological assembly of truncated tau protein into paired helical filaments in Alzheimer's disease. *Acta Neuropathol.*, **91**, 633–41.

Morishima-Kawashima, M., Hasegawa, M., Takio, K., Suzuki, M., Titani, K. & Ihara, Y. (1993). Ubiquitin is conjugated with amino-terminally processed tau in paired helical filaments. *Neuron*, **10**, 1151–60.

Mukaetova-Ladinska, E. B., Harrington, C. R., Roth, M. & Wischik, C. M. (1993). Biochemical and anatomical redistribution of tau protein in Alzheimer's disease. *Am. J. Pathol.*, **143**, 565–78.

Novak, M., Kabat, J. & Wischik, C. M. (1993). Molecular characterization of the minimal protease resistant tau unit of the Alzheimer's disease paired helical filament. *EMBO J.*, **12**, 365–70.

Perry, R. H., Irving, D., Blessed, G., Fairbairn, A. & Perry, E. K. (1990). Senile dementia of the Lewy body type. A clinically and neuropathologically distinct form of Lewy body dementia in the elderly. *J. Neurol. Sci.*, **95**, 119–39.

Roses, A. D. (1995). On the metabolism of apolipoprotein E and the Alzheimer diseases. *Exp. Neurol.*, **132**, 149–56.

Wischik, C. M., Novak, M., Thøgersen, H. C. et al. (1988). Isolation of a fragment of tau derived from the core of the paired helical filament of Alzheimer disease. *Proc. Natl. Acad. Sci. USA*, **85**, 4506–10.

Wischik, C. M., Edwards, P. C. & Harrington, C. R. (1995a). The tau protein amyloidosis of Alzheimer's disease: its mechanisms, potential triggers and consequences. In *Neurobiology of Alzheimer's Disease*, ed. D. Dawbarn, & S. J. Allen, pp. 89–148. Oxford: BIOS Scientific.

Wischik, C. M., Edwards, P. C., Lai, R. Y. K. et al. (1995b). Quantitative analysis of tau protein in paired helical filament preparations: implications for the role of tau phosphorylation in PHF assembly in Alzheimer's disease. *Neurobiol. Aging*, **16**, 409–31.

Yan, S. D., Yan, S. F., Chen, X. et al. (1995). Non-enzymatically glycated tau in Alzheimer's disease induces neuronal oxidant stress resulting in cytokine gene expression and release of amyloid β-peptide. *Nature Med.*, **1**, 693–9.

26

Cytoskeletal pathology in Alzheimer's disease and Lewy body dementia – an epiphenomenon?

J. CARTER, D. HANGER
and S. LOVESTONE

Summary

Cortical Lewy bodies are the defining pathological feature of Lewy body dementia. Ultrastructural, immunocytochemical and direct biochemical analysis confirm that Lewy bodies represent intraneuronal perikaryal accumulations of phosphorylated neurofilament proteins. Lewy bodies are thus a marker that the normal architecture of the neuronal cytoskeleton is disrupted.

Considerable evidence points to cytoskeletal disruption as a constituent part of the molecular pathogenesis of neurodegeneration. In terms of these cytoskeletal-related changes, Lewy body diseases appear to result from a disorder of neurofilament accumulation, in contrast to Alzheimer's disease in which the microtubule-associated protein, tau, accumulates. The two diseases appear to be distinct at a molecular level and evidence is amassing for a distinction at the genetic level. It seems that for both Alzheimer's disease and Lewy body dementia phosphorylation of cytoskeletal proteins is altered.

Experimental models have shown that changes in expression of neurofilaments lead to disruption of neurofilament assembly, neurofilament pathology and neuronal loss. Evidence is reviewed here that changes in neurofilament processing are intrinsic to the neurodegenerative process in Lewy body dementia.

26.1 Introduction

Alzheimer's disease (AD) is characterized by the pathological lesions of amyloid plaques and neurofibrillary tangles. In addition to plaques and tangles however, AD brains often contain cortical Lewy bodies which are also found in a subset of dementia patients with relatively few or even no discernible tangles. Neurofibrillary tangles are composed principally of abnormally phosphorylated tau assembled into paired helical filaments (PHF-tau), structures not confined to intracellular tangles but widely distributed in the brain as neuropil threads, extracellular tangles and in plaque associated neurites. How do these pathological lesions relate to each other – if at all? It has been persuasively argued that as amyloid precursor protein (APP) mutations unequivocally cause a rare form of AD, that β-amyloid deposition is central to the neurodegeneration of AD and furthermore that as transgenic mice expressing these APP mutations have plaques but no tangles, the neurofibrillary tangle and associated cytoskeletal changes in AD may be epiphenomena unimportant to an understanding of pathogenesis. Are Lewy bodies also an epiphenomena or do they represent an important neuropathological process. If β-amyloid deposition is exclusively the cause of neuronal loss then it might be hypothesized that all brains with amyloid plaques should contain similar cytoskeletal changes. On the other hand, if β-amyloid deposition triggers a multiplicity of neurodegenerative cascades then distinct patterns of neuronal loss and cytoskeletal changes might be discerned. Furthermore, if these distinct patterns describe different clinical syndromes or treatment strategies then the question is of considerable clinical importance. Indeed, the question as to whether there is clear blue water between Lewy body disease and AD becomes central to neurodegeneration research.

26.2 A proportion of Lewy body disease brains contain no PHF-tau

The composition of the Lewy body has not been fully determined and some reports have suggested that both neurofilament (Goldman et al., 1983) and tau (Galloway et al., 1988; Pollanen et al., 1992) epitopes are present in the Lewy body itself. PHF-tau is widely distributed throughout the cortex in AD. Therefore, whether or not the Lewy body contains tau, PHF-tau should be detectable in the diseased brain if the neurodegenerative processes of AD and Lewy body dementia are similar.

We have recently examined a large series of brains of patients with dementia for evidence of PHF-tau (Strong et al., 1995). The sample of 48 brains consisted of 12 with AD, 12 with senile dementia Lewy body type (SDLT), 13 with Parkinson's disease (PD) and 11 controls. The SDLT cases all contained large numbers of Lewy bodies, variable densities of plaques and relatively few tangles. There was no correlation between the density of plaques and that of either tangles or Lewy bodies. Samples from the same cortical area were homogenized and tau protein extracted and examined by Western blot analysis using a polyclonal antibody to tau and a monoclonal antibody to tau that discriminates between normal and PHF-tau. Using this procedure we confirmed that, as expected, all AD brains and no control or PD brains contained PHF-tau. Of the 12 SDLT brains only one contained moderate amounts of PHF-tau and this subject had a relatively large density of tangles ($144/mm^2$ compared with less than $1/mm^2$ for all other samples). Three SDLT brains produced faint bands of tau on the Western blot that comigrated with PHF-tau although these were not strongly reactive with tau antibodies. We interpret this as indicating a small amount of phosphorylated tau in these samples which also had significant, although low numbers of tangles (less than $1/mm^2$ compared with less than $0.2/mm^2$ for all other samples). The experimental procedures and analysis were at all times blind to the neuropathological findings.

This study demonstrates that PHF-tau is not present in SDLT brains unless neurofibrillary tangles are present and therefore that a subset of pure or PHF-tau free Lewy body dementias can be described. Furthermore, there was no numerical correlation between the density of plaques and either tangles, Lewy bodies or PHF-tau. It follows that the process of neurodegeneration of Lewy body disease is not identical to that of AD and moreover, that as large numbers of senile plaques were present in all the SDLT cases examined, that the cascade from amyloid deposition to tau phosphorylation is not obligatory.

26.3 The association of apolipoprotein E with Lewy body dementia is weaker than with Alzheimer's disease

Untangling these distinct neurodegeneration cascades may prove productive. The $\epsilon 4$ allele of the apolipoprotein E (Apo E) gene has been described as a risk factor for AD and other dementias although this genetic finding might be due to a protective effect of the Apo E $\epsilon 2$ or $\epsilon 3$ alleles at this locus. The mechanisms whereby Apo E exerts a risk or protective effect are yet to be determined but in vitro studies suggest isoform specific effects of Apo E binding to both β-amyloid and tau. One hypothesis that has emerged suggests that the binding of Apo E2 and Apo E3 to tau protects tau from phosphorylation. It becomes important then to determine the role of Apo E in non-PHF-tau dementias such as Lewy body disease.

An association between Lewy body dementia and the Apo E ε4 allele has been described (Benjamin et al., 1994 and others), although some reports note that the association is lower than for AD (Hardy et al., 1994). Interestingly the ε4 frequency is lower in diffuse Lewy body disease (possibly corresponding to the PHF-tau free dementia described above) than in the Lewy body variant of AD (Galasko et al., 1994). In a sample of Lewy body dementia subjects the ε4 frequency was related to neuritic pathology (Hansen et al., 1994) and to hippocampal CA2/CA3 neuritic degeneration – itself an early marker of cytoskeletal changes (Lippa et al., 1995).

In the sample of patients described in the study by Strong et al. (1995) the ε4 frequency in the Alzheimer cases (0.5) was significantly higher than for controls (0.2) or PD patients (0.22) (Perry et al., personal communication). The ε4 frequency for SDLT subjects (0.35) is mid-way between that for controls and Alzheimer cases. However, when only the pure and PHF-tau free subset of SDLT cases are considered then the ε4 frequency is not significantly different from that of controls (0.29). The number of subjects available for this study was small; relatively tangle free SDLT cases are rare, PHF-tau free subjects are rarer still, and a larger group needs to be examined for this finding to be taken with confidence. Also, these results appear to be somewhat contradictory to that of Harrington et al. (1994). These studies need to be repeated with larger and different populations. However, failure to find an association between Apo E allelic variation and PHF-tau free Lewy body disease might add weight to the suggestion that the Apo E risk factor in AD is mediated through tau phosphorylation.

26.4 Lewy bodies contain disrupted neurofilaments

Detailed ultrastructural examination of cortical and subcortical Lewy bodies has shown that they consist of neurofilament-like fibrils surrounding an amorphous central region. A proportion of Lewy bodies are labelled by antibodies to neurofilaments, particularly by those to phosphorylated neurofilaments, although the number of labelled Lewy bodies varies according to the antibody used (Goldman et al., 1983). Epitopes from all three neurofilament subunit proteins have been found in both the core and the periphery of Lewy bodies although not all antibodies exhibit the same pattern of labelling and some show regional distinctions within individual Lewy bodies. Recently, sufficient amounts of cortical Lewy bodies have been isolated from postmortem human brain to begin a biochemical analysis of their protein constituents (reviewed in Pollanen et al., 1993). The phosphorylation status of the neurofilaments in Lewy bodies may be accurately determined once sufficient neurofilament proteins can be isolated and analysed directly. The presence of neurofilament proteins in Lewy bodies has thus been established by immunological techniques but has yet to be confirmed by direct protein chemical analysis of the isolated proteins.

Within the neuronal cytoskeleton, axonal and dendritic neurofilaments form parallel arrays. The wider spacing of axonal neurofilaments is probably caused by the increased phosphorylation of neurofilaments in axons generating a charge repulsion between adjacent filaments. In contrast, neurofilaments appear to be radially orientated in the periphery of nigral Lewy bodies and more randomly organized in cortical Lewy bodies. This apparent disruption of neurofilament organization has led to investigations focusing on neurofilament processing and phosphorylation.

26.5 Neurofilament processing and phosphorylation

The presence of different cortical lesions in Alzheimer's disease and Lewy body dementia but containing phosphorylated cytoskeletal proteins in both, suggests that phosphorylation may be an important mechanism in disease pathogenesis. The majority of cytoskeletal proteins are phosphorylated, indeed some of them are amongst the most highly phosphorylated proteins present in neurones. The neurofilaments in neurones are key filaments that determine the calibre of axons. Although they appear to be relatively stable, neurofilaments are dynamic structures that are continuously being produced, modified and metabolized. Axonal neurofilaments exist as relatively insoluble heteropolymers of the three soluble neurofilament protein subunits: NF-H (110 kDa, but 200 kDa apparent molecular mass by sodium dodecyl sulphate-polyacrylamide gel electrophoresis, SDS-PAGE); NF-M (100 kDA, 160 kDa by SDS-PAGE) and NF-L (62 kDa, 68 kDa by SDS-PAGE). Neurofilaments are amongst the most highly phosphorylated of the cytoskeletal proteins and NF-H and NF-M in particular become highly phosphorylated in their carboxy-terminal domains in axonal neurofilaments compared with their counterparts in the neuronal cell body. NF-L is less highly phosphorylated than the other two subunits although the sites and amount of phosphorylation on NF-L also vary according to its subcellular location. As the axon extends away from the cell body, the degree of neurofilament phosphorylation increases, particularly in the carboxy-termini of NF-H and NF-M. This gives rise to two types of phosphorylated neurofilament protein, axonal (highly phosphorylated in carboxy-terminal regions) and perikaryal (usually less highly phosphorylated), that can be distinguished by phosphate-dependent antibodies.

A disruption of phosphorylation could result in a lack of appropriate neurofilament degradation, influence neurofilament transport or the stoichiometry of neurofilament triplet proteins available for assembly into neurofilaments. There is some evidence that decreases in neurofilament phosphorylation, particularly NF-H, increase their susceptibility to degradation by the calcium-dependent protease, calpain. Alterations in neurofilament phosphorylation in the perikaryon such as that found in Lewy bodies, might therefore protect the protein from being metabolized normally. It is not yet known whether in Lewy bodies the neurofilaments deposit in the cell body as a consequence of phosphorylation or whether phosphorylation occurs as a consequence of neurofilament accumulation.

Neurofilaments are phosphorylated by different protein kinases in their amino- and carboxy-terminal domains and this phosphorylation may be a mechanism for the control of neurofilament polymerization. There appear to be two distinct types of kinases involved in neurofilament phosphorylation: second-messenger-dependent protein kinases that are primarily responsible for phosphorylation at the amino-terminal end and proline-directed protein kinases that phosphorylate the carboxy-terminal regions of the neurofilament subunits.

Several protein kinases have been shown to phosphorylate neurofilaments in vitro but it is not yet known which are the relevant in vivo kinases. Two protein kinases have been linked to Lewy bodies by immunocytochemical studies. Ca^{2+}/calmodulin-dependent protein kinase II (Ca/Cam kinase II) immunoreactivity has been shown to be associated with filaments (possibly neurofilaments) in Lewy bodies (Iwatsubo et al., 1991). Given that neurofilament proteins are able to bind to calmodulin and that Ca/CaM kinase II can phosphorylate neurofilaments, this may be a physiologically important observation. More recently, an antibody to cyclin-dependent kinase 5 (cdk5), but not antibodies to p34 cyclin-dependent kinase 2 or to the extracellular regulated kinase 1, has also been shown to label both cortical and nigral Lewy bodies (Brion & Couck, 1995). The majority of Lewy bodies in tissue sections are strongly labelled by antibodies to the small heat-shock protein, ubiquitin. An important observation in both the studies on protein kinase immunoreactivity was that the number of Lewy bodies immunoreactive with the antibodies to Ca/CaM kinase II and cdk5 was approximately the same as that for Lewy bodies labelled by antibodies to ubiquitin. It remains to be seen how tight is the association between these protein kinases and Lewy bodies in vivo and whether these enzymes are responsible for normal or aberrant phosphorylation of neurofilaments. Neurofilament phosphorylation is a dynamic process in neurones so it seems likely that the association of protein kinases with Lewy bodies may be balanced by the presence of protein phosphatases. To date there have been no reports of phosphatases specifically associated with Lewy bodies and it is possible that these and other protein kinases are yet to emerge as enzymes involved in Lewy body pathogenesis.

Neurofilaments may be one of a number of proteins in Lewy bodies that are linked to ubiquitin. For example, another small heat-shock protein, α B crystallin, is normally associated with intermediate filaments and in Lewy bodies α B crystallin is itself ubiquitinated (Lowe, 1994). However, studies on isolated nigral Lewy bodies have shown that ubiquitin immunoreactivity is reduced following detergent extraction whereas neurofilament immunoreactivity is increased (Pollanen et al., 1993). The covalent attachment of a protein such as ubiquitin to neurofilaments may produce an effect on the polypeptides that prevents their normal assembly and leads to the formation of neurofilament aggregates.

Neurofilaments normally interact with several other cytoskeletal proteins, and it is likely that some of these interactions have an effect on the stability and organization of neurofilaments. For example, neurofilaments are linked by crossbridges to microtubules and this probably enhances their stability. Simply mixing neurofilaments with certain charged proteins leads to the formation of neurofilament bundles. Hence, it is possible that a disruption in neurofilament binding to an associated protein, possibly by a prior defect in neurofilament phosphorylation, may lead to the deposition of neurofilaments in Lewy bodies.

26.6 Experimental models of neurofilament abnormalities

Animal and cellular models can be used to investigate neurofilament accumulations as a result of abnormal synthesis, assembly, degradation and transport.

26.6.1 Neurofilament synthesis

During development neurofilaments appear shortly after terminal neuronal differentiation increasing in late embryonic and early postnatal life when neurites are growing but have not reached their targets. The expression of subunits NF-L and NF-M precedes that of NF-H with a final burst of expression of all three subunits during neuronal maturation and axonal calibre expansion. Initial synthesis in the cell body is of soluble neurofilament proteins but within 6–12 h of synthesis there is a shift in solubility reflecting polymerization of the subunits as they enter the axon as assembled filaments.

Recently neurofilament accumulations have been reproduced in transgenic mice by overexpressing mouse (m) NF-L and human (h) NF-H subunits. The NF-L (m) transgenic mice expresses four times the normal level of NF-L, associated with a concomitant increase in NF-H and large accumulations of densely packed 10 nm neurofilaments in motor neurone cell bodies together with proximal axonal swellings (Xu et al., 1993). Skeletal muscles showed signs of denervation atrophy although neuronal loss was not a prominent feature. The abnormality was fatal by three to four weeks of age. In contrast, the NF-H (h) transgenic mice had a slow onset progressive neuronopathy at three to four months of age although perikaryal neurofilament accumulations were present in motor and sensory neurones (Cote et al., 1993). The accumulations within both NF-L and NF-H transgenics contain phosphorylated NF-H as confirmed by immunocytochemistry such that the morphological effects of forcing increased neurofilament synthesis bears a striking resemblance to that observed in motor neurone disease. Consistent with this is another recent observation that neurofilament accumulation in cell bodies of motor neurones (caused by the expression of a mutant NF-H (m)) is accompanied by 25% loss of axons in the ventral roots (Eyer & Peterson, 1994).

Disappointingly for Lewy body dementia research, although phosphorylated accumulations of neurofilaments are reproduced in these mice transgenic for neurofilaments they lack the structural appearance of Lewy bodies and there is no cerebral pathology. More encouraging are recent reports that on re-examination of transgenic mice overexpressing NF-L (h) aberrant accumulations of NF-L are detectable in several non-specific thalamic nuclei which project diffusely to the cerebral cortex (Matthieu et al., 1995). Moreover, cell counts show most neuronal loss in the parietal cortex and thalamus in the oldest animals. The authors suggest that NF-L overexpression here results in a chronic dysregulation of NF-L eventually leading to neuronal degeneration. Although the results of the above experiments indicate that a significant overexpression of neurofilament synthesis can reproduce the pathology of neurofilament accumulations other studies find neurofilament abnormalities at relatively low levels of expression of transgenic proteins. For example, mice expressing the human NF-M subunit at only low levels (2–25%) of the endogenous NF-M develop spherical inclusions of phosphorylated neurofilament in selective neuronal populations within the cortex (Vickers et al., 1994). These are similar in their location and morphology to cortical Lewy bodies. This is an age-dependent phenomenon occurring only in transgenic mice older than 12 months.

26.6.2 Neurofilament assembly

In vivo and in vitro techniques have been used to establish how the head, tail and rod domains of the neurofilaments may influence assembly (reviewed in Lee & Cleveland, 1994). In vitro purified NF-L is capable of self assembly into 10 nm filaments but NF-M and NF-H form only short, kinked filaments. Using transfection of individual neurofilament subunits into cell lines which lack an endogenous intermediate filament network, it has been shown that none of the neurofilament subunits are capable of independent de novo self assembly. Filaments are observed only if NF-L is coexpressed with NF-M or NF-H, demonstrating conclusively that neurofilaments are obligate heteropolymers. In non-neuronal cells a point mutation in the α-helical rod domain of mouse NF-L induced collapse of the normal intermediate filament network into perinuclear aggregates containing endogenous and mutant NF-L. Transgenic mice expressing the same construct produced neurofilament accumulations containing NF-L and phosphorylated NF-H in motor neurones with selective lower motor neurone death (Lee et al., 1994). This is perhaps the most convincing evidence to date that direct disruption of neurofilament assembly can lead to neurofilament pathology and neuronal loss.

Although neurofilaments are very stable structures with long half lives in axons, once assembled, they are not entirely static. Recent investigations support a two pool hypothesis in which neurofilaments move at two different velocities, one relatively fast equivalent to slow axonal transport and the other much slower as to be stationary with exchange of subunits between the two pools.

A defect in slow axonal transport has been suggested by many authors to be the most plausible mechanism underlying neurofilament accumulation. In neurotoxic models β,β'-iminodipropionitrile (IDPN) administration produces large neurofilament accumulations in rat proximal motor axons (Griffin et al., 1978). Ultrastructural studies of radiolabelled proteins confirm that neurofilaments in these axons move at a rate corresponding to slow axonal transport. After IDPN addition, however, the neurofilament proteins are retained in axonal swellings. The pathology of neurodegenerative disease is therefore reproduced in these models by direct inhibition of slow axonal transport. It may be that the neurofilament accumulations described above arise from defects of axonal transport, possibly because slow axonal transport is saturated by overexpression or because of changes in the filament structure resulting from altered ratios of NF-L, NF-M and NF-H.

26.7 Conclusions

Pathological and biochemical investigations confirm that there exists a subset of patients with Lewy body dementia lacking the tangles and PHF-tau characteristic of AD. In these individuals it follows that the route from β-amyloid deposition to neuronal loss does not necessarily involve tau phosphorylation. It is not yet clear whether or not an increase in the frequency of the Apo E $\epsilon4$ allele is associated with Lewy body dementia. In contrast to AD, Lewy body dementia appears to be a disorder of neurofilament disruption. Analysis of Lewy bodies by immunocytochemistry suggests that one defect associated with neurofilament disruption might be aberrant phosphorylation. Significant advances have been made, using animal and cellular models, into the nature of the abnormalities that produce the neurofilament accumulations in Lewy bodies. Caution must be exercised when extrapolating from experimental models but it seems clear that a number of factors, such as increased neurofilament synthesis, mutations in neurofilament subunits and/or impairment of axonal transport of neurofilaments can lead to a common pathogenic sequence that includes neurofilament accumulation as a central intermediary leading to neuronal degeneration. The significance of this to Lewy body research cannot be ignored. The specific mechanisms remain to be determined but it is apparent that primary changes in the cytoskeleton account for some of the pathological changes encountered in neurodegenerative diseases, including Lewy body dementia, and the suggestion that they are an epiphenomenon should be firmly dismissed.

References

Benjamin, R., Leake, A., Edwardson, J. A. et al. (1994). Apolipoprotein E genes in Lewy body and Parkinson's disease. *Lancet*, **343**, 1565.

Brion, J.-P. & Couck, A.-M. (1995). Cortical and brainstem-type Lewy bodies are immunoreactive for the cyclin-dependent kinase 5. *Am. J. Pathol.* (in press).

Cote, F., Collard, J. F. & Julien, J. P. (1993). Progressive neuronopathy in transgenic mice expressing the human neurofilament heavy gene: a mouse model of Amyotrophic Lateral Sclerosis. *Cell*, **73**, 35–46.

Eyer, J. & Peterson, A. (1994). Neurofilament-deficient axons and perikaryal aggregates in viable transgenic mice expressing a neurofilament β-Galactosidase fusion protein. *Neuron*, **12**, 389–405.

Galasko, D., Saitoh, T., Xia, Y. et al. (1994). The apolipoprotein E allele $\epsilon 4$ is overrepresented in patients with the Lewy body variant of Alzheimer's disease. *Neurology*, **44**, 1950–1.

Galloway, P. G., Grundke-Iqbal, I., Iqbal, K. & Perry, G. (1988). Lewy bodies contain epitopes both shared and distinct from Alzheimer neurofibrillary tangles. *J. Neuropath. Exp. Neurol.*, **47**, 654–63.

Goldman, J. E., Yen, S.-H., Chiu, F.-C. & Peress, N. S. (1983). Lewy bodies of Parkinson's disease contain neurofilament antigens. *Science*, **221**, 1082–4.

Griffin, J. W., Hoffman, P. N., Clark, A. W., Carroll, P. T. & Price, D. L. (1978). Slow axonal transport of neurofilament proteins: Impairment by β, β'-Iminodipropionitrile administration. *Science*, **202**, 633–5.

Hansen, L. A., Galasko, D., Samuel, W., Xia, Y., Chen, X. & Saitoh, T. (1994). Apolipoprotein-E $\epsilon 4$ is associated with increased neurofibrillary pathology in the Lewy body variant of Alzheimer disease. *Neurosci. Lett.*, **182**, 63–5.

Hardy, J., Crook, R., Prihar, G., Roberts, G., Raghavan, R. & Perry, R. (1994). Senile dementia of the Lewy body type has an apolipoprotein E $\epsilon 4$ allele frequency intermediate between controls and Alzheimer's disease. *Neurosci. Lett.*, **182**, 1–2.

Harrington, C. R., Louwagie, J., Rossau, R. et al. (1994). Influence of apolipoprotein E genotype on senile dementia of the Alzheimer and Lewy body types. Significance for etiological theories of Alzheimer's disease. *Am. J. Pathol.*, **145**, 1472–4.

Iwatsubo, T., Nakano, I., Fukunaga, K. & Miyamoto, E. (1991). Ca2 + / calmodulin-dependent protein kinase II immunoreactivity in Lewy bodies. *Acta Neuropathol. (Berl.)*, **82**, 159–63.

Lee, M. K. & Cleveland, D. W. (1994). Neurofilament function and dysfunction: involvement in axonal growth and neuronal disease. *Curr. Opin. Cell. Biol.*, **6**, 34–40.

Lee, M. K., Marszalek, J. P. & Cleveland, D. W. (1994). A mutant neurofilament subunit causes massive, selective motor neuron death: Implications for human motor neuron disease. *Neuron*, **13**, 975–88.

Lippa, C. F., Smith, T. W., Saunders, A. M. et al. (1995). Apolipoprotein E genotype and Lewy body disease. *Neurology*, **45**, 97–103.

Lowe, J. (1994). Lewy bodies. In *Neurodegenerative diseases*, ed. D. B. Calne, pp. 51–69. Philadelphia, PA: W. B. Saunders.

Matthieu, J. F., Ma, D., Descarries, L., Vallee, A., Parent, A., Julien, J. P. Douchet, G. (1995). CNS distribution and overexpression of neurofilament

NF-L in mice transgenic for Human NF-L: aberrant accumulation in thalamic perikarya. *Exp. Neurol.*, **132**, 134–46.

Pollanen, M. S., Bergeron, C. & Weyer, L. (1992). Detergent-insoluble cortical Lewy body fibrils share epitopes with neurofilament and tau. *J. Neurochem*, **58**, 1953–6.

Pollanen, M. S., Dickson, D. W. & Bergeron, C. (1993). Pathology and biology of the Lewy body. *J. Neuropathol. Exp. Neurol.*, **52**, 183–91.

Strong, C., Anderton, B. H., Perry, R. H., Perry, E K., Ince, P. G. & Lovestone, S. (1995). Abnormally phosphorylated tau protein in Senile Dementia of Lewy Body Type and Alzheimer's disease: evidence that the disorders are distinct. *Alz. Dis. Assoc. Disord*, **9**(4), 218–22.

Vickers, J. C., Morrison, J. H., Friedrich, V. L. et al. (1994). Age-associated and cell type specific neurofibrillary pathology in transgenic mice expressing the human midsized neurofilament subunit. *J. Neurosci.*, **14**, 5603–12.

Xu, Z., Cork, L. C., Griffin, J. W. & Cleveland, D. W. (1993). Increased expression of neurofilament subunit NF-L produces morphological alterations that resemble the pathology of human motor neuron disease. *Cell*, **73**, 23–33.

27

Genetic correlations in Lewy body disease

T. SAITOH[†] and R. KATZMAN

Summary

A subpopulation of Alzheimer's disease (AD) patients with neocortical
Lewy bodies (LB) and subtle extrapyramidal signs, a clinical-pathological
phenotype that we have termed the Lewy body variant of AD (LBV), has
an increased allele frequency of APO E ϵ4 allele, similar to that observed
in AD subjects without LB (pure AD), although individuals homozygous
for the APO E ϵ4 allele are overrepresented in pure AD as compared with
age-matched controls, but not as markedly in subjects with LBV.
Furthermore, we have found that the CYP2D6B mutant allele, a risk
factor for Parkinson's disease (PD), is overrepresented in LBV, a finding
that has been controversial. To further evaluate the involvement of the
CYP2D6 locus in LBV, the *Xba*I restriction fragment length polymorphisms (RFLP) of CYP2D6, 44 kb, 15/9 kb, and 13 kb (D mutation), were
examined for association with LBV. The 15/9-kb RFLP was found in
pure AD or in non-AD individuals but was not found in LBV. On the
other hand, the 44-kb *Xba*I RFLP in the presence of the concomitant
CYP2D6B mutant allele was strongly associated with LBV. The tightest
association with LBV was found in the combination of the 44-kb RFLP
and CYP2D6B mutant allele in the absence of the 15/9-kb RFLP. A
CYP2D6 deletion mutation D, detected as 13-kb RFLP, was not linked
to LBV. Taken together, these findings suggest that the inactivation of
CYP2D6 represented by the B or D mutation may not per se be the risk
factor for LBV but that an independent mutation or allele linked to the
CYP2D6B mutation and the 44-kb *Xba*I RFLP (such as NF-H or PDGfb
genes) might be associated with LB formation in AD. These results however remain consistent with the hypothesis that LBV is related by genetic
risk factors to both AD and PD.

[†] Deceased

27.1 Introduction

The Lewy body variant of AD (LBV; Hansen et al., 1989, 1990), also sometimes referred to as Lewy body dementia (Gibb et al., 1987) or senile dementia of the Lewy body type (Perry et al., 1990), has become recognized as the second most common neuropathologic correlate of late-onset dementia, after neuropathologically pure AD. In our cohort of neuropathologically confirmed AD patients, about 25% are identified as LBV after autopsy examination (Hansen et al., 1990). The brains from LBV subjects have neurofibrillary tangles in hippocampal structures and neocortical senile plaques, including both diffuse and neuritic plaques, to fully meet diagnostic criteria for AD (Khachaturian, 1985), although whether LBV is a subtype of AD or a separate dementing disorder has been a matter of debate (Pollanen et al., 1993).

27.2 Apolipoprotein E gene allele 4 is highly represented in LBV

We and others recently found that the APO E ϵ4 allele – which is linked with AD with onset after age 60 years (Corder et al., 1993; Saunders et al., 1993a,b; Strittmatter et al., 1993 – is also a risk factor for LBV (Galasko et al., 1994; Hardy et al., 1994; Harrington et al., 1994; Pickering-Brown et al., 1994; St. Clair et al., 1994; Lippa et al., 1995b) suggesting that LBV is genetically classified as AD (Table 27.1). This classification is further supported by the finding that some patients with the early-onset familial form of AD associated with the 717 mutation of the amyloid precursor protein (APP) is associated with LB in the neocortex and mild extrapyramidal features during life (Mann et al., 1992) as well as subjects from early-onset families with chromosome 14 mutations (Lippa et al., 1995a). Since different groups utilize different names for the same entity, which we call LBV, it is worth commenting on the basis of our tabulating Lippa's data and Harrington's data as LBV. We defined LBV as the combination of clinical dementia and neuropathological detection of numerous neocortical amyloid plaques (both diffuse and neuritic) and neocortical LB. Lippa and associates have differentiated diffuse plaque cases and neuritic plaque cases (Lippa et al., 1995b), and we agree that the biological/pathological significance of diffuse vs neuritic plaques must be pursued further in the future. It would be extremely valuable to identify genes that dictate the development of neuritic plaques.

Table 27.1. *Apolipoprotein E genotype*

Health status and reference	Total	APO E genotype					
		$\epsilon2/\epsilon2$	$\epsilon2/\epsilon3$	$\epsilon2/\epsilon4$	$\epsilon3/\epsilon3$	$\epsilon3/\epsilon4$	$\epsilon4/\epsilon4$
Control							
Menzel et al. (1983)	1000	8	110	30	627	202	23
Harrington et al. (1994)	58	1	7	1	33	16	0
Marder et al. (1994)	44	1	4	0	31	7	1
Koller et al. (1995)	78	2	10	0	46	19	1
Maestre et al. (1995)	59	0	8	1	42	7	1
Total	1239	12	139	32	779	251	26
(%)	(100)	(1.0	(11.2)	(2.6)	(62.9)	(20.3)	(2.1)
AD							
Rebeck et al. (1993)	39	0	1	1	14	17	6
Schmechel et al. (1993)	143	0	3	6	47	64	23
Galasko et al. (1994)	74	0	3	0	24	35	12
Harrington et al. (1994)	67	0	2	2	27	30	6
Maestre et al. (1995)	43	0	1	1	22	16	3
Total	366	0	10	10	134	162	50
(%)	(100)	(0)	(2.7)	(2.7)	(36.6)	(44.3)	(13.7)
LBV							
Galasko et al. (1994)	40	0	1	1	18	18	2
Harrington et al. (1994)	26	0	3	0	6	15	2
Lippa et al. (1995a)	40	2	2	0	18	15	3
Total	106	2	6	1	42	48	7
(%)	(100)	(1.9)	(5.7)	(0.9)	(39.6)	(45.3)	(6.6)
PD							
Harrington et al. (1994)	51	0	8	1	33	9	0
Marder et al. (1994)	79	2	4	1	55	17	0
Koller et al. (1995)	113	1	12	5	67	26	2
Total	243	3	24	7	155	52	2
(%)	(100)	(1.2)	(9.9)	(2.9)	(63.8)	(21.4)	(0.8)

All the available published data demonstrate that the APO E genotype frequencies in LBV subjects (Galasko et al., 1994; Hardy et al., 1994; Harrington et al., 1994; Pickering-Brown et al., 1994; St. Clair et al., 1994; Lippa et al., 1995) are similar to those in AD (Saunders et al., 1993a,b; Strittmatter et al., 1993), and that the APO E $\epsilon4$ allele frequency is increased to a similar extent in pure AD and LBV compared with nondemented elderly subjects (Table 27.1). Recent reports have attributed much or all of the dementia in LBV patients to the LB, claiming that the AD lesions are more scanty than in pure AD and are compatible with aging rather than AD. However, our LBV patients had enough cortical plaques (counting both neuritic and diffuse plaques) to meet the NIH criteria of AD (Khachaturian, 1985). Regarding APO E allele frequencies, LBV is closely related to pure AD. The APO E ε4 allele is associated with AD lesions, but not with LB (see PD in Table 27.1). The finding that LBV and pure AD patients share this genetic marker provides another line of evidence linking the clinical and pathological picture of LBV to the AD lesions.

Compared with the pure AD group, relatively fewer subjects in the LBV group were homozygous for APO E ε4. This might suggest that the ε4/ε4 state predisposes so strongly to AD that the expression of LB lesions is muted. This genetic finding, together with the fact that LBV has somehow blunted neurofibrillary pathology, suggests that biochemical and cellular traits associated with AD, some of which may be affected by APO E ε4 and those associated with PD, exemplified by the presence of LB, may interact with each other. We hypothesize that molecular and cellular alterations in AD promoted by genetic (APP, APO E, chromosome 1 mutation, chromosome 14 mutation) and environmental factors may be affected by the presence of another set of genetic factors associated with PD and that the combination will manifest as LBV. One of this second set of genetic factors might be associated with CYP2D6 (or close gene).

27.3 Cytochrome P_{450} debrisoquine 4-hydroxylase in PD and LBV

Like AD, PD is likely to be a multifactorial disease having both genetic and environmental components. A number of investigators have hypothesized that PD may result from exposure to environmental toxins, and abnormalities in detoxifying enzymes may contribute to the expression of PD. A cytochrome P_{450} family of the enzyme debrisoquine 4-hydroxylase is responsible for detoxifying many drugs and environmental toxins. Recent molecular genetic studies have identified several molecular variants of the gene, CYP2D6, that encodes debrisoquine 4-hydroxylase. Depending on race, 1% to 12% of the population lacks the ability to metabolize debrisoquine and other drugs containing β-blockers, antidysrhythmic agents, neuroleptics, and tricyclic antidepressant drugs and are termed poor metabolizers (Alvan et al., 1990).

Several mutant CYP2D6 alleles were found to correlate with the phenotype of 'poor metabolizer', and the presence of a genetic marker for the poor metabolizer phenotype has been found to increase the risk for PD about twofold (Armstrong et al., 1992; Smith et al., 1992; Kondo & Kanazawa, 1993; Kurth & Kurth, 1993). Since the presence of LBs is a hallmark of PD, and allele B of the CYP2D6 gene is associated with PD (Armstrong et al., 1992; Smith et al., 1992; Kondo & Kanazawa, 1993; Kurth & Kurth, 1993), we questioned whether allele B of the CYP2D6 gene might also be associated with LBV. In our study with LBV, we found the increased representation of CYP2D6B mutant allele in association with LBV.

27.4 CYP2D6B mutant allele is highly represented in LBV

Our study suggested that the CYP2D6B mutant allele is overrepresented in the LBV (Saitoh et al., 1995). In late 1994, there was a letter from Dr John Hardy's group claiming the absence of an overrepresentation of the CYP2D6B allele in LBV (Rempfer et al., 1994). The combined result is shown in Table 27.2. The Fisher's exact test shows that in the combined data, the representation of individuals having at least one B allele in LBV is higher than that in non-AD controls ($p = 0.0499$) and higher than that in pure AD ($p = 0.0161$). Thus, the higher representation of the CYP2D6B mutant allele in LBV holds with the combined cases. Further, this association became much stronger when, as described later, we combined CYP2D6B and the nearby marker *Xba*I RFLP.

27.4.1 In 'pure' AD, subjects with wild-type CYP2D6 alleles have more synaptic alterations than those with the CYP2D6B mutant allele as measured by choline acetyltransferase (ChAT)

The association of the CYP2D6B mutant allele with LBV is reported (Saitoh et al., 1995). It appears that the presence of the CYP2D6B allele not only is associated with LB formation, but also affects some pathological feature(s) of AD. Individuals with the CYP2D6B allele have milder synaptic pathology in pure AD than those without this allele (Chen et al., 1995).

The two hallmarks of AD neuropathology that we focused on were the formation of senile plaques and tangles and the decline of two synaptic markers synaptophysin and ChAT, which are consistently found in AD.

Table 27.2. *Representation of CYP2D6B mutation in AD and LBV*

	Number of subjects (no-B/with-B)		
	UCSD	Newcastle	Total
Non-AD	37 (28/9)	17 (13/4)	54 (41/13)
Pure-AD	83 (58/25)	17 (16/1)	100 (74/26)
LBV	44 (20/24)	19 (16/3)	63 (36/27)[*]

The UCSD study is from Saitoh et al. (1995). The Newcastle study is from Rempfer et al. (1994). The CYP2D6B mutation is significantly more represented in LBV as compared to 'Non-AD' or 'Pure AD' (*$p < 0.05$, by Fisher's exact test).

Our analysis was focused on pure AD since we have more than triple the number of pure AD than LBV cases. Because of the small number of cases, similar analyses were not performed among LBV patients.

The consistently found neurotransmitter deficit in AD is associated with the cholinergic projection to the frontal cortex. This can be shown in the decline in ChAT-containing nerve terminals morphologically and in the activity of this enzyme in homogenates of cortex tissue from AD patients. Choline acetyltransferase activity in the midfrontal region of cerebral cortex in pure AD individuals with ($N = 26$) and without ($N = 58$) the CYP2D6B mutant allele were analyzed. ChAT activity in individuals with the CYP2D6B allele was significantly higher ($p = 0.037$ by the two-tailed Student's t test). The two groups compared are matched for age, duration of disease, severity of dementia and representation of APO E ϵ4.

27.4.2 The presence of the CYP2D6B mutant allele is associated with a less-remarkable decline in a generic presynaptic marker, synaptophysin, in 'pure' AD brains

Frontal ChAT activity reflects the integrity of cholinergic nerve terminals that are minor fractions relative to total nerve terminals. In order to evaluate the intactness of total nerve terminals, synaptophysin concentration in the midfrontal region of cerebral cortex in pure AD individuals with ($N = 18$) and without ($N = 34$) the CYP2D6B mutant allele was analyzed. Synaptophysin levels in individuals with the CYP2D6B allele was significantly higher ($p = 0.049$ by the two-tailed Student's t test). However, this value was lower than normal levels of synaptophysin. It should be noted that synaptic density has not yet been measured morphologically in this series.

27.4.3 In 'pure' AD, in the absence of Lewy bodies, the two hallmark lesions of AD, senile plaques and neurofibrillary tangles, were not significantly affected by the presence of the CYP2D6B mutant allele

The pathology that characterizes AD is the presence of senile plaques and neurofibrillary tangles. The comparison of plaque numbers in the frontal cortex between individuals with and without the CYP2D6B mutant allele did not reveal significant differences. Likewise, the comparison of tangle numbers in frontal cortex between individuals with and without the CYP2D6B mutant allele did not reveal significant differences.

Thus, a subpopulation of AD patients with neocortical Lewy bodies (LBV) has a higher representation of the CYP2D6B mutant allele, a risk factor for PD, than those without LB (pure AD) and that individuals with this CYP2D6B allele in pure AD have reduced synaptic pathology. Because approximately 25% of the AD population is LBV and 25% of pure AD individuals have the CYP2D6B allele with reduced synaptic pathology, knowledge of the accurate molecular mechanisms of LB development and molecular/cellular mechanisms by which the CYP2D6B mutant allele or a closely linked gene affect synaptic pathology and LB formation should be important for the development of therapeutic strategies for treatment of AD. It is possible that medications which are effective in alleviating the symptoms in pure AD without the CYP2D6B allele might not be effective in treating the LBV or pure AD with the CYP2D6B allele and vice versa. Therefore, it is important to keep in mind the presence of heterogeneity of AD in developing a therapeutic strategy of this disease, and the genotyping of CYP2D6 may help this process. However, it will be imperative to identify the actual mutations located in the CYP2D6 region of chromosome 22 that are responsible for the symptoms.

27.5 XbaI polymorphisms 44 kb and 15/9 kb are linked to CYP2D6B mutant allele

Association of the CYP2D6B mutant allele, previously shown to be linked to PD, with LBV (Saitoh et al., 1995) was further reinforced by our recent study where the CYP2D6 RFLP with *Xba*I was investigated in order to gain further insight as to the mutation linked to LBV. It was found that both the 44-kb *Xba*I RFLP and 15/9-kb RFLP were linked to the CYP2D6B mutant allele. It is important to note that our study is a case-control study and that the subjects are unrelated; we are using restriction enzyme fragments as markers of unknown alleles rather than as linkage markers within families or between siblings. In our subjects, CYP2D6B with the concomitant 15/9-kb *Xba*I RFLP was excluded from LBV whereas a strong association of LBV with CYP2D6B in the presence of the concomitant 44-kb *Xba*I RFLP was found. Furthermore, LBV was not associated with the deletion mutant D of CYP2D6, as detected by the 13-kb *Xba*I RFLP. Therefore, although the CYP2D6B mutant allele results in a loss of debrisoquine 4-hydroxylase activity, this may not be the biochemical explanation for the predisposition to LBV. These findings point to the presence of a mutation linked to both CYP2D6B and 44-kb *Xba*I RFLP that is responsible for the phenotype of LBV.

A southern blot of *Xba*I-digested genomic DNA probed with CYP2D6 cDNA detected several RFLPs. In our collection of 208 autopsied brains from the Caucasian population, at least one 29-kb wild-type allele was found in all cases whereas 14.9% (31 cases) had one 44-kb allele, 6.3% (13 cases) had one 13-kb allele, and 4.3% (9 cases) had one 15/9-kb allele. The representation of three RFLP alleles (44 kb, 15/9 kb, and 13 kb) among individuals with and without CYP2D6B mutant allele is uneven. Sixty-eight percent of 44-kb RFLP carriers, 100% of 15/9-kb RFLP carriers, and 15% of 13-kb RFLP carriers had at least one CYP2D6B mutation allele. Since only 28% of individuals without these three mutant RFLPs have one or two CYP2D6B mutations, 44-kb and 15/9-kb RFLPs are overrepresented among CYP2D6B mutation carriers ($p < 0.0001$). The CYP2D6D deletion represented by the *Xba*I 13-kb RFLP was not associated with CYP2D6B mutation.

27.6 15/9-kb *Xba*I Polymorphism is not present in our LBV brains

The strong association of the 15/9-kb *Xba*I RFLP with the CYP2D6B mutation, which is more highly represented in LBV than in pure AD, prompted us to analyze the association of the 15/9-kb RFLP with LBV. A survey of CYP2D6B individuals as to the presence of the 15/9-kb *Xba*I RFLP revealed that the 15/9-kb *Xba*I RFLP is excluded from LBV. DNA samples from individuals with the CYP2D6B mutant allele were tested for the presence of the 15/9-kb *Xba*I RFLP in three diagnostic categories. The 15/9-kb *Xba*I RFLP was never found among individuals without the CYP2D6B mutant allele. Although in the pure AD or non-AD population the 15/9-kb *Xba*I RFLP was found in individuals with the CYP2D6B mutant allele, no 15/9-kb RFLP was found in CYP2D6B individuals with LBV. This distribution of the 15-kb *Xba*I RFLP in LBV is significantly different from that in non-AD ($p = 0.0406$) and marginally different from that in pure AD ($p = 0.0826$).

27.7 The 44-kb *Xba*I polymorphism is tightly associated with the CYP2D6B allele in LBV

The 44-kb *XBa*I polymorphism, which is also linked to the CYP2D6B mutant allele, was analyzed next in the three categories of individuals, non-AD, pure AD, and LBV. The 44-kb *Xba*I RFLP was found to be strongly associated with the CYP2D6B mutant allele in LBV, mildly associated in pure AD, and not associated in non-AD individuals.

Therefore, the association of CYP2D6B with LBV is affected by concomitant presence of *Xba*I RFLP. The tightest association of CYP2D6B mutation with LBV is found in the presence of the 44-kb RFLP and in the absence of the 14/9-kb RFLP. Among those individuals with the 44-kb and without the 15/9-kb *Xba*I RFLP (5 non-AD, 17 pure AD, and 8 LBV) 100% of LBV (8/8) have CYP2D6B mutation, whereas 52.9% of pure AD (9/17), and 60% of non-AD (3/5) individuals have this mutant allele. Even with this small number of sample size, the overrepresentation of CYP2D6B allele in LBV as compared with pure AD was significant ($p = 0.0261$ by Fisher's exact test) within this subclass of subjects. Further numbers are needed to confirm this finding.

27.8 The deletion mutant CYP2D6D as detected by the 13-kb *Xba*I RFLP is not linked to LBV

The CYP2D6B mutation eliminates the splicing signal at the exon 3/4 boundary, resulting in the lack of enzyme activity (Hanioka et al., 1990). If the association of the CYP2D6B mutant allele with LBV is due to the deficient enzyme activity of debrisoquine 4-hydroxylase, it is expected that the independent CYP2D6 mutation that causes deficient enzyme activity is also associated with LBV. To test this possibility a deletion mutant CYP2D6D, which can be detected as 13-kb *Xba*I RFLP, was analyzed for its association with LBV. This allele which is present in only 3% of the non-AD population was found to be present in 7% of the 'pure' AD brains and 5% of the LBV brains; hence this allele was not overrepresented in LBV.

27.9 Discussion

CYP2D6 is an extremely small gene spanning only 15 kb. Thus, linkage or association of the B mutant allele with any phenotype such as PD or LBV may actually reflect the presence of an as yet unknown mutation near the CYP2D6 gene. This possibility is suggested by the current observations that the CYP2D6D mutation associated with poor metabolism of drugs, which is similar to the CYP2D6B mutation, is not associated with LBV brains. Moreover, the presence of the 44-kb and 15/9-kb *Xba*I RFLP of the CYP2D6 gene affects the association of CYP2D6B mutation with LBV. The potential genes associated with LBV include, in addition to CYP2D6, the genes for platelet derived growth factor b (PDGFb) and neurofilament-H (NF-H), which are mapped close to one another on chromosome 22. All three are suspected to be involved in PD or LBV. The CYP2D6B mutation has been found to be associated with PD (Armstrong et al., 1992; Smith et al.; 1992; Kondo & Kanazawa, 1993; Kurth & Kurth, 1993) and LBV (Saitoh et al., 1995). Because this mutation eliminates a splicing signal in the debrisoquine 4-hydroxylase gene, the resulting inactivation of this enzyme and the consequent poor metabolizer phenotype have been considered to be responsible for these LB-associated diseases. However, this explanation is not satisfactory because the deletion mutant CYP2D6D is not associated with LBV and the CYP2D6B mutation with concomitant 15/9-kb RFLP is not associated with LBV. Therefore, if a mutation responsible for LBV is within the CYP2D6 gene, this mutation does not result in a simple inactivation of the enzyme but is likely to result in a gain of a new function. This explanation better fits the autosomal dominant effect of the CYP2D6B-linked mutation. One possibility is the creation of the dominant-negative form of debrisoquine 4-hydroxylase. This possibility needs to be tested in the future.

Lewy bodies, the spherical inclusions found in PD and in LBV, appear to be largely composed of neurofilaments (NF), some of which are abnormally phosphorylated (Goldman et al., 1983; Schmidt et al., 1991; Arai et al., 1992; Pollanen et al., 1993). PDGF-bb (the homodimer of two b chains) supports the survival of nigral dopaminergic neurons, which develop LB (Nikkah et al., 1993). Antibodies against both PDGFb and NF-H immunolabel LB. Transgenic animals with overexpression of NF or expression of a mutated NF were found to undergo neurodegeneration (Côté et al., 1993; Xu et al., 1993; Eyer & Peterson, 1994). Interestingly, in the case of transgenic mice expressing an NF-H-β-galactosidase fusion protein, LB-like abnormal aggregates of filaments developed (Eyer & Peterson, 1994). NF-H or PDGFb mutations linked to CYP2D6B might be responsible for biochemical alterations in individuals with CYP2D6B.

To conclude this portion of the study, *Xba*I RFLP analysis of CYP2D6 gene revealed that: (1) 25% of brains in our ADRC brain bank have the mutant alleles 44-kb, 15/9-kb, or 13-kb RFLP; (2) the presence of 44-kb and the absence of 15/9-kb RFLP in addition to the presence of the CYP2D6B mutant allele is the best predictor of LBV; and (3) the deletion of the CYP2D6 gene detected by the 13-kb RFLP (CYP2D6D) is not associated with LBV. Therefore, it is likely that the simple inactivation of the CYP2D6 gene is not enough or not linked to LBV. Instead either an allele or mutation in an independent gene adjacent to CYP2D6B (such as NF-H or PDGFb genes) or an additional mutation within the CYP2D6 gene might be required for the LB formation to manifest. Future investigation needs to clarify the nature of this potential mutation.

27.10 Conclusion

Previous genetic data along with the new data presented in this communication clearly demonstrate that there are two genetic risk factors for LBV, APO E and CYP2D6 (or a closely linked genetic variant). The identification of the actual mutation in or near the CYP2D6 gene is a next step and will require a much larger sample of subjects. One aspect which is left to future study is the way the cellular and biochemical reactions affected by APO E (AD cascades), particularly those leading to the development of neurofibrillary tangles, and those affected by CYP2D6 or a nearby gene (PD cascades) interact. It is likely that two cascade reactions interfere with each other in regard to alteration of intraneuronal fibrils. A better understanding of both cascade reactions will be required to clarify the nature of the interactions.

Acknowledgements

We thank Robert Davignon and Patty Melendrez for their help in the preparation of this manuscript. The current research has been supported by the National Institutes of Health (AG08205 and AG05131).

References

Alvan, G., Bechtel, P., Iselius, L. & Gundert-Remy, U. (1990). Hydroxylation polymorphisms of debrisoquine and mephenytoin in European population. *Eur. J. Clin. Pharmacol.*, **39**, 533–7.

Arai, H., Lee, V. M., Hill, W. D., Greenberg, B. D. & Trojanowski, J. Q. (1992). Lewy bodies contain β-amyloid precursor proteins of Alzheimer's disease. *Brain Res.*, **585**, 386–90.

Armstrong, M., Daly, A. K., Cholerton, S., Bateman, D. N. & Idle, J. R. (1992). Mutant debrisoquine hydroxylation genes in Parkinson's disease. *Lancet*, **399**, 1017–18.

Chen, X., Xia, Y., Alford, M. et al. (1995). The CYP2D6B allele is associated with a milder synaptic pathology in Alzheimer's disease. *Ann. Neurol.* **38**, 653–8.

Corder, E. H., Saunders, A. M., Strittmatter, W. J. et al. (1993). Gene dose of apolipoprotein E type 4 allele and the risk of Alzheimer's disease in late onset families. *Science*, **261**, 921–3.

Côté, F., Collard, J.-F. & Julien, J.-P. (1993). Progressive neuronopathy in transgenic mice expressing the human neurofilament heavy gene: A mouse model of amyotrophic lateral sclerosis. *Cell*, **73**, 35–46.

Eyer, J. & Peterson, A. (1994). Neurofilament-deficient axons and perikaryal aggregates in viable transgenic mice expressing a neurofilament-β-galactosidase fusion protein. *Neuron*, **12**, 389–405.

Galasko, D., Saitoh, T., Xia, Y. et al. (1994). The apolipoprotein E allele ε4 is over-represented in patients with the Lewy body variant of Alzheimer's disease. *Neurology*, **44**, 1950–1.

Gibb, W. R., Esiri, M. M. & Lees, A. J. (1987). Clinical and pathological features of diffuse cortical Lewy body disease (Lewy body dementia). *Brain*, **110**, 1131–53.

Goldman, J. E., Yen, S. H., Chiu, F. C. & Peress, N. S. (1983). Lewy bodies of Parkinson's disease contain neurofilament antigens. *Science*, **221**, 1082–4.

Hanioka, N., Kimua, S., Meyer, U. A. & Gonzalez, F. J. (1990). The human *CYP2D* locus associated with a common genetic defect in drug oxidation: a G_{1934} to A base change in intron 3 of a mutant *CYP2D6* allele results in an aberrant 3' splice recognition site. *Am. J. Hum. Genet.*, **47**, 994–1001.

Hansen, L. A., Masliah, E., Terry, R. D. & Mirra, S. S. (1989). A neuropathological subset of Alzheimer's disease with concomitant Lewy body disease and spongiform change. *Acta Neuropathol.*, **78**, 194–201.

Hansen, L., Salmon, D., Galasko, D. et al. (1990). The Lewy body variant of Alzheimer's disease: A clinical and pathological entity. *Neurology*, **40**, 1–8.

Hardy, J., Crook, R., Prihar, G., Roberts, G., Raghavan, R. & Perry, R. (1994). Senile dementia of the Lewy body type has an apolipoprotein E epsilon 4 allele frequency intermediate between controls and Alzheimer's disease. *Neurosci. Lett.*, **182**, 1–2.

Harrington, C. R., Louwagie, J., Rossau, R. et al. (1994). Influence of apolipoprotein E genotype on senile dementia of the Alzheimer and Lewy body types. Significance for etiological theories of Alzheimer's disease. *Am. J. Pathol.*, **145**, 1472–84.

Khachaturian, Z. S. (1985). Diagnosis of Alzheimer's disease. *Arch. Neurol.*, **42**, 1097–105.

Koller, W. C., Glatt, S. L., Hubble, J. P. et al. (1995). Apolipoprotein E genotypes in Parkinson's disease with and without dementia. *Ann. Neurol.*, **37**, 242–5.

Kondo, I. & Kanazawa, I. (1993). Debrisoquine hydroxylase and Parkinson's disease. *Adv. Neurol.*, **60**, 338–42.

Kurth, M. C. & Kurth, J. H. (1993). Variant cytochrome P_{450} CYP2D6 allelic frequencies in Parkinson's disease. *Am. J. Med. Genet. (Neuropsych. Genet.)*, **48**, 166–8.

Lippa, C. F., Smith, T. W., Nee, L. et al. (1995a). Familial Alzheimer disease and cortical Lewy bodies: Is there a genetic susceptibility factor? *Dementia*, **6**, 191–4.

Lippa, C. F., Smith, T. W., Saunders, A. M. et al. (1995b). Apolipoprotein E genotype and Lewy body disease. *Neurology*, **45**, 97–103.

Maestre, G., Ottman, R., Stern, Y. et al. (1995). Apolipoprotein E and Alzheimer's disease: Ethnic variation in genotype risks. *Ann. Neurol.*, **37**, 254–9.

Mann, D. M. A., Jones, D., Snowden, J. S., Neary, D. & Hardy, J. (1992). Pathological changes in the brain of a patient with familial Alzheimer's disease having a missense mutation at codon 717 in the amyloid precursor protein gene. *Neurosci. Lett.*, **137**, 225–8.

Marder, K., Maestre, G., Cote, L. et al. (1994). The apolipoprotein epsilon 4 allele in Parkinson's disease with and without dementia. *Neurology*, **44**, 1330–1.

Menzel, H. J., Kladetzky, R. G. & Assmann, G. (1983). Apolipoprotein E polymorphism and coronary artery disease. *Arteriosclerosis*, **3**, 310–15.

Nikkhah, G., Odin, P., Smits, A. et al. (1993). Platelet-derived growth factor promotes survival of rat and human mesencephalic dopaminergic neurons in culture. *Exp. Brain Res.*, **92**, 516–23.

Perry, R. H., Irving, D., Blessed, G., Fairbairn, A. F. & Perry, E. K. (1990). Senile dementia of Lewy body type. A clinical and neuropathologically distinct form of Lewy body dementia in the elderly. *J. Neurol. Sci.*, **95**, 119–39.

Pickering-Brown, S. M., Mann, D. M., Bourke, J. P. et al. (1994). Apolipoprotein E4 and Alzheimer's disease pathology in Lewy body disease and in other β-amyloid-forming diseases [letter]. *Lancet*, **343**, 1155.

Pollanen, M. S., Dickson, D. W. & Bergeron, C. (1993). Pathology and biology of the Lewy body. *J. Neuropathol. Exp. Neurol.*, **52**, 183–91.

Rebeck, G. W., Reiter, J. S., Strickland, D. K. & Hyman, B. T. (1993). Apolipoprotein E in sporadic Alzheimer's disease: Allelic variation and receptor interactions. *Neuron*, **11**, 575–80.

Rempfer, R., Crook, R., Houlden, H. et al. (1994). Parkinson's disease, but not Alzheimer's disease, Lewy body variant associated with mutant alleles at cytochrome P_{450} gene. *Lancet*, **344**, 815.

Saitoh, T., Xia, Y., Chen, X. et al. (1995). The CYP2D6B mutant allele is overrepresented in the Lewy body variant of Alzheimer's disease. *Ann. Neurol.*, **37**, 110–12.

Saunders, A. M., Schmader, K., Breitner, J. C. et al. (1993a). Apolipoprotein E epsilon 4 allele distributions in late-onset Alzheimer's disease and in other amyloid-forming diseases. *Lancet*, **342**, 710–11.

Saunders, A. M., Strittmatter, W. J., Schmechel, D. et al. (1993b). Association of apolipoprotein E allele ∈4 with late-onset familial and sporadic Alzheimer's disease. *Neurology*, **43**, 1467–72.

Schmechel, D. E., Saunders, A. M., Strittmatter, W. J. et al. (1993). Increased amyloid β-peptide deposition in cerebral cortex as a consequence of apolipoprotein E genotype in late-onset Alzheimer disease. *Proc. Natl. Acad. Sci. USA*, **90**, 9649–53.

Schmidt, M. L., Murray, J., Lee, V. M., Hill, W. D., Wertkin, A. & Trojanowski, J. Q. (1991). Epitope map of neurofilament protein domains in cortical and peripheral nervous system Lewy bodies. *Am. J. Pathol.*, **139**, 53–65.

Smith, C. A. D., Gough, A. C., Leight, P. N. et al. (1992). Debrisoquine hydroxylase gene polymorphism and susceptibility to Parkinson's disease. *Lancet*, **339**, 1375–7.

St. Clair, D., Norrman, J., Perry, R., Yates, C., Wilcock, G. & Brookes, A. (1994). Apolipoprotein E ∈4 allele frequency in patients with Lewy body dementia, Alzheimer's disease and age-matched controls. *Neurosci. Lett.*, **176**, 45–6.

Strittmatter, W. J., Saunders, A. M., Schmechel, D. et al. (1993). Apolipoprotein E: High avidity binding to β-amyloid and increased frequency of type 4 allele in late onset familial Alzheimer disease. *Proc. Natl. Acad. Sci. USA*, **90**, 1977–81.

Xu, Z., Cork, L. C., Griffin, J. W. & Cleveland, D. W. (1993). Increased expression of neurofilament subunit NF-L produces morphological alterations that resemble the pathology of human motor neuron disease. *Cell*, **73**, 23–33.

Résumé of pathology workshop sessions

P. G. INCE, S. LOVESTONE, J. S. LOWE
and R. H. PERRY

The Workshop on Pathology addressed the following questions and objectives.

1. Lesions which need to be distinguished in the pathological assessment of Lewy body dementia and the methods which should be used in their pathological evaluation.
2. Pathological diagnostic criteria and assessments which should:
   (a) be applicable to general diagnostic work
   (b) facilitate clinical correlative research studies
   (c) anticipate developments in identification of genetic linkages with disease
   (d) be nonjudgemental in relation to clinical syndromes
3. Key areas for future pathological investigation.
4. The relationship between the different terms which have been used to describe this condition (diffuse Lewy body disease, senile dementia of Lewy body type, Lewy body variant of Alzheimer's disease, cortical Lewy body disease, Lewy body dementia).

Terms of reference

It was agreed that the area of discussion comprised the neuropathology of patients who have cognitive decline associated with the presence of Lewy bodies (LB). For the purposes of the discussion the term 'dementia with Lewy bodies' (DLB) was considered most appropriate.

What lesions are significant?

The workshop identified the following pathological features as being relevant to DLB:

Pathological features associated with DLB
1. **Essential** for diagnosis of DLB
   Lewy bodies
2. **Associated** but not essential
   Lewy-related neurites
   Plaques (all morphological types)
   Neurofibrillary tangles
   Regional neuronal loss – especially brain stem (substantia nigra and locus coeruleus) and nucleus basalis of Meynert
   Microvacuolation (spongiform change) and synapse loss
   Neurochemical abnormalities and neurotransmitter deficits

The nature of the Lewy body

It was agreed that Lewy bodies were, in general, easily identifiable intra-cytoplasmic eosinophilic inclusion bodies, being usually spherical but displaying other morphological forms. The terms brainstem, or classical Lewy bodies, were endorsed to describe the inclusions with a hyaline core and pale halo typically seen in nigral and locus coeruleus neurons. The term cortical Lewy body (CLB) was endorsed to describe the less well defined spherical inclusions seen in cortical neurons. The term pale body was endorsed to describe the granular spherical inclusions seen in brain stem neurons for which there is some evidence for a precursor or early form of classical Lewy body (Dale et al., 1992). The different appearances of brain stem and CLB were recognized and discussed and the contribution of electron microscopy to understanding Lewy body disease, including the value of continued ultrastructural immunochemical studies, agreed.

Immunohistochemical and protein chemical studies which have characterized the composition of Lewy bodies were discussed. It was agreed that both classical and cortical Lewy bodies are based on neuronal intermediate filaments. All three neurofilament (NF) subunits are found but NF-L is present in greater quantity than NF-M or N-H, probably reflecting the normal stoichiometry (Pollanen et al., 1993). Using the currently available although somewhat limited antibodies to neurofilaments in immunocytochemical studies of Lewy bodies, NF subunits are found which are phosphorylated and unphosphorylated at different epitopes. In addition to neurofilaments, LBs contain α B crystallin, ubiquitin, and enzymes of the ubiquitin cycle. A variety of other proteins have been identified in Lewy bodies using well-characterized antibodies. The value of the concept of dividing constituent proteins into 'constitutional' and 'associated' elements was raised. However, this concept will require continuing re-evaluation as new data accumulate. There was a consensus that tau protein was not found in Lewy bodies and that this was a feature that could be used to distinguish CLB from small spherical tangles. The importance of biochemical work on purified CLB was recognized and it was noted that extraction procedures may strip the Lewy body of some associated proteins. It was agreed that the dense, hyaline, spherical core of Lewy bodies probably results from covalent crosslinking of constituent protein(s).

The exact pathobiology of the Lewy body remains enigmatic. While there is indirect evidence that this may be a manifestation of a cell stress response this is not yet certain.

Models for Lewy bodies

The absence of neuronal models for Lewy bodies was considered a serious handicap to research at present. MPTP-related eosinophilic inclusions are of interest but are not exactly equivalent to Lewy bodies. It was agreed that Lewy bodies have biochemical similarities to other intermediate filaments, ubiquitinated inclusions, and that insights gained from models of hepatic Mallory bodies were of value.

Techniques for identification of cortical Lewy bodies

The detection of LBs probably represents the single most important factor in the prominence of DLB. It was noted within the workshop that conventional H/E and other aniline dye techniques are generally extremely helpful although lacking sensitivity in determining the presence of CLBs. Anti-ubiquitin staining is more sensitive but is by no means specific for CLBs. Whilst the workshop agreed that ubiquitin staining was helpful, as is anti-tau and silver stain techniques, distinguishing rounded tangles and dystrophic neurites from LBs remains problematic in cases of combined cortical neurofibrillary tangle and LB involvement.

CLBs must clearly be distinguished from small ballooned neurons and, after discussion, it was noted that this could be achieved by noting lack of cellular extensions, lack of vacuolation, and the use of antineurofilament antibodies.

A consensus emerged that conventional staining supplemented by stains to detect plaques and tangles as well as immunochemical staining to detect tau protein and ubiquitin had a place in arriving at a diagnosis of DLB. It was noted that in many cases the identification of CLB posed little problem. In other cases with severe Alzheimer-changes and age-related pathology, clearly identifying spherical inclusions as Lewy bodies requires several special techniques supplemented by diagnostic experience.

For the future the participants emphasized the need for an improved, more sensitive marker for CLB. Although certain antineurofilament antisera were sensitive for the detection of Lewy bodies they were not sufficiently robust for general diagnostic use.

Regional distribution of cortical Lewy bodies

The location of Lewy bodies is important both macroscopically within defined anatomical regions of brain, and microscopically with respect to neurons. It was noted that both neuronal and non perikaryal forms are recognized and that Lewy bodies occur both in the brainstem and the cortex with a preference for certain nuclei or regions. It was agreed that the published meticulous work of Kosaka et al. (1994) accurately reflected the regional location of LBs in typical cases (Kosaka, 1990; Kosaka et al., 1989; see also Perry et al., 1990).

The work of Braak and Braak (1991) in proposing a staged model for Alzheimer's disease was discussed in relation to Lewy body disease. Consideration was given to the concept that Lewy body pathology might also be a staged process with a selective hierarchy of disease severity. After some discussion it emerged that there is no substantial evidence for a staged disease process. On the contrary, cases were commonly encountered which demonstrate a clear lack of regional hierarchy of progression. Lewy body diseases therefore represent a spectrum of multifocal pathology with different regions being affected in differing severity in different patients.

It was noted that certain cortical areas are preferentially involved in Lewy body pathology, and that it was possible to divide regions into those that were consistently affected, less consistently affected, and rarely affected. A ranking of entorhinal = cingulate > temporal > frontal > parietal was accepted. All patients with brainstem Lewy bodies have some

CLB but in most cases associated solely with clinical Parkinson's disease these may be sparsely distributed.

Further consideration was given to the concept of a 'spectrum' of Lewy body disorders. While certain general patterns of Lewy body distribution are commonly encountered (as typified by the groupings proposed by Kosaka (Kosaka, 1990; Kosaka et al., 1994; Perry et al., 1989)) there are sufficient cases with atypical or overlapping features to make a rigid classification on the basis of regional distribution difficult to apply in practice. Again, the concept of Lewy body disease as a multifocal pathology was felt to be compelling.

The need for conventional pathological studies of Lewy body disease to relate density of inclusions to other pathological and clinical features was stressed. This includes the need to study prospectively assessed cohorts from random community-based samples.

The question was posed as to whether regional differences in the pattern of nigral cell loss should be assessed and whether this may then explain patients with tremor-dominant or rigidity-dominant patterns of extrapyramidal movement disorder. It was felt that this hypothesis should not comprise part of a routine assessment but should be addressed in prospective research studies.

It was considered that a semi-quantitative rating for CLB density was desirable and a scheme was devised based around the CERAD protocol for assessment of AD pathology (see Appendix 2). This scheme generates a score which would be a measure of the 'cortical Lewy body burden'. It would be desirable for this scheme to be validated against clinical and other features of disease. It was felt that inter-laboratory comparisons of different patient cohorts would be possible by adopting this approach.

Lewy-related neurites

The neuritic abnormality originally described by Dickson et al. (1991) was accepted to be a distinctive part of Lewy body pathology which represents an abnormality in neural processes invisible on H/E but highlighted by ubiquitin staining. Lewy-related neurites contain neurofilament proteins and that these are present in a diffuse or filamentous form but are not condensed as in LBs. Whilst some of the composition of these neurites are similar to those of LBs they do not contain α B crystallin. These lesions are found in the CA2/CA3 region of the hippocampus, amygdala, nucleus basalis of Meynert (nbM), the dorsal vagal nucleus, and other brain stem nuclei.

In neuropathological assessment the presence of these neurites in the hippocampus, nbM and brainstem nuclei should be documented. The possibility of using a standard reference set of pictures allowing subjective assessment of density in defined regions was considered but no role in routine assessment was proposed.

Aβ plaques, neurofibrillary tangles and associated tau pathology

While it was noted that some cases have no associated Alzheimer-type pathology (ATP), ATP was a common feature of most cases of DLB and the validated CERAD protocol was proposed as the most appropriate for the documentation of these changes.

In this connection it was noted that the dominant plaque type in dementia with CLB lacks tau-immunoreactive dystrophic neurites (Dickson et al., 1991). If the diagnosis of Alzheimer's disease is made according to criteria which place a weighting on the presence of large numbers of neocortical plaques irrespective of morphology then it can be considered that most cases of Lewy body dementia also have Alzheimer's disease. If the diagnosis of Alzheimer's disease is based on the presence of tangles in neocortex and tau-immunoreactive neuritic plaques then a much smaller proportion of patients with cortical Lewy bodies can be said to have Alzheimer's disease. It was observed that the diagnostic status of Alzheimer cases with minimal neocortic tangle formation was unresolved and that previous studies of DLB show increased densities of archicortical tangles compared with patients presenting with Parkinson's disease alone (Ince et al., 1991). For this reason it was conceded that some workers would be very resistant to not making a pathological diagnosis of Alzheimer's disease in cases with associated CLBs. Further work will be needed to clarify these issues. The precise terminology individuals use for the disease was considered less important than establishing a common framework for the evaluation of the pathological lesions present.

In view of the advances in molecular pathology of AD some attempt should be made to document the presence or absence of the following plaque types in LBD:

Diffuse
Neuritic: tau immunoreactive
       :   ubiquitin immunoreactive

which would facilitate correlation with emerging insights into risk factors for plaque development.

Spongiform change (microvacuolation)

It was noted that spongiform change in a restricted pattern of distribution was a feature of some patients with dementia associated with cortical Lewy bodies, and that the possibility that this was a prion-related phenomenon has been excluded. However, not enough was known about this phenomenon and further work, particularly electron microscopy (EM) will be required to characterize it. It was postulated that this feature is associated with patients who have rapid clinical progression and this was highlighted as an issue in need of resolution.

Synaptic loss

Work on the evaluation of synaptic density using immunochemical staining for synaptophysin and other synaptic proteins was discussed. This was a useful line of enquiry of relevance to DLB but not something to be undertaken as part of routine assessment. Validation and reproducibility of synaptophysin immunochemical staining should be encouraged.

Biochemical assessments

The abnormal phosphorylation and truncation of neurofilament protein was considered to be a key element of the Lewy body phenomenon and future work should look for fundamental defects in neurofilament function/metabolism. Appropriate preservation of tissues at autopsy for these studies was encouraged.

Neurochemical assessments

A profound neocortical cholinergic deficit was a key element of many patients with DLB. Use of this observation as a component of a diagnostic profile was discussed. It was felt that it would be important to preserve tissue from key brain areas for neurochemical analysis but this need not form part of the routine documentation of pathological material.

It had been suggested that cortical neurons containing LB were tyrosine hydroxylase immunoreactive. This hypothesis is not yet

confirmed and it was recognized that few investigations on the transmitter content of neurons bearing CLB had been performed.

Existing nomenclature for dementia associated with cortical Lewy bodies

Dr Hansen proposed a 'Rosetta stone' which would allow translation of
nomenclature used by the various groups working on DLB. It was agreed
that the terms used by different groups had both overlaps and exclusions,
and that patients encountered in the series from different centres were not
always comparable. The difficulties thus posed by reconciling data from
different centres reinforced the idea of moving towards a common set of
descriptive pathological criteria. The extent to which the referral patterns
of differing groups of clinicians (especially neurologists vs psychiatrists)
has an effect on the composition of autopsy cohorts was emphasized.

Pathological criteria for diagnosis of Lewy body disorders

A detailed discussion was held throughout the workshop on the useful-
ness of pathological criteria. Clearly clinicians wish neuropathologists to
categorize, whereas neuropathologists, faced with the complexity of neurodegeneration in the brain, often prefer to detail the pathology present.
There seems to be a constant interplay between those who tend to group
disorders together, the 'lumpers' and those who tend to divide phenomena into smaller groups, the 'splitters'. Despite these problems and with
encouragement from the clinicians the pathology workshop agreed to
neuropathological criteria (see Appendix 2). The workshop agreed on a
mechanism to assign a descriptive diagnosis, evaluating and rating the
severity of significant pathological lesions. This allows individual groups
to correlate clinical and pathological findings in individual cases and issue
a definitive diagnosis according to existing published criteria.

It was accepted that the CERAD protocol represents a useful advance
in systematically and reproducibly categorizing neuropathological correlates of dementia and that this should be encouraged. The full CERAD
protocol is a considerable undertaking and the group did not accept the
need to complete it in full for each case. CERAD have approached not
only Alzheimer's disease but also Lewy body and vascular dementia and
the aim of the pathological workshop was to contribute towards a revision of CERAD rather than setting up entirely independent criteria.

Molecular genetics and dementia with cortical Lewy bodies

It was noted that there are overlaps between Alzheimer's disease and DLB and it was desirable to study the relationship between the genetic factors which have been associated with AD and PD and the pathological lesions found in the Lewy body disorders. This should be advanced by promoting re-evaluation of cases according to the newly proposed diagnostic assessment criteria and by sharing material between research groups. In particular it was felt important to study the influence of the APO E ε4 allele on cytoskeletal pathology in defined pathological subgroups of Lewy body disorders. This would address questions related to whether this is a tau, amyloid or NF-related risk factor. Sharing material should be encouraged, particularly in view of the relative scarcity of patients with 'pure' cortical Lewy body pathology in the absence of AD changes.

References

Braak, H. & Braak, E. (1991). Neuropathological staging of Alzheimer-related changes. *Acta Neuropathol. (Berl.)*, **82**, 239–59.

Dale, G. E., Probst, A., Luthert, P., Martin, J., Anderton, B. H. & Leigh, P. N. (1992). Relationship between Lewy bodies and pale bodies in Parkinson's disease. *Acta Neuropathol (Berl.)*, **83**, 525–9.

Dickson, D. W., Ruan, D., Crystal, H. et al. (1991). Hippocampal degeneration differentiates diffuse Lewy body disease (DLBD) from Alzheimer's disease: Light and electron microscopic immunocytochemistry of CA2-3 neurites specific to DLBD. *Neurology*, **41**, 1402–9.

Ince, P. G., Irving, D., MacArthur, F. & Perry, R. H. (1991). Quantitative neuropathological study of Alzheimer-type pathology in the hippocampus: comparison of senile dementia of Alzheimer type, senile dementia of Lewy body type, Parkinson's disease and non-demented elderly control patients. *J. Neurol. Sci.*, **106**, 142–52.

Kosaka, K. (1990). Diffuse Lewy body disease in Japan. *J. Neurol.*, **237**, 197–204.

Kosaka, K., Tsuchiya, K. & Yoshimura, M. (1989). Lewy body disease with and without dementia: a clinicopathological study of 35 cases. *Clin. Neuropathol.*, **7**, 299–305.

Kosaka, K., Iseki, E., Odawara, T. et al. (1994). A proposal of a cerebral type of Lewy body disease. *Abst. 12th International Congress of Neuropathology*, Toronto.

Perry, R. H., Irving, D., Blessed, G., Perry, E. K. & Fairbairn, A. F. (1989). Senile dementia of Lewy body type and the spectrum of Lewy body disease. *Lancet*, **1**, 1108.

Perry, R. H., Irving, D., Blessed, G., Fairbairn, A. F. & Perry, E. K. (1990). Senile dementia of Lewy body type: a clinically and neuropathologically distinct form of Lewy body dementia in the elderly. *J. Neurol. Sci.*, **95**, 119–39.

Pollanen, M. S., Dickson, D. W. & Bergeron, C. (1993). Pathology and biology of the Lewy body. *J. Neuropathol. Exp. Neurol.*, **52**, 183–91.

Part three

Treatment issues

28

Psychopharmacology of cognitive impairment in Parkinson's disease

H. J. SAGAR

Summary

Dementia occurs in PD and lesser cognitive deficits, of 'frontal-lobe' type, are detectable in nondemented patients even at diagnosis. Cortical Lewy bodies, Alzheimer changes and vascular disease have been considered to underlie clinical dementia in PD but, in nondemented cases, attention has been more focused on the neurochemical changes. Dopamine deficiency causes disruption to frontostriatal circuits but noradrenergic, cholinergic and serotonergic defects also occur and are involved in cognitive and affective disturbance in other conditions.

Modulation of these transmitter systems in PD using drugs with specific neurochemical effects suggests that dopamine deficiency causes selective impairment in 'frontal lobe' functions, such as working memory and planning, but many functions are unaffected. Noradrenergic modulation also affects frontal-lobe function although both facilitatory and inhibitory effects occur. Cholinergic deficits render patients sensitive to the effects of anticholinergic therapy, particularly on memory. Serotonergic deficits are related to depression.

Our longitudinal studies show that a subgroup of patients dement early. Risk factors for dementia include greater age at diagnosis and rapidly progressive motor disability. CT scans at diagnosis show a high incidence of abnormality, suggesting that structural rather than neurochemical pathology is responsible for the cognitive deficits. Predictive factors for dementia can be established from the neuropsychological profile at diagnosis.

The pathology of cognitive impairment in PD is multifaceted. Neurochemical deficits are more amenable to therapy through standard pharmacological means but another challenge is to identify early risk factors for the development of cortical pathology so that neuroprotection can be developed and targeted at appropriate patients.

28.1 Cognitive impairment in Parkinson's disease

Although motor deficits are the most consistent signs of Parkinson's disease (PD), cognitive dysfunction also occurs. Thus, the incidence of clinical dementia is significantly higher in PD than in the general population and specific cognitive deficits are recognized in clinically nondemented, nondepressed patients, even early in the course of the disease. Comparison of cognitive test results between patients with PD and patients with other neurodegenerative diseases, such as Alzheimer's disease (AD), has shown that some deficits are disproportionately severe in PD, and are thus related to the specific pathology of that condition. The affected cognitive domains include aspects of attentional control, short-term memory and immediate recall, conditional visuospatial memory and planning. Many of these impairments are thought to be due to frontal-lobe dysfunction but the neurochemical and neuropathological substrates remain unclear (Sagar & Sullivan, 1988; Brown & Marsden, 1988).

PD is associated with dopamine (DA) depletion from the caudate nucleus and putamen, and other structures, including the hypothalamus, nucleus accumbens and prefrontal cortex. Depletion has, however, also been shown in other neurotransmitter systems, notably the noradrenergic locus coeruleus, leading to loss of cortical noradrenaline (NA). Cholinergic cells of the nucleus basalis of Meynert are also involved, leading to degeneration of cholinergic cortical afferents. Central NA and acetylcholine (ACh), in particular, have been linked with cognitive processes, such as memory and attention (Agid et al., 1987; Robbins & Everitt, 1987; Sagar & Sullivan, 1988).

Converging lines of evidence from clinical studies (Kopelman, 1985), human psychopharmacology (Frith et al., 1985) and experimental studies in animals (Robbin & Everitt, 1987) suggest that these transmitter changes, separately or conjointly, could be involved in cognitive disturbance. However, because of the multivariate nature of these changes in PD, it is difficult to identify the critical pathology underlying the cognitive deficits. Other candidate processes include intrinsic frontal lobe pathology from diffuse cortical Lewy body disease, coexistent Alzheimer's disease and vascular changes (reviewed at this conference).

If the origin of cognitive disturbance in PD lies in intrinsic frontal lobe pathology or nondopaminergic subcortico-frontal afferents, the cognitive deficits are unlikely to respond in any major way to dopamine replacement or dopaminergic drugs. Moreover, the extent of cognitive impairment is unlikely to correlate well with the severity of dopamine-responsive motor deficits, although the correlation may be somewhat better with motor disability resistant to levodopa since this may depend on nondopaminergic pathology (discussed in Agid et al., 1987).

28.2 Pharmacological treatment of cognitive impairment

One way of investigating the neurochemical basis of impaired cognition in PD is to attempt reversal of the deficits using drugs with relatively specific pharmacological actions. Just as the dopaminergic involvement in the motor symptoms of PD was confirmed by the efficacy of levodopa therapy, successful treatment of the cognitive deficits would provide valuable information about their neurochemical substrates. Few studies have attempted to identify links between specific cognitive processes and neurochemical pathology in PD. This is particularly surprising because, in motor control, PD has been shown as an excellent model of a neurochemical deficiency disease in humans and both the cognitive deficits and the neurochemical pathology (dopaminergic and nondopaminergic) are better characterized than in other dementing conditions.

28.2.1 Dopamine

Alexander, De Long and colleagues have described five parallel but independent circuits between the striatum and frontal cortex; two of these loops are of particular relevance to PD: one 'motor', which links the putamen with the supplementary motor cortex and the second, 'complex', which links the caudate and prefrontal cortex (reviewed by Flaherty and Graybiel, 1994). Some authors have suggested that disruption of the complex loop, from dopamine deficiency in the caudate nucleus, is the critical lesion responsible for the cognitive disturbance. Others have suggested that the dysfunction arises from loss of mesocortical dopaminergic afferents to the prefrontal cortex. Both of these hypotheses predict that cognitive function would be sensitive to adequate dopamine replacement in PD; in addition, aspects of cognitive capacity would tend to correlate with motor disability since both functions would be affected, albeit perhaps to different degrees, by the extent of dopamine depletion corresponding to the severity of the disorder (discussed in Cooper et al., 1992).

Relatively few studies have examined directly the effect of manipulation of dopamine levels on cognitive function in PD. Gotham et al. (1988) studied the performance of a group of PD patients, on and off levodopa medication, on a series of tasks sensitive to frontal lobe damage. In the treated state, performance of patients differed from that of control subjects on tasks for which no difference was observed in the untreated state. The authors concluded that dopamine replacement adequate to produce optimal motor control had noxious effects on other dopamine pathways that governed cognition. In elderly subjects, levodopa selectively facilitated effortful, as opposed to automatic, memory processes, that is, those processes that are most compromised in PD. Other studies have reported improvement in delayed verbal recall, choice reaction time and vigilance from levodopa in PD. Those studies that have studied patients longitudinally, before and after the institution of levodopa therapy, have in general reported an initial mild improvement in cognitive performance that gradually declines to pretreatment levels (discussed in Cooper et al., 1992).

In general, no consistent pattern of benefit has emerged from studies of cognitive function in PD, possibly partly because of the limited and varied nature of the tasks employed and partly because of differences in the PD population under study. Few studies have examined a wide range of cognitive domains or compared the effects of different drug therapies; thus, further study is required to evaluate the specificity of the observations, both with respect to the cognitive domain affected and the nature of the drug employed (for further discussion, see Sagar, 1991). Some of the apparently specific changes in cognition resulting from change in dopamine status in PD may, for example, be attributable to changes in affect/arousal which appears to fluctuate in parallel with indices of cognition. Moreover, many studies have examined chronically medicated patients, who may show different response to levodopa replacement from early patients, owing to the chronic effects of levodopa therapy on dopamine receptors.

In a study of newly diagnosed, never treated PD patients, Cooper et al. (1991) showed that cognitive deficits were present at a disease duration of as little as 16 months and in subjects who scored normally on a Mini-Mental State test (MMST). The deficits, involving particularly short term and working memory, cognitive sequencing, set formation and semantic fluency, showed only weak correlations with physical disability. Only those tests requiring motor control or visuomotor coordination associated significantly with scores on a test of fine finger movements;

motor control, on the other hand, correlated significantly with an index of depression. In that paper, we suggested the presence of two sets of dissociable processes in the earliest clinical stages of the disease: one involving motor control and affect in which deficits produce psychomotor retardation and the second serving cognition in which deficits lead to impaired working memory and attention. The evidence suggested that the former are related to dopaminergic pathology but the latter principally to nondopaminergic lesions.

In order to investigate the neurochemical pathology of the cognitive impairment in early PD, a longitudinal study of these patients was undertaken, after treatment (Cooper et al., 1992). Patients were reassessed after randomization to levodopa, bromocriptine or benzhexol. All treatments except bromocriptine produced a significant improvement in motor control. However, improvements in the cognitive domain, over and above practice effects, were minimal. The only neuropsychological deficit, which showed significant improvement, was the Digit Ordering Test of working memory which appeared to benefit from dopaminergic but not anticholinergic therapy (Fig. 28.1). This improvement is particularly interesting because Digit Ordering demonstrated one of the most prominent deficits of PD in the untreated state. Dopamine treatment appears to attenuate the deficit of untreated patients in the reordering of items in short-term memory.

The results of assessment on treatment showed that affect continued to dissociate from cognitive performance. Change in depressive symptoms from one phase to the next did not correlate significantly with change in cognitive test performance over the same assessments; neither did severity of depression correlate significantly with the cognitive test scores achieved on treatment. Conversely motor control, which had shown only weak association with cognition in the untreated state, correlated with performance on a wide range of cognitive tasks on treatment. A similar finding was shown by Pillon et al. (1989) who reported stronger associations between cognitive test results and physical disability when patients were treated than when their symptoms were unalleviated. The authors claimed that cognitive deficits associated most strongly with axial symptoms and that both were largely independent of dopaminergic dysfunction. Thus, in a treated state the patients' axial symptoms represented a greater proportion of their disability (since they had not responded to levodopa) and hence correlations between cognition and motor control increased. Taken together, the evidence suggests that, in general, motor and cognitive impairments are mediated by different

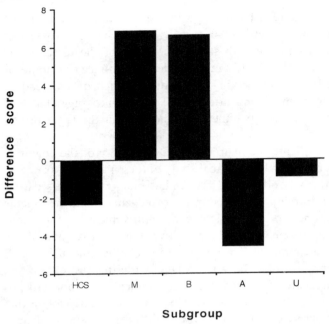

Fig. 28.1 Performance on the Digit Ordering Test of working memory in patients with PD, expressed as a difference score (performance on treatment minus performance off treatment). Patients receiving levodopa (Madopa; M) or bromocriptine (B) showed a significant improvement in performance but healthy control subjects tested twice (HCS) and those receiving antiocholinergic therapy (A) or no treatment (U) showed no change in response.

pathologies. The conflicting observations of relationships between cognition and motor disability in PD probably relate to the multifactorial nature of the neuropathology: dopamine appears critical for motor control but not cognition; cognitive impairment is caused by noradrenergic and cholinergic neurochemical deficits and intrinsic cortical pathology which may also underlie motor disability that is resistant to levodopa therapy.

Other studies have shown a heterogeneous effect of levodopa on cognition in PD with, overall, selective improvement in some tests of frontal lobe function in PD patients with severe clinical disability but no effect on other cognitive functions (Lange et al., 1992). The dissociation between the dopaminergic influences on cognition and motor control may be due in part to the production of supraoptimal levels of DA in structures serving cognition, such as the caudate-frontal circuits, in conjunction with optimal DA replacement in structures serving motor control, such as the putamen (Gotham et al., 1988). Some cognitive processes seem to be independent of levodopa treatment, however, and other evidence implicates nondopaminergic pathology in the aetiology of these impairments.

28.2.2 Acetylcholine

Pharmacological treatment of human cognitive deficits has been demonstrated in AD and Korsakoff's syndrome (KS). Although the effects of cholinergic agonists and anticholinesterases in AD have been small and not always beneficial, most recent, controlled large-scale studies have reported improvements (reviewed by Kopelman, 1987). Moreover, these small successes have to be regarded positively in the context of treating severely demented patients with the cholinergic drugs currently available. A recent series of studies (Jones et al., 1992; Sahakian et al., 1989) has also shown clearly beneficial effects of subcutaneous nicotine in a test of rapid information processing in normal elderly subjects and patients with AD. The actions of nicotine are quite complex, with both pre- and post-synaptic effects on cholinergic neurons and stimulatory actions on the coeruleo-cortical NA and the mesolimbic DA systems. Some studies have highlighted the potential of the new class of 5-HT3 receptor antagonists, including ondansetron, in the treatment of cognitive deficits. The mechanism of action of these compounds may be through an enhancement of release of cortical ACh by the blockade of inhibitory presynaptic 5-HT3 receptors on the cholinergic terminals, although other effects, such as antagonism to mesolimbic DA, and other effects of 5-HT3 antagonism may also occur. This indirect means of boosting ACh release has special advantages in the treatment of cognitive dysfunction in PD because the action will not affect ACh release in the dorsal striatum owing to the paucity of 5-HT3 binding sites in that region. Consequently, this form of cholinergic treatment is very unlikely to lead to extrapyramidal motor complications.

In the Cooper et al. (1992) study, anticholinergic treatment of PD appeared to exacerbate deficits in those aspects of memory that were most compromised in the untreated state. These deficits largely comprised an 'acquisition' deficit but not an accelerated rate of forgetting, an effect similar to that found with cholinergic blockade in normal subjects (Fig. 28.2). It seems likely therefore that any effect of anticholinergic medication is to exacerbate a preexisting deficit in processes of registration that underlie immediate memory. This effect may occur because anticholinergic drugs impair attentional control, especially for effort-

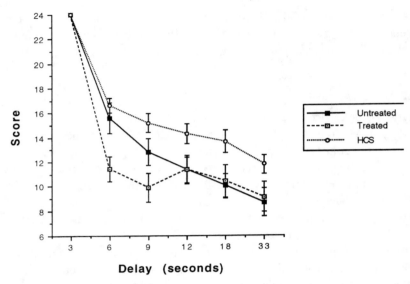

Fig. 28.2 Performance on the Brown-Peterson Test of short-term memory in patients with PD before and after treatment with anticholinergic drugs. Treatment produced an initial registration deficit but no change in forgetting rate.

demanding tasks (Dunne & Hartley, 1986) at which PD patients perform particularly poorly.

A previous investigation of cholinergic function in PD has shown that scopolamine (a cholinergic blocking agent) impairs recognition memory, in doses insufficient to affect cognition in age matched controls (Dubois et al., 1987). Perry et al. (1985) found extensive reductions of choline acetyltransferase and moderate reductions of acetylcholinesterase in all four cortical lobes. These levels correlated significantly with the number of neurons in the nucleus basalis of Meynert, possibly indicating the primary site of neuron degeneration and hence one cause of declining cognitive function in PD. Memory loss and confusional states commonly occur in PD patients following anticholinergic treatment. Nondemented PD patients show less reduction in cortical ChAT activity than do demented PD patients (Perry et al., 1985).

28.2.3 *Noradrenaline*

Korsakoff patients showed surprising cognitive benefit in two controlled trials using clonidine, which has adrenergic agonist actions at pre- and post-synaptic alpha-2, and post-synaptic alpha-1 receptors (Mair & McEntee, 1983, 1986). Analogous effects have been observed in frontal-lobe tests of memory in aged rhesus monkeys or in young animals with lesions of the noradrenergic innervation of the cortex; adrenergic receptor mapping in these animals suggests that the key site of action of clonidine is at post-synaptic alpha-2 binding sites (Arnsten & Goldman-Rakic, 1985). The neurochemical specificity of the action of clonidine is, however, highly questionable and effects on cognition may be severely compounded by its nonspecific effects on cortical arousal. A recent extension of the clonidine study has shown comparable results using the drug guanfacine, which is a more selective agonist at alpha-2 receptors and causes less sedation and hypotension than clonidine. Guanfacine had a more potent effect on memory facilitation than did clonidine at doses lower than those that produce hypotension (Arnsten & Goldman-Rakic, 1987). Reaction times of PD patients in continuous performance tasks correlate positively with cerebrospinal fluid concentrations of the NA metabolite, 3-methoxy-4-hydroxy-phenylene glycol, although the concentrations of the metabolite were normal (Stern et al., 1984). In the covert orienting paradigm of Posner, PD patients showed normal engagement but reduced maintenance of attention (Wright et al., 1990); the similarity to the pattern produced by reduced catecholamine neurotransmission suggested that noradrenergic deficiency underlies at least some of the attentional deficits in PD (although the specificity of the catecholamine effect has been challenged). The alpha-2 antagonist idazoxan releases NA in the CNS in human subjects and increases blood flow to the frontal lobes in normal subjects. In frontal lobe dementia, idazoxan produced improvement in performance on tests of executive capacity, compatible with a relatively specific effect on frontal lobe function (Sahakian et al., in press).

These observations encouraged us recently to undertake a controlled study of the effects of guanfacine on cognitive performance in PD (Tidswell et al., unpublished observations). Patients were selected on the basis of a minimum level of cognitive impairment on one of two screening tests, the Blessed Dementia Scale (BDS) and the Wisconsin Card Sorting Test (WCST). Patients were excluded if taking psychoactive medication, scoring 13 or more on the BDS, scoring 26 or more on the Beck Depression Inventory (BDI), suffering severe on/off motor fluctuations, or if onset of PD symptoms was after 70 years of age. All patients were taking levodopa preparations, and many were taking other drugs for PD; these medications and doses were kept constant during the study.

Patients were randomized double-blind to one of four treatment groups, namely guanfacine 0.1 mg, 0.2 mg, or 0.4 mg daily or matching placebo. Before treatment, the four patient groups did not differ significantly from each other with respect to age, duration of disease, premorbid or current intelligence, motor disability or global cognitive impairment (as measured by the BDS). A comprehensive battery of tests to assess intelligence, memory, executive, visuospatial and motor functioning and mood was administered by the same observer off treatment, after 4 weeks guanfacine and after one week wash-out.

Treatment effects were calculated as the mean baseline score subtracted from the scores on treatment. In addition, in order to reduce the within-subject variance across tests, and to reduce the risk of chance significant observations, a pooled cognitive score was obtained for each subject for tests determined a priori to be of 'executive' or 'memory' type. Scores on each type of test were converted to standard Z-scores (the number of standard deviations from the mean) and summed for each subject to give two cognitive measures: standard executive score and a standard memory score. Finally, in order to examine the possibility of heterogeneity of response within the group of patients treated with guanfacine, the variance of the difference scores for patients treated with guanfacine were compared with those from patients treated with placebo using the F ratio statistic.

On the WCST, the between-patient variance of the treated difference score for total categories sorted (F ratio $= 2.98$, $p < 0.05$) and for perseverative responses (F ratio $= 2.98$, $p < 0.05$) was significantly greater in the guanfacine-treated group than the placebo group, reflecting an improvement in performance with guanfacine treatment in some patients but a deterioration in others. Thus, 18% of treated patients fell outside the placebo range on total categories (with treatment showing equal positive and negative effects), and 30% on perseverative responses (with all but a single patient showing improvement on treatment). An increase in the population variance on guanfacine treatment was also seen for scores on verbal fluency, using the category of animals (F ratio $= 4.94$, $p < 0.01$: Fig. 28.3). The reduction in mean perseverative response score was significantly greater with 0.2 mg guanfacine than placebo (Fisher, $p < 0.05$) but no other comparison of mean performance between treatment groups was significant for performance on either WCST or verbal fluency.

On the Digit Ordering Test of working memory, the treated difference score was significantly less on guanfacine than placebo, reflecting a net deterioration at all doses of guanfacine (placebo vs all treated patients,

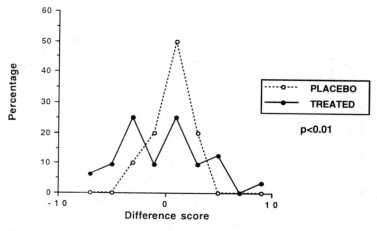

Fig. 28.3 Frequency distribution of treatment difference scores for category fluency (animals) in patients taking guanfacine or placebo. Guanfacine produced a significant change in the population variance of difference scores; i.e. some patients improved whilst others deteriorated on guanfacine treatment.

$t = 2.92$, $p < 0.01$). Guanfacine did not produce any specific change in performance on any of the other individual executive tests.

The overall 'executive standard score' was calculated as the sum of the standard (Z) scores from each of the following tests:

- Wisconsin card sorting test – four measures: categories, total errors, perserverations and cards to first category
- Verbal fluency – three measures: objects, animals, birds/colours
- Digit ordering – one measure: total score
- Picture arrangement – one measure: Mcfie error score
- Verbal temporal ordering – one measure: mean score on recency discrimination.
- MIT verbal recency test – one measure: excess of order errors over content errors

Guanfacine produced a clear dose-related effect on the frontal standard score. 0.1 mg guanfacine produced an improvement in executive performance; 0.4 mg caused a decline in performance and 0.2 mg produced an intermediate effect (Fig. 28.4). The change in score between the 0.1 and 0.4 mg groups was significant (Fisher, $p < 0.05$).

In summary of the executive tests, guanfacine produced clear increases in the variance of scores on WCST and category fluency, indicating both

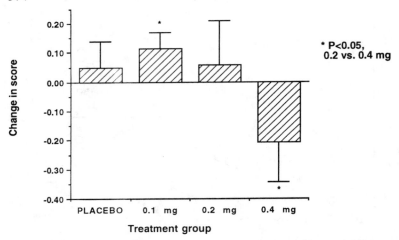

Fig. 28.4 Change in the 'frontal standard score' on guanfacine treatment expressed as a difference score (performance on treatment minus performance off treatment). Performance on tests sensitive to frontal lobe dysfunction improved on 0.1 mg guanfacine daily but deteriorated on guanfacine 0.4 mg daily.

positive and negative effects on performance on these tasks. Digit ordering was sensitive to an inhibitory effect of drug at all doses. The results, particularly when pooled into the executive standard score, indicate dose- and patient-related effects of guanfacine on performance. In general, low doses (0.1 mg) produced benefit whereas higher doses (0.4 mg) produced impairment.

On matching-to-sample from the CANTAB battery, significant treatment effects on per cent correct score were seen at the Os delay condition of the test with a significant effect in favour of increasing treatment level ($F = 2.48$, $p < 0.02$) but no specific effect was seen on a number of other standard memory tests.

An overall 'memory standard score' was derived from the sum of the standard (Z) scores of each of the following tests:

- Wechsler memory scale – one measure: memory quotient
- Wechsler memory scale – one measure: Logical Memory immediate score
- Brown – Peterson short term memory test – one measure: total score
- Rey complex drawing – one measure: delay/immediate score
- pattern recognition – one measure: total score
- spatial recognition – one measure: total score

- delayed matching to sample – three measures: 0, 4 and 12 second delay

Changes in performance in the direction of both improvement and deterioration were seen at different doses of guanfacine. Although 1-factor ANOVA of the treated difference scores by treatment group did not show any significant difference, post-hoc tests (Fisher $p < 0.05$) indicated a difference in memory performance between patients on 0.1 mg and 0.2 mg of guanfacine (Fig. 28.4). Patients on the lower dose *improved* in performance.

Guanfacine had a significant beneficial effect on intentional but not incidental spatial recall. This effect is of considerable interest, as we have shown that PD patients are disproportionately impaired compared to healthy control subjects at item recall on the intentional dual task, which involves the most effortful processing. Dopaminergic treatment does not correct this impairment.

No significant effect of guanfacine on motor performance was observed. Guanfacine 0.2 mg daily had a detrimental effect on mood, compared with placebo or 0.1 mg.

In summary, these results showed both small dose-related improvements on certain tests and impairments on others and, overall, significantly greater variability in performance amongst subjects on treatment compared with those on placebo. This latter observation may reflect a dual action of guanfacine at pre- and post-synaptic alpha-2 receptors. Thus some executive deficits in PD may be due to alteration in noradrenergic function.

28.2.4 Serotonin

Studies of 5-HT involvement in cognitive function are meagre. In AD, serotonergic treatment generally produces little improvement in cognition. However, cognitive effects of alcohol were attenuated by the selective 5-HT reuptake inhibitors, zimelidine (Weingartner et al., 1983) and fluvoxamine (Linnoila et al., 1987); fluvoxamine-associated improvement correlated with reduction in CSF levels of 5-HIAA, the major metabolite of serotonin.

The relationship between depression and cognitive impairment in PD is unclear. Depression has been considered an integral feature of 'subcortical dementia' and a complex functional relationship between depression and specific cognitive deficits of PD has been proposed (reviewed by

Sagar & Sullivan, 1988). Depression has been linked to ascending mono-amine systems and may benefit from treatment that modulates these systems. 5-HT has also been strongly implicated in the pathogenesis of depression and deficits in 5-HT neurotransmission have been demon-strated in PD. Furthermore, concentrations of 5-HIAA, the main meta-bolite of serotonin, are lower in the cerebrospinal fluid of depressed, as compared with non-depressed, PD patients. Although antidepressant medication has been used effectively in the treatment of depression in PD, its action on cognitive function has been little explored. However, the study of Cooper et al. (1991) on 60 newly diagnosed, untreated patients indicated dissociations between motor impairment, cognitive deficits and depression in PD. Specifically, depressed and nondepressed patients did not differ in their performance on cognitive tests except where speed of response was critical to performance whereas depression and motor impairment were strongly associated. The relationship between cognition and depression may, however, differ between early and chronic PD cases (Starkstein et al., 1989), implying different patho-physiological bases for depression according to duration of disease and nature of treatment.

28.3 Structural pathology and predictors of dementia

In an extension of our studies on the acute effects of psychopharmaco-logical manipulation, we have monitored the cognitive profile of de novo patients in relation to their advancing motor disability, long-term drug therapy and neuropathophysiology to ascertain which factors are most significantly involved in the cognitive decline of the disease and to estab-lish risk factors at diagnosis for the development of dementia. These factors include CT scan appearances as well as demographic variables and neuropsychological test results.

CT scans were carried out on all patients at diagnosis and the findings were classified qualitatively into three groups: normal or with mild gen-eralized atrophy but no focal lesions; focal or multifocal abnormality which was not directly relevant to the development of parkinsonism, for example, lacunar infarcts not involving the basal ganglia; and focal, generalized or multifocal abnormality which was considered directly re-levant, for example, basal ganglia infarcts or hydrocephalus. Patients in the third group were excluded from the study.

An interim analysis has been carried out on the first 149 patients admitted to the study (Collinson et al., unpublished observations) and

35 healthy control subjects who were monitored in parallel. The groups were matched in age (mean PD 59.9, control 59.5 years), premorbid IQ as assessed by the NART (mean PD 108, control 110) and years of education (mean PD 10.3, control 10.4). All PD patients fulfilled the PDS Brain Bank criteria for the diagnosis of idiopathic PD. Subjects in either group were excluded if they had a past or current history of any medical condition that may impair cognition or if they were taking psychoactive medication. After evaluation at diagnosis and after the institution of medication, subjects were followed at approximately annual intervals for up to eight assessments over six years.

Thirty-four patients have dropped out from further follow-up. Of these, 14 refused and 8 were geographically or physically unable. Four died, of whom three were demented; the remaining eight were too demented to undertake cognitive testing. The findings *at diagnosis* in these 11 patients who later demented were compared with the nondemented patients still in the study.

At diagnosis, the demented patients differed significantly from the nondemented in age of onset of PD (mean demented 65.3, nondemented 57.3 years) score on the BDS (mean demented 5.89, nondemented 2.8 years) and motor disability which was higher on all measures in the demented group. The demented group also tended to higher depression scores (BDI mean demented 13.2, nondemented 9.1). However, the groups did not differ on any other demographic variable. Importantly, there was no difference in duration of symptoms; in fact, the demented group tended to have a *shorter* duration of symptoms at diagnosis (mean demented 13.2, nondemented 19.2 months). This latter observation shows that the differences between the groups at diagnosis are not simply due to having detected the demented patients at a later chronological stage but rather that the demented cases form a subgroup with more rapid progression of cognitive disability and probably motor and affective disability as well. Initial response to treatment did not differ between the groups (in fact, was slightly better in the demented group).

CT scans at diagnosis were available in 114 cases (10 demented and 80 nondemented). The incidence of scans showing abnormality (but not directly relevant to parkinsonism) was significantly higher in the demented group than the nondemented group (demented 70%, nondemented 33.8%). In most cases, the abnormalities were generalised atrophy and multiple, tiny white matter low density areas of uncertain pathology.

An analysis was carried out to determine the predictive value of cognitive test results at diagnosis, independent of age, in those patients showing abnormal CT scans (Tooth et al., unpublished observations). Subgroups of 7 demented and 16 nondemented cases were selected from the patients with abnormal scans to match for age of onset (mean demented 64.1, nondemented 62.8 years). Comparison of these groups showed the cases who later demented to have inferior performance at diagnosis than those who did not on the Digit Ordering Test of working memory, immediate memory tests from the Wechsler Memory Scale, the Picture Arrangement subtest of the WAIS, category fluency, and visuo-motor coordination (copy of the Rey figure) but not motor disability. The Digit Ordering Test was the most sensitive in predicting dementia (sensitivity 0.86, specificity 0.67) and had a high negative predictive value (0.95) but a low positive predictive value (0.4). However, abnormal performance (less than two standard deviations from the control mean) on two of three tests – Digit Ordering, copy of the Rey figure and immediate Logical Memory from the Wechsler Memory Scale – had a sensitivity of 0.71, specificity 0.93, positive predictive value 0.71 and negative predictive value 0.93.

Results of this study suggest that a subgroup of patients with a high risk of dementia can be identified at diagnosis. These patients have a higher age, incidence of ill-defined, multifocal CT changes, greater motor disability and, allowing for age, inferior performance on cognitive tests, particularly those sensitive to frontal lobe dysfunction. These patients probaby have widespread cerebral pathology, including cortical Lewy body disease. However, the contribution of cerebral pathology to the cognitive impairment of those cases which fall short of a clinical diagnosis of dementia remains to be established; our preliminary observations suggest that cognitive decline also occurs in this group over time, albeit at a slower rate.

28.4 Conclusions

The pathology of cognitive impairment in PD is almost certainly multi-faceted. Depletion in the major subcortical neurochemical systems, dopamine, acetylcholine, noradrenaline and serotonin all contribute to cognitive decline in PD, probably in qualitatively different ways. The importance of these pathologies is that they are more amenable to therapy through standard pharamacological means than structural changes in the cerebral cortex. Cortical neuronal loss, notably from cortical Lewy body disease but also Alzheimer pathology and multi-infarction, are the major causes of severe dementia, and may occur much earlier in the disease than has been generally recognized. One challenge is to identify early risk factors for these pathologies so that specific protective therapy can be developed and targeted at appropriate patients. The ability to identify reliably patients at risk may well be possible by sophisticated use of existing neuroimaging and neuropsychological tests.

References

Agid, Y., Ruberg, M., Dubois, B. & Pillon, B. (1987). Anatomoclinical and biochemical concepts of subcortical dementia. In *Cognitive Neurochemistry*, ed. S. Stahl et al., pp. 248–71. Oxford: Oxford University Press.

Arnsten, A. F. T. & Goldman-Rakic, P. S. (1985). Alpha-2-adrenergic mechanisms in prefrontal cortex associated with cognitive decline in aged nonhuman-primates. *Science*, **230**, 1273–6.

Arnsten, A. F. T. & Goldman-Rakic, P. S. (1987). Noradrenergic mechanisms in age-related cognitive decline. *J. Neural Transm. (Suppl.)*, **24**, 317–24.

Brown, R. & Marsden, C. D. (1988). Subcortical dementia: the neuropsychological evidence. *Neuroscience*, **25**, 363–87.

Cooper, J. A., Sagar, H. J., Jordan, N., Harvey, N. S. & Sullivan, E. V. (1991). Cognitive impairment in early untreated Parkinson's disease and its relationship to motor disability. *Brain*, **114**, 2095–122.

Cooper, J. A., Sagar, H. J., Doherty, S. M., Jordan, N., Tisdwell, P. & Sullivan, E. V. (1992). Different effects of dopaminergic and anticholinergic therapies on cognitive and motor function in Parkinson's disease: a follow-up study of untreated patients. *Brain*, **115**, 1701–25.

Dubois, B., Danze, F., Pillon, B., Cusimano, G., Lhermitte, F. & Agid, Y. (1987). Cholinergic-dependent cognitive deficits in Parkinson's disease. *Ann. Neurol.*, **22**, 26–30.

Dunne, M. P. & Hartley, L. R. (1986). Scopolamine and the control of attention in humans. *Psychopharmacology*, **89**, 94–7.

Flaherty, A. W. & Graybiel, A. M. (1994). Anatomy of the basal ganglia. In *Movement Disorders*, Vol. 3, ed. C. D. Marsden & S. Fahn. Oxford: Butterworth Heinemann.

Frith, C. D., Dowdy, J., Ferrier, I. N. & Crow, T. J. (1985). Selective impairment of paired-associated learning after administration of a centrally-acting adrenergic agonist (clonidine). *Psychopharmacology*, **87**, 490–3.

Gotham, A. M., Brown, R. G. & Marsden, C. D. (1988). Frontal cognitive function in patients with Parkinson's disease on and off levodopa. *Brain*, **111**, 299–321.

Jones, G. M., Sahakian, B. J., Levy, R., Warburton, D. M. & Gray, J. A. (1992). Effects of acute subcutaneous nicotine on attention, information processing and short-term memory in Alzheimer's disease. *Psychopharmacology*, **108**, 485–94.

Kopelman, M. D. (1985). Multiple memory deficits in Alzheimer-type dementia-implications for pharmacotherapy. *Psych. Med.*, **15**, 527–41.

Kopelman, M. D. (1987). How far could cholinergic depletion account for the memory deficits of Alzheimer-type dementia or the alcoholic Korsakoff syndrome? In *Cognitive Neurochemistry*, ed. S. Stahl et al., pp. 303–27. Oxford: Oxford University Press.

Lange, K. W., Robbins, T. W., Marsden, C. D., James, M., Owen, A. M. & Paul, G. M. (1992). L-dopa withdrawal in Parkinson's disease selectively impairs cognitive performance in tests sensitive to frontal lobe dysfunction. *Psychopharmacology (Berl.)*, **107**, 394–404.

Linnoila, M., Eckardt, M., Durcan, M., Lister, R. & Martin, P. (1987). Interactions of serotonin with ethanol – clinical and animal studies. *Psychopharm. Bull.*, **23**, 452–7.

Mair, R. G. & McEntee, W. J. (1983). Korsakoff's psychosis – noradrenergic systems and cognitive impairment. *Behav. Brain Res.*, **9**, 1–32.

Mair, R. G. & McEntee, W. J. (1986). Cognitive enhancement in Korsakoff's psychosis by clonidine – a comparison with L-dopa and ephedrine. *Psychopharmacology*, **88**, 374–80.

Perry, E. K., Curtis, M., Dick, D. J. et al. (1985). Cholinergic correlates of cognitive impairment in Parkinson's disease: comparisons with Alzheimer's disease. *J. Neurol. Neurosurg. Psychiatry*, **48**, 413–21.

Pillon, B., Dubois, B., Cusimano, G., Bonnet, A., Lhermitte, F. & Agid, Y. (1989). Does cognitive impairment in Parkinson's disease result from non-dopaminergic lesions? *J. Neurol. Neurosurg. Psychiatry*, **52**, 201–6.

Robbins, T. W. & Everitt, B. J. (1987). Psychopharmacological studies of arousal and attention. In *Cognitive Neurochemistry*, ed. S. Stahl et al., pp. 135–70. Oxford: Oxford University Press.

Sagar, H. J. (1991). Specificity of cognitive impairment in neurological disease: methodological critique of Parkinson's disease. *Behav. Neurol.*, **4**, 89–102.

Sagar, H. J. & Sullivan, E. V. (1988). Patterns of cognitive impairment in dementia. In *Recent Advances in Clinical Neurology*, Vol. 5, ed. C. Kennard, pp. 47–86. Edinburgh: Churchill Livingstone.

Sahakian, B., Jones, G., Levy, R., Gray, J. & Warburton, D. (1989). The effects of nicotine on attention, information processing and short-term memory in patients with dementia of the Alzheimer type. *Br. J. Psychiatry*, **154**, 797–800.

Sahakian, B. J., Coull, J. T. & Hodges, J. R. (in press). Selective enhancement of executive function by idazoxan in a patient with dementia of the frontal lobe type. *J. Neurol. Neurosurg. Psychiatry*.

Starkstein, S. E., Berthier, M. L., Bolduc, P. L., Preziosi, T. J. & Robinson, R. G. (1989). Depression in patients with early versus late onset of Parkinson's disease. *Neurology*, **39**, 1441–5.

Stern, Y., Mayeux, R. & Cote, L. (1984). Reaction-time and vigilance in Parkinson's-disease – possible role of altered norepinephrine metabolism. *Arch. Neurol.*, **41**, 1086–9.

Weingartner, H., Rudorfer, M. V., Buchsbaum, M. S. & Linnoila, M. (1983). Effects of serotonin on memory impairments produced by ethanol. *Science*, **221**, 472–4.

Wright, M. J., Burns, R. J., Geffen, G. M. & Geffen, G. M. (1990). Covert orientation of visual attention in Parkinson's disease: an impairment in the maintenance of attention. *Neuropsychologia*, **28**, 151–9.

29

Management of the noncognitive symptoms of Lewy body dementia

I. G. McKEITH, A. FAIRBAIRN
and R. HARRISON

Summary

Noncognitive symptoms, particularly visual hallucinations and system-atized delusions, are frequent symptoms in patients with Lewy body dementia (LBD) and may dominate the clinical picture. The neurobio-logical basis for these symptoms appears to be an imbalance in cortical monoaminergic:cholinergic function.

Because these psychotic symptoms are distressing and may precipitate requests for institutionalization, clinicians frequently attempt pharmaco-logical management, usually with neuroleptic medication. Abnormal sen-sitivity of LBD patients to neuroleptic medication has been established in two retrospective casenote studies in Newcastle. The increased mortality associated with neuroleptic medication is two- to threefold, 50% of neu-roleptic treated patients being susceptible. Review of the case literature suggests that similar neuroleptic sensitivity responses have been noted in other centres but their clinical significance has not been appreciated. The mechanism underlying neuroleptic sensitivity in LBD appears to be nigrostriatal dopaminergic depletion, associated with a failure of adap-tive upregulation of postsynaptic striatal D2 receptors.

These early reports of neuroleptic sensitivity in LBD have already had an impact upon UK regulatory recommendations about the need for caution in neuroleptic prescribing in elderly patients with dementia. A systematic approach to the management of noncognitive symptoms in patients with LBD is described, and novel approaches including the use of atypical antipsychotics and cholinergic enhancers are discussed.

381

29.1 What are the 'noncognitive' symptoms of dementia?

It is the behavioural changes associated with dementia, rather than impairment of memory or other intellectual functions per se, which are the most frequent source of distress to sufferers and carers, and which act as major determinants of outcome, including the rate of cognitive decline, the probability of institutionalization and the survival time until death (Rabins, 1994). 'Noncognitive symptom' is an unsatisfactory generic term which is often used to describe psychotic features (delusions and hallucinations), mood disorders (predominantly anxiety, depression or lability), alterations in personality, and a variety of other miscellaneous behavioural changes such as sleep disturbance or motor over/under activity. Other closely related symptoms such as misidentification syndromes or false beliefs which are based upon misinterpretation of events are usually considered as part of the same cluster, but seem more obviously secondary to impairments in perception, memory and judgement and as such the term 'noncognitive' appears less appropriate for them. Support for making such distinctions between different types of symptoms comes from findings that in AD patients, hallucinations and delusions are more frequent in those with higher cognitive test scores (Burns et al., 1990), less cortical atrophy on CT scan (Jacoby & Levy, 1980), and relative preservation of neurons in the parahippocampal gyrus (Förstl et al., 1994). Patients with misidentification symptoms are more severely impaired on each of these parameters.

29.2 How frequent are noncognitive symptoms in Lewy body and other dementias?

Noncognitive symptoms may be of particular importance in patients with Lewy body dementia (LBD) who as a group appear to have higher rates of psychosis than Alzheimer's disease (AD) and multi-infarct dementia (MID) patients. For example, in one autopsy confirmed series (McKeith et al., 1992b), 80% of 20 LBD patients had visual hallucinations, in contrast to 19% of 21 AD and none of 9 MID patients. The corresponding percentages for auditory hallucinations were 45%, 0% and 11% and for delusions, 80%, 19% and 11% respectively, each diagnostic group-wise comparison being highly significant ($p < 0.001$, Fisher's exact test). Recent data from the Newcastle MRC prospective study (see Chapter 6) suggests that the more frequent psychotic experiences of LBD patients do not substantially differ in form or content from those of AD patients (usually visual, realistic, animate but mute figures) but they are more intense and persistent, and often dominate the clinical picture. They may sometimes occur as the first symptom of the illness in the absence of sustained cognitive impairment, an initial diagnosis of delusional disorder (late paraphrenia) or psychotic depression often being made and revised only when cognitive decline becomes apparent. At the other end of the diagnostic spectrum there is also a group of patients with established Parkinson's disease (PD) who develop hallucinations and delusions after many years of motor impairment. The objective of this chapter is to consider potential management strategies, pharmacological and non-pharmacological for noncognitive and behavioural disturbances in this clinically heterogenous population.

29.3 What are the causes of noncognitive symptoms in Lewy body dementia?

The neuropathological and biochemical correlates of the clinical symptoms and neuropsychological deficits of LBD are considered in detail elsewhere in this volume and might be expected to give a lead to the formulation of treatment strategies. Although the distribution of LB in limbic structures and the deep layers of the temporal neocortex is consistent with the generation of complex perceptual disturbances, the density of LB in limbic cortex bears no simple relationship to the incidence of hallucinations (Perry et al., 1995). Other groups have found a correlation between LB burden and severity of cognitive impairment (Lennox et al., 1989; Chapter 2), which was not seen in the Newcastle series. Significant associations were found however between reduced cholinergic activity and decreasing mental test scores in parietal neocortex (Perry et al., 1993). An extensive comparison of cholinergic, serotin- (5HT) and dopamine- (DA) -ergic activities between hallucinating and nonhallucinating LBD cases showed choline acetyltransferase to be reduced to below 20% of normal in temporal and parietal cortex in the hallucinators, compared to around 50% in nonhallucinators. In contrast, 5HT and 5-hydroxyindoleacetic acid levels were higher in hallucinating cases, suggesting that this symptom is associated with a 5HT:cholinergic imbalance. An analogous situation may occur for DA:cholinergic interactions. This neurochemical data is consistent with the observed effects of psychoactive compounds. Anticholinergic drugs are known to be potent hallucinogens which also cause impairments in attention and consciousness – reports of such experiences appear qualitatively similar to those in LBD. 5HT and

DA agonists similarly can cause psychotic phenomena. Promising pharmacological treatment strategies should therefore include cholinergic enhancement of 5HT/DA antagonism. No controlled studies have been carried out to date and information about the effects of drug treatment in LBD can only be derived from retrospective review of case records of patients treated in a clinical setting and some recent reports of systematic, but uncontrolled, drug trials.

29.4 The response of LBD patients to prescribed medication – a literature review

One hundred and one individual case reports of patients with neuropathologically confirmed LBD and with sufficient clinical details were identified by literature review (McKeith, 1993). Eighty-five of these had coexisting Alzheimer type pathology and will be referred to as 'common' cases (after Kosaka, 1990), and 13 were 'pure' cases with LB as the only positive pathological finding. The 'common' group were as expected significantly older 73.8 (95% Cl = 71.5–76.1) years vs. 57.4 (45.9–67.9) years. Hallucinations were recorded in 24.7% and delusions in 13% of the common cases; in the pure cases the figures were similar at 31% and 23% respectively. These absolute rates for psychotic symptoms are much lower than the 50–75% or greater rates which are described in more recent series (e.g. the Newcastle cohorts; McKeith et al., 1992a, 1992b), and illustrate that estimates of symptom frequency are highly determined by the methods of detection. Nevertheless, this limited data does suggest that delusions and hallucinations in LBD are primarily related to LB pathology with associated neuronal loss and neurochemical deficits, and are not simply a consequence of coexisting Alzheimer type lesions.

Details of antipsychotic medication could be found in only 12 of the 101 case reports. One patient (male, 65 years presenting with poor concentration and aphasia, later developing hallucinations) received haloperidol and another (male, 70 years with memory loss, irritability and hallucinations) haloperidol, chlorpromazine and thiothixene, each without relief of symptoms and with no apparent adverse effects. A further patient in the same small series (male, 75 years presenting with episodic confusion and hallucinations – Burkhardt et al., 1988) received haloperidol following which there appeared to be a rapid decline with agitation, fluctuating alertness, blepharospasm and myoclonic jerking.

Gibb et al. (1989) reported a 69-year-old male who presented with memory loss and later received 'a few doses of haloperidol (1.5 mg)'.

Three months later he was unable to communicate with all his limbs 'very rigid'. Two other cases were described by Gibb et al. (1989) – a 71-year-old man with memory loss and wandering who developed a parkinsonian syndrome complicated by venous and pressure ulcerations of the legs and flexion contractions of the knees following a single (20 mg) dose of flupenthixol, and a 66-year-old woman presenting with memory loss and hallucinations who tolerated thioridazine 50 mg daily, but who deteriorated rapidly in the month after being prescribed chlorpromazine 100 mg 'as required'.

Byrne et al. (1989) remarked upon the marked deterioration in extrapyramidal function produced by neuroleptic treatment in 3 of her 15 cases – a 74-year-old female presenting with falls, bradykinesia and rigidity, a 71-year-old woman presenting with forgetfulness and visual hallucinations and an 83-year-old man with memory failure accompanied by overvalued ideas. Crystal et al. (1990) similarly noted dramatic gait deterioration in three patients given low-dose neuroleptics. These case reports suggest that the outcome of neuroleptic administration to LBD patients is of limited clinical efficacy and a high incidence of adverse events.

The literature review also provides an opportunity to look for evidence of precipitation or exacerbation of psychotic or behavioural symptoms by anticholinergic and dopamine agonists which were prescribed to treat parkinsonism – details are available for 17 patients. A 30-year-old man with no cognitive impairment made a dramatic response to levodopa but died suddenly age 38 – no reference is made to him developing any psychiatric features (Ikeda et al., 1978). A 33-year-old woman initially responded to a combination of levodopa and a peripheral decarboxylase inhibitor, in conjunction with amantadine and benzhexol (Gibb et al., 1987). The substitution of bromocriptine for the levodopa combination led to the emergence of paranoid delusions and auditory hallucinations which remitted only temporarily when the bromocriptine was withdrawn. A 60-year-old man presenting with orthostatic hypotension (Yoshimura et al., 1980) later developed parkinsonism which transiently responded to levodopa before he demented, and a 73-year-old man with dementia and a shuffling gait improved slightly with levodopa and bromocriptine (Tiller-Borcich & Forno, 1988). No treatment response to levodopa was seen in two other patients – a 65-year-old man presenting with dementia and developing parkinsonism and depression (Mitsuyama et al., 1984) and a 69-year-old woman presenting with parkinsonism and later dementing, (Sima et al., 1986). In these last four cases adverse effects including the emergence of psychotic symptoms were not mentioned – this is consistent with Byrne et al.'s (1989) experience in their detailed description of a series of 15 LBD cases in Nottingham. Eleven of the 15 received levodopa; ten were assessed as showing definite improvement and one probable. Adverse effects were not mentioned as a significant factor.

Taken together these reports suggested that noncognitive symptoms in LBD patients are not particularly related to dopamine agonist treatments, and even when there was an apparent association (see Gibb et al., 1987 and above) the psychosis persisted despite drug withdrawal suggesting that the effect of medication was to precipitate a symptom to which the patient was already predisposed. This reflects our own clinical experience in this population.

Reference in the literature to the effects of anticholinergic drugs is so sparse as to make interpretation difficult. Byrne et al. (1989) is the only informative source. Orphenadrine may have precipitated postural instability, falling and confusion in an 82-year-old man with parkinsonism and mild forgetfulness; benzhexol had little effect on a 72-year-old woman with parkinsonism progressing through fluctuating confusion to dementia, and withdrawal and anticholinergics did not relieve the fluctuating confusion of a 70-year-old woman with auditory and visual hallucinations.

29.5 Neuroleptic sensitivity in Lewy body dementia

The hypothesis made by the Newcastle group, of an abnormal sensitivity of LBD patients to the extrapyramidal side effects of neuroleptic medication, is based upon two sets of independent observations. In each of these, retrospective case note reviews of patients with autopsy confirmed dementias (LBD and AD) were compared by clinicians blind to the neuropathological diagnosis. In the first series of patients, who reached autopsy between 1982 and 1989 (McKeith et al., 1992a), 67% (14/21) of LBD and 57% (21/37) of AD patients received neuroleptics – prescribing rates similar to those generally reported for elderly demented patients in contact with medical services. Fifty-seven per cent (8/14) of the neuroleptic treated LBD patients deteriorated rapidly after either, receiving neuroleptics for the first time, or following an increase in dose from a previously low or intermittent regime. The mean survival time from presentation to death for these eight patients was 7.4 months (95% Cl = 3.5–11.3), significantly less than that of the six patients who had only mild or no adverse reactions, 28.5 months (12.9–44.1), and of the seven never receiving neuroleptics who survived 17.8 months (−7.4 to 43.0). The characteristic description of neuroleptic sensitivity was of initial sedation (often thought to be therapeutically beneficial in the first instance), but followed by the sudden onset of rigidity accompanied by postural instability and falls. A rapid deterioration with increased confusion, immobility, rigidity, fixed flexion posture and decreased food and fluid intake was not reversed by anticholinergic medication when used. Death was usually by complications of immobility and/or reduced fluid intake in this already physically frail elderly group.

In a later study (McKeith et al., 1992b), a separate population of patients was examined for evidence of neuroleptic sensitivity and a survival analysis was performed to estimate the magnitude of its effect upon mortality risk. Possible predictors of severe neuroleptic sensitivity were also analysed. The general observations were strikingly similar to those for the earlier cohort. Eighty per cent (16/20) of LBD and 67% (14/21) of AD patients reaching autopsy between 1990 and 1992 received neuroleptics. Fifty-four per cent (7/16) of neuroleptic treated LBD patients showed severe neuroleptic sensitivity and their increased mortality risk compared with the remainder of the LBD group was 2.7 at the first survival endpoint which was six months after presentation to services. This fell gradually to 2.09 at 36 months ($p < 0.05$ – logrank test for all endpoints). The maximum period of increased risk is within the first six months of presentation to clinical services, during which 3/7 LBD patients died with severe neuroleptic sensitivity reactions. None of the remainder of the group died ($p = 0.031$, Fisher's exact test).

29.6 Minimizing treatment risks – the Committee on Safety of Medicine guidelines

A wide variety of different neuroleptics were implicated in sensitivity reactions (presented in detail in McKeith et al., 1992a, 1992b). Two of the seven severe sensitivity reactions in the 1990–92 LBD patients were associated with depot preparations as was the only case of severe neuroleptic related deterioration in an AD patient, a 79-year-old man who developed marked extrapyramidal features for the first time after receiving three consecutive depot injections and who died 8 weeks after the last dose. A similar pattern had already been noted in the earlier cohort – 4/8 severe neuroleptic sensitivity reactions occurred in association with intramuscular administration and in one of these a depot had been used. Intramuscular and depot preparations avoid first pass hepatic metabolism and it is likely that the increased incidence of severe adverse reactions is partly due to a increased dose effect, although it should be recognized that severe behavioural disturbance and noncompliance with oral medication, which are the usual indications for parenteral administration, may themselves be associated with increased morbidity. We were unable to find retrospective evidence for pharmacokinetic differences between neuroleptic sensitive and tolerant LBD cases – CYP2D6 allele frequencies being similar in each group (the B allele variant is associated with slow hepatic metabolism of a variety of psychotropics, including neuroleptics, by the enzyme-debrisoquine hydroxylase).

The impact in the UK which these reports of neuroleptic sensitivity in LBD has had is reflected in the contents of a recent circular issued to all doctors and dentists in the UK by the Committee on the Safety of Medicines (CSM, 1994). This advises that 'if neuroleptic medications are used in elderly patients with dementia, **very low doses** (sic) should be given with cautious titration against the clinical state. Particular care should be taken in patients with features suggestive of the newly described Lewy body dementia because sudden life-threatening deterioration may occur'.

29.7 How valid is the neuroleptic sensitivity hypothesis?

Is the statement circulated by the CSM justified by the evidence currently available (i.e., the Newcastle data and the literature review summarized above) and if so, are there any potentially less hazardous alternatives for treating the noncognitive symptoms of LBD? Given the clinical restraints imposed by the proposition of neuroleptic sensitivity in LBD, additional and independent supportive evidence of its incidence, disease specificity and magnitude of effect would seem desirable. A Catch 22 situation may however have been created if opinion has already changed such that the prescription of neuroleptics to LBD patients is generally viewed as a hazardous practice (with possible medico-legal consequences). If this is the case it may prove difficult to do further 'naturalistic' studies of neuroleptic prescribing in LBD, since not only will the number of patients exposed in the future be small, but they will be a highly selected group, probably with extreme levels of behavioural disturbance and already having a worse prognosis than those patients in whom neuroleptics can be successfully avoided. A randomized double blind placebo controlled trial of low dose neuroleptics in LBD might obtain ethical approval, but it is unclear what the outcome measures would be. Even a marginally raised mortality risk would appear to be a substantial disincentive for all patients except those with the most severe psychotic symptoms or behavioural disturbance. Not only would this produce sampling biases of the type already described, but the acceptability of and compliance with a placebo regime would prove extremely difficult.

An alternative validation strategy is to look for neuropathological and neurochemical differences between neuroleptic sensitive and neuroleptic tolerant cases. Data from the two Newcastle cohorts are presented and discussed in detail by Piggott in Chapter 34. In summary neuroleptic sensitivity in LBD appears to be based upon a loss of substantia nigra dopaminergic neurons almost into the PD range, with an associated impairment of compensatory upregulation of post-synaptic D2 receptors in the striatum (Piggott et al., 1994). At least some LBD patients therefore appear to have nigrostriatal dopaminergic neurotransmission which is at, or just slightly above, a critical functional threshold and which is lacking in adaptive potential. The D2 receptor blockade produced by even low doses of neuroleptic medication is sufficient to suddenly render the system sub-functional, thereby producing acute extrapyramidal symptoms. Even if this is only a partial explanation, it suggests that all D2 antagonists will have the potential to provoke such reactions and that these may be critically dose dependent.

29.8 Can LBD patients at risk of neuroleptic sensitivity be identified pre-treatment?

Within the neuroleptic sensitivity literature there is a clear indication that some patients meeting clinical (Lee et al., 1994; Allen et al., 1995) and pathological criteria (McKeith et al., 1992a,b) for LBD, can tolerate a variety of neuroleptics in dosage (albeit low), which causes some improvement in psychotic symptoms. In the Newcastle series, 50% of treated cases fell into this category and given the biases of an autopsy sample it is likely that an even greater proportion of LBD patients in clinical practice might be in this lower risk group. In the absence of alternative treatments it seems a pity to deny effective neuroleptic therapy to those patients who are able to tolerate it, and their pretreatment identification would be a useful advance in management. Unfortunately age at time of treatment, sex, severity of cognitive impairment and presence or absence of hallucinations, delusions or pre-existing parkinsonism did not predict the risk of adverse neuroleptic response in the Newcastle series. Although clinical prognostic indicators may yet emerge under the rigorous conditions of controlled trials, more direct measures of nigrostriatal function may be needed to identify those already on the brink of a dopaminergic crisis. Striatal D2 receptors can, for example, be labelled, visualized and quantified in vivo, using iodinated raclopride in conjunction with single photon emission computed tomography (SPECT). Neuroendocrine challenge tests (e.g. rise in prolactin levels following a single dose of a D2 antagonist) may also provide useful information about the functional integrity of central dopaminergic function. Whether or not such tests will be developed for clinical use largely depends on whether successful non-neuroleptic based treatments for non-cognitive symptoms are identified.

Until further information is available to guide clinicians, it would seem sensible to adopt the cautious approach to neuroleptic prescribing in LBD which the CSM have recommended (see above). We would additionally suggest that pretreatment baseline measures of cognitive, non-cognitive and extrapyramidal function should be recorded using standardized scales, and these should be repeated once or twice weekly during the initial period of dose titration. In this way the relative benefits and adverse consequences of treatment are monitored and the earliest signs of deterioration should be reliably detected. Neuroleptics should be stopped if extrapyramidal symptoms appear for the first time in an LBD patient who previously displayed no evidence of parkinsonism, and should be substantially reduced or stopped in patients whose pre-existing parkinsonism worsens. A reintroduction of the drug at a lower dose probably should only be contemplated once extrapyramidal function has returned to pretreatment level. Since the majority of severe sensitivity reactions probably occur within a week or two of receiving medication, it may be wise to admit patients with a suspected diagnosis of LBD into hospital during initiation of neuroleptic therapy and to ensure that very regular clinical assessments are recorded.

29.9 Other pharmacological strategies

Other potential pharmacological treatment strategies for LBD patients have recently been reviewed (Harrison & McKeith, 1995) and only those for which clinical data exist will be considered here.

29.10 Reduction or withdrawal of antiparkinsonian medication

The precise role of antiparkinsonian medication in causing, precipitating or exacerbating confusional and psychotic symptoms in LBD patients is unknown. Anticholinergic and dopaminergic drugs would each be expected to predispose to the ACh/DA imbalance which is associated with hallucinations in LBD and the first step in managing such symptoms probably should be a reduction in any antiparkinsonian drugs the patient is taking. The effects on motor and mental function should be recorded on standard scales as described previously in relation to neuroleptic prescribing. In patients who are taking several different antiparkinsonians, the preferred order of reduction/withdrawal is probably L-deprenyl, anticholinergics, followed by direct, then indirect, dopamine agonists. If psychotic symptoms persist despite withdrawal of antiparkinsonians to a level where further motor impairment becomes unacceptable, an antipsychotic should be added as previously described.

In these circumstances where the clinician is walking a therapeutic tightrope between parkinsonism and psychosis, the best outcome is invariably a compromise between a relatively mobile but psychotic patient and a nonpsychotic but immobile individual. The patient and his carer(s) may only be able to decide which is the lesser of these evils after experiencing both states.

29.11 Novel (atypical) antipsychotics

Early case reports of the efficacy and safety of novel antipsychotics such as risperidone (Lee et al., 1994; Allen et al., 1995) in LBD patients may need to be treated with caution, since in addition to its 5HT2 antagonism it is also a potent D2 blocker (Owens, 1994). We have seen several severe exacerbations of parkinsonism in LBD patients after only two or three days of receiving low doses (0.5–1.0 mg daily) of risperidone (McKeith et al., 1995). Similar observations have been made in relation to the use of risperidone for patients with advanced PD and psychosis (Ford et al., 1994). The 5HT2 antagonist properties of risperidone are thought to explain the reduced incidence of extrapyramidal side-effects in treating schizophrenic psychoses, and it is quite possible that it may have demonstrable advantages over conventional neuroleptics in LBD. The anecdotal evidence available suggests that the maximum tolerated dose in many LBD patients will be 0.5–1.0 mg daily or less – whether or not a useful antipsychotic effect will be seen at such low dosage needs to be demonstrated in a suitably designed open study.

Clozapine, a dibenzazepine, which has relatively low D2 antagonism, may have a higher therapeutic index in LBD than other atypical antipsychotics. Several case reports and small series have documented an antipsychotic effect of clozapine in PD (Factor et al., 1994). Clozapine also has potent antimuscarinic activity which may exacerbate confusion and cognitive impairment and limit its use in many LBD patients. The maximum tolerated dose range for such individuals appears to be only 12.5–50 mg daily, and as with risperidone, antipsychotic efficacy needs to be established at such low dosage. The attendant risks of neutropenia and agranulocytosis associated with clozapine therapy are well documented, but with regular blood count monitoring should not be a particular contraindication.

29.12 Acetylcholinesterase inhibitors

An alternative treatment strategy has been proposed based upon evidence that cholinergic dysfunction is more pronounced in hallucinated vs. non-hallucinated LBD patients (Perry et al., 1993, 1995), particularly those in whom indices of dopaminergic and serotonergic function are relatively preserved. Certainly, the delirious and hallucinatory experiences reported by some LBD patients are reminiscent of the signs of exogenously administered cholinergic poisoning. Cummings et al. (1993), recently showed that oral physostigmine was better tolerated than haloperidol by two patients clinically diagnosed as AD, and had equivalent antipsychotic effects. In this context it is interesting to note the reports of clinical improvement in patients given tacrine (another cholinesterase inhibitor) who despite clinical diagnoses of AD, were found at autopsy to have cortical LB (Perry et al., 1994). Cholinergic failure is likely to form a substrate for deficits in level of consciousness, selective attention, memory and perception and may account not only for the persistent cognitive deficits of LBD but also for the fluctuating delirium commonly seen, often in association with prominent hallucinatory states. Again caution is needed since LBD patients may be at risk of worsening extrapyramidal symptoms when given cholinergic agonists. The dose range in which cognitive and noncognitive improvements occur in LBD will not necessarily be the same as that for AD and dose finding studies are required.

29.13 Serotonergic antagonists

Zoldan et al. (1995) showed marked to moderate improvement in visual hallucinations, paranoid delusions and confusion in 15/16 patients with advanced PD, given the selective 5HT3 antagonist ondansetron (12–24 mg daily) in an open-label, 4–8 week trial. No major adverse side effects were seen and parkinsonism did not worsen. Relative serotonergic overactivity characterizes hallucinated LBD cases (Perry et al., 1993) and further controlled studies of 5HT2 and 5HT3 antagonists would seem desirable.

29.14 Sedatives and antidepressants

A variety of other psychotropic drugs currently available may be of considerable value in the management of LBD patients and with less adverse potential than neuroleptics. Agitation, anxiety and insomnia are common symptoms and may respond well to benzodiazepine sedatives. Drowsiness and unsteadiness are the major unwanted effects. Chlormethiazole may provide a useful sedative effect particularly for patients with troublesome nightmares and nocturnal hallucinations. Major depression seems to occur as commonly in LBD as in AD and there is no specific information about response or side effects of different classes of antidepressants, although one might expect the anticholinergic effects of tricylics to be disadvantageous in both disorders.

29.15 Nonpharmacological treatments

Although the majority of this chapter has been focused on the drug treatment of noncognitive symptoms of LBD, there is no doubt that until safe and effective medications become available, the mainstay of clinical management is to educate patients and carers about the nature of their symptoms and suggest ways to cope with them. The fluctuating nature of confusional and hallucinatory states in LBD present particular problems since patients frequently retain quite vivid recollections of their experiences during their lucid periods, in contrast to AD sufferers whose severe memory impairment often renders them largely unaware of (and therefore less persistently distressed by) their experiences. LBD patients usually need frequent reassurance that their visions and nightmares are part of a physical illness affecting their brain and not evidence of madness. Carers are similarly better able to respond to the patient's behavioural disturbance once they understand its underlying cause. Explanations of the risks and benefits associated with changes in medication are also helpful and enable patients to make decisions about their optimal balance between motor and mental symptoms and side-effects.

29.16 Conclusion

Lewy body dementia provides a newly recognized therapeutic challenge in geriatric psychiatry. Faced with the particular hazards of typical neuroleptic medication for the treatment of psychosis in this disorder, new avenues using atypical neuroleptics, cholinergic therapy or serotonergic antagonists need to be explored.

References

Allen, R. L., Walker, Z., D'Ath, P. J. & Katona, C. L. E. (1995). Risperidone for psychotic and behavioural symptoms in Lewy body dementia. *Lancet*, **346**, 185.

Burkhardt, C. R., Filley, C. M., Kleinschmidt-DeMasters, B. K., de la Monte, S., Norenberg, M. D. & Schneck, S. A. (1988). Diffuse Lewy body disease and progressive dementia. *Neurology*, **38**, 1520–8.

Burns, A., Jacoby, R. & Levy, R. (1990). Psychiatric phenomena in Alzheimer's disease. *Br. J. Psychiatry*, **157**, 72–94.

Byrne, E. J., Lennox, G., Lowe, J. & Godwin-Austen, R. B. (1989). Diffuse Lewy body disease: clinical features in 15 cases. *J. Neurol. Neurosurg. Psychiatry*, **52**, 709–17.

Committee on Safety of Medicines. (1994). Neuroleptic sensitivity in patients with dementia. *Curr. Probl. Pharmacovigilance*, **20**, 6.

Crystal, H. A., Dickson, D. W., Lizardi, J. E., Davies, P. & Wolfson, L. I. (1990). Antemortem diagnosis of diffuse Lewy body disease. *Neurology*, **40**, 1523–8.

Cummings, J. L., Gorman, D. G. & Schapira, J. (1993). Physostigmine ameliorates the delusions of Alzheimer's disease. *Biol. Psychiatry*, **33**, 536–41.

Factor, S. A., Brown, D., Molho, E. S. & Podskalny, G. D. (1994). Clozapine: a 2-year open trial in Parkinson's disease patients with psychosis. *Neurology*, **44**, 544–6.

Ford, B., Lynch, T. & Greene, P. (1994). Risperidone in Parkinson's disease. *Lancet*, **344**, 681.

Förstl, H., Burns, A., Levy, R. & Cairns, N. (1994). Neuropathological correlates of psychotic phenomena in confirmed Alzheimer's disease. *Br. J. Psychiatry*, **165**, 53–9.

Gibb, W. R. G., Esiri, M. M. & Lees, A. J. (1987). Clinical and pathological features of diffuse cortical Lewy body disease. *Brain*, **110**, 1131–53.

Gibb, W. R. G., Luthert, P. J., Janota, I. & Lantos, P. (1989). Cortical Lewy body dementia: clinical features and classification. *J. Neurol. Neurosurg. Psychiatry*, **52**, 185–92.

Harrison, R. W. S. & McKeith, I.G. (1995). Senile dementia of Lewy body type – A review of clinical and pathological features: Implications for treatment. *Int. J. Geriatr. Psychiatry*, **10**, 919–26.

Ikeda, K., Ikeda, S., Yoshimura, T., Kato, H. & Namba, M. (1978). Idiopathic Parkinsonism with Lewy type inclusions in cerebral cortex. *Acta Neuropathol. (Berl.)*, **41**, 165–8.

Jacoby, R. & Levy, R. (1980). Computed tomography in the elderly – 2. Senile dementia. *Br. J. Psychiatry*, **136**, 256–9.

Kosaka, K. (1990). Diffuse Lewy body disease in Japan. *J. Neurol. (Japan)*, **237**, 197–204.

Lee, H., Cooney, J. M. & Lawlor, B. A. (1994). Case report: The use of Risperidone, an atyptical neuroleptic in Lewy body disease. *Int. J. Geriatr. Psychiatry*, **9**, 415–17.

Lennox, G., Lowe, J., Morrell, K., Landon, M., & Mayer, R. J. (1989). Anti-ubiquitin immunocytochemistry is more sensitive than conventional techniques in the detection of diffuse Lewy body disease. *J. Neurol. Neurosurg. Psychiatry*, **52**, 67–71.

McKeith, I. G. (1993). The clinical diagnosis of Lewy body dementia. MD thesis. University of Newcastle upon Tyne.

McKeith, I. G., Perry, R. H., Fairbairn, A. F., Jabeen, S. & Perry, E. K. (1992a). Operational criteria for senile dementia of Lewy body type. *Psychol. Med.*, **22**, 911–22.

McKeith, I. G., Fairbairn, A. F., Perry, R. H., Thompson, P. & Perry, E. K. (1992b). Neuroleptic sensitivity in patients with senile dementia of Lewy body type. *BMJ*, **305**, 673–8.

McKeith, I. G., Harrison, R. W. S. & Ballard, C. G. (1995). Neuroleptic sensitivity to Risperidone in Lewy body dementia. *Lancet*, **346**, 699.

Mitsuyama, Y., Fukunaga, H. & Yamashita, M. (1984). Alzheimer's disease with widespread presence of Lewy bodies. *Folia Psychiatrica et Neurologica Japonica*, **38**, 81–8.

Owens, D. G. C. (1994). Extrapyramidal side effects and tolerability of Risperidone: a review. *J. Clin. Psychiatry*, **55** (suppl), 29–35.

Perry, E. K., Irving, D., Kerwin, J. M. et al. (1993). Cholinergic neurotransmitter and neurotrophic activities in Lewy body dementia. Similarity to Parkinson's and distinctions from Alzheimer's disease. *Alzheimer Dis. Assoc. Disord.*, **7**(2), 62–79.

Perry, E. K., Haroutunian, V., Davis, K. L. et al. (1994). Neocortical cholinergic activities differentiate Lewy body dementia from classical Alzheimer's disease. *Neuroreport*, **5**, 747–9.

Perry, E. K., Perry, R. H., McKeith, I. G., Piggott, M. A., Smith, P. & Marshall, E. (1995). Clinical pathological and neurochemical features of Lewy body dementia. In *Alzheimer and Parkinson's diseases*, ed. I. Hanin et al., pp. 77–86. New York: Plenum Press.

Piggott, M. A., Perry, E. K., McKeith, I. G., Marshall, E. & Perry, R. H. (1994). Dopamine D_2 receptors in demented patients with severe neuroleptic sensitivity. *Lancet*, **343**, 1044–5.

Rabins, P. V. (1994). Noncognitive symptoms in Alzheimer's disease. Definitions, treatment and possible etiologies. In *Alzheimer's Disease*, ed. R. D. Terry, R. Katzman, & K. L. Bick, pp. 415–29. New York: Raven Press.

Sima, A. A. F., Clark, A. W., Sternberger, N. A. & Sternberger, L. A. (1986). Lewy body dementia without Alzheimer changes. *Can. J. Neurol. Sci.*, **13**, 490–7.

Tiller-Borcich, J. K. & Forno, L. S. (1988). Parkinson's disease and dementia with neuronal inclusions in the cerebral cortex: Lewy bodies or Pick bodies. *J. Neuropathol. Exp. Neurol.*, **47**, 526–35.

Yoshimura, M., Shimada, H., Nagura, H. & Tomonaga, M. (1980). Two autopsy cases of Parkinson's disease with Shy–Drager syndrome. *Trans. Jpn. Pathol. Soc. (Japan)*, **4**, 568–70.

Zoldan, J., Friedberg, G., Livneh, M. & Melamed, E. (1995). Psychosis in advanced Parkinson's disease: Treatment with ondansetron, a 5HT3 receptor antagonist. *Neurology*, **45**, 1305–8.

30

Altered consciousness and transmitter signalling in Lewy body dementia

E. K. PERRY and R. H. PERRY

Summary

Neurochemical pathology associated with alterations in consciousness in Lewy body dementia (LBD) is discussed in relation to cholinergic and monoaminergic systems projecting to the cortex. Extensive loss of cholinergic activity from neocortical areas in hallucinating LBD cases is consistent with the ability of anticholinergic drugs (antimuscarinics such as scopolamine) to induce similar types of hallucinations in normal individuals. Evidence is reviewed which suggests the M_4 muscarinic subtype, which is particularly high in primate visual cortex and is activated by the atypical neuroleptic clozapine, may be involved in atropine psychosis. The possible role of non-cortical areas such as the brainstem reticular activating system in abnormal conscious activity in LBD is also considered, as is the involvement of the cholinergic system in schizophrenic psychosis. Amongst a range of potential approaches to cholinergic therapy in LBD, it is argued that stimulation of the nicotinic cholinergic receptor may be particularly useful since this may benefit both cognitive and motor dysfunction and also provide some degree of neuroprotection.

30.1 Introduction

'Consciousness: the having of perceptions, thoughts, and feelings; awareness. The term is impossible to define except in terms that are unintelligible, without a grasp of what consciousness means. Consciousness is a fascinating but elusive phenomenon: it is impossible to specify what it is, what it does or why it evolved. Nothing worth reading has been written about it' (Sutherland, 1989).

The bridge between mind and brain in dementing disorders such as Alzheimer's disease (AD), has generally been supported by objective

397

measures of memory loss and related cognitive impairment, or psychotic features such as depression and aggression which also have overt behavioural counterparts. Subjective experiences such as hallucinations have received far less attention in dementia, being reported in only a small proportion (up to 20%) of AD patients.

The subject of consciousness is not generally considered in neurobiological research into degenerative diseases of the brain such as dementia. Given the current focus of much research in Alzheimer's disease on molecular genetics, cytoskeletal and other protein abnormalities, discussion of consciousness might be considered at least premature and at most irrelevant. However in dementia associated with Lewy bodies it is not so much memory loss that initially presents patients and their carers with a major problem, but rather alterations in consciousness in which images are perceived in the waking state for which there is no recognizable external reality. As will be discussed, these hallucinations resemble certain drug-induced experiences which are sought for 'cultural', ritualistic or recreational purposes. With few exceptions, patients with Lewy body dementia do not consider the hallucinations as a positive experience and react with fear and aggression. There is then a need in relation to potential therapy to investigate the phenomenon in terms of brain mechanisms affected by the disease. Such research might additionally provide some insights of certain aspects of consciousness which could ultimately challenge Sutherland's viewpoint.

Hallucinations in dementia originally came to the attention of clinicians in Newcastle as a result of a retrospective survey of the case histories of a group of elderly demented patients, classified as senile dementia of Lewy body type, in which Lewy bodies were identified in the cortex and brainstem (Perry et al., 1989, 1990a). The incidence of hallucinations in this series was found to be 57%. Interestingly, with the increasing attention of psychogeriatricians, this incidence in a larger, including prospectively assessed, autopsy confirmed series of Lewy body dementia patients has risen to 80% compared with 20% in AD (Perry et al., in press). Obviously the identification of such alterations in consciousness depends on the ability and inclination of the patient to describe the experiences in response to appropriate interrogation. Neurochemical investigations of the postmortem brain in Lewy body dementia (LBD) provide opportunities to search for functional counterparts of such subjective experiences and indicate that hallucinations may be related to derangement of neocortical neurotransmitter systems.

Disturbances of consciousness such as hallucinations can be considered as qualitative, involving changes in the contents of the conscious 'stream' of awareness. There are, in addition, other alterations in consciousness in LBD which might more appropriately be described as quantitative changes in the level of consciousness. These include periodic mental 'absences' when the patient is awake but is not apparently aware of, or interacting with, the surroundings (Perry et al., 1990a). More catastrophic than these are episodes of syncope, accompanied by falling and injury. The biological basis of such disturbances in consciousness – which may last from a few seconds to several hours and occur in up to 50% of LBD patients (McKeith et al., 1992) – has not yet been fully investigated. A cardiovascular basis (episodic hypotension or dysrythmia) seems unlikely since with one exception in 10 affected cases, blood pressure and cardiac rhythm were normal. The exception was an 83-year-old female with Stokes Adams attacks (Perry, R., unpublished). 'Absences' are said to be a common feature of cingulotomy and since the anterior cingulate cortex is one of the most affected areas in terms of cortical Lewy bodies (Perry et al., 1989), clinical correlates of cingulate pathology in LBD cases would be worth investigating. Pathology of the brainstem reticular activating system is also worth exploring in this context.

30.2 Contribution of the cortical cholinergic system to hallucinations

The idea that cortical acetylcholine may be involved in hallucinations experienced by patients with senile dementia of Lewy body type originated from three observations:

1. Neocortical cholinergic deficits are more extensive in hallucinating compared to nonhallucinating cases of Lewy body dementia (LBD) (Perry et al., 1990b).
2. There is a higher prevalence of psychotic features, especially visual hallucinations, and lower neocortical cholinergic activity in LBD compared with classical Alzheimer's disease (AD) (see below).
3. Anticholinergic drugs (e.g. scopolamine or atropine) induce hallucinations in normal individuals similar to those reported in LBD (reviewed Perry & Perry, 1995).

30.3 Hallucinations in LBD and cortical monoaminergic:cholinergic imbalance

Activity of the cholinergic enzyme, choline acetyltransferase, is lower in the neocortex (particularly temporal or parietal) in diffuse Lewy body disease, Lewy body variant of AD or LBD compared with AD (Dickson et al., 1987; Langlais et al., 1993; Perry et al., 1994; see also Fig. 30.1). LBD patients with, as opposed to without hallucinations have significantly lower activity (over 80% reductions compared with the normal, Perry et al., 1990b). Basal nucleus of Meynert neuron numbers which are consistently reduced in diffuse Lewy body disease (Dickson et al., 1987, see also Chapter 22) were also lower in a small number of hallucinating

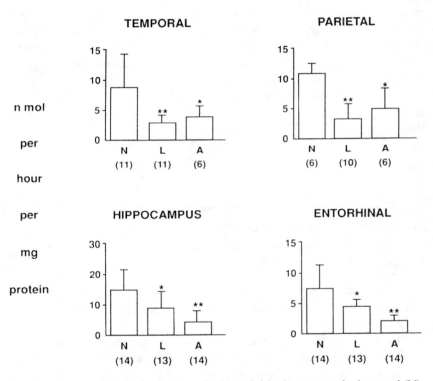

Fig. 30.1 Levels of choline acetyltransferase activities in age-matched normal (N), Lewy body dementia (L) and Alzheimer's disease (A) cases. Data are mean ± SD with case numbers. Significant differences compared with the normal *$p < 0.05$, **$p < 0.01$. Temporal and parietal cortex were derived from Brodmann areas 21 and 39/40. In these neocortical areas (but not in hippocampus or entorhinal cortex) activities in hallucinating cases were approximately 50 per cent of those in hallucinating cases (Perry et al., 1990b).

compared with nonhallucinating cases (Perry et al., 1993a). However 5-HT or an index of 5-HT turnover (the ratio 5HIAA:5HT) is higher in nonhallucinating patients (Perry et al., 1990b, 1993b), and 5-HT$_2$ receptor binding which diminishes in AD, is normal in hallucinating LBD cases (Cheng et al., 1991). These data suggest that hallucinations may be related to a neocortical transmitter imbalance based on hypocholinergic and relatively hypermonoaminergic function and are consistent with the recent conclusion of Lipowski (1990) based on a review of the literature on chemically induced delirium (see also Chapter 5). A recent survey of cholinergic activities in archicortex (hippocampus and entorhinal cortex) has indicated less extensive (30–50%) reductions in choline acetyltransferase compared with neocortex and no distinction between hallucinators and nonhallucinators (Melrose et al., in preparation).

In Parkinson's disease (PD), the archetypal Lewy body disease, neocortical cholinergic activities (of choline acetyltransferase but apparently not of the high affinity choline uptake carriers, Rodriguez et al., 1994) are also low and hallucinations are frequently induced by higher doses of levodopa. This suggests that in unmedicated Parkinson patients cholinergic deficits may be offset by dopaminergic deficits. However, a recent survey suggests the prevalence of hallucinations in PD may have been underestimated. If questioned diplomatically (patients are often reluctant to admit to hallucinating), 44% of Parkinson patients reported these experiences (Haeske-Dewick, 1995) which were associated with increasing age, decreasing cognitive function but surprisingly not with levodopa medication.

Subcortical regions influence interactions between cortical cholinergic and monoaminergic systems. Dopamine in the septum inhibits acetylcholine release in the hippocampus (Durkin et al., 1986), scopolamine induced deficits in spatial working memory in rats are reversed by D_1 receptor blockade (Levin et al., 1990), and destruction of the A–10 septal dopaminergic pathways in mice results in increased choline acetyltransferase (Yanai et al., 1993). Degeneration of the mesolimbic dopaminergic system may thus offset hypocholinergic activity in some archicortical areas. This may possibly account for the relative sparing of archicortical cholinergic activities and lack of severe dementia and memory loss in LBD. Mesolimbic dopaminergic systems are affected to a moderate extent in PD although activities remain to be investigated in LBD. In the neocortex, by contrast, there may be no compensatory upregulation of cholinergic function due to dopaminergic degeneration. Neocortical association areas (in, e.g. temporal lobe) which are most likely involved in complex hallucinations, do not receive a major cholinergic input from the septum and mesocortical (e.g. frontal) dopamine and HVA are normal in LBD and PD (Perry et al., 1993b).

This concept of a clinical symptom associated with degeneration in one system being naturally 'rectified' by degeneration in another system, is also exemplified in a recent comparison of the striatum in PD, LBD and an unusual case of corticobasal degeneration (CBD) (Chapter 34). Anticholinergics reduce the severity of extrapyramidal movement disorder in PD, loss of cholinergic activity in the putamen in LBD may partly account for the absence or minimal signs of motor dysfunction in LBD, and in an atypical CBD case the absence of parkinsonism despite severe substantia nigra and striatal dopamine loss could be related to extensive loss of putamen cholinergic activities. Clinicopathological correlations thus enter a new realm of complexity as multiple transmitter indices need to be considered simultaneously.

30.4 Anticholinergic drugs induce hallucinations

The ritualistic use of extracts of solanaceous plants (such as belladonna, mandrake, henbane or datura which contain the antimuscarinic chemicals scopolamine and/or atropine) to induce altered conscious states including hallucinatory visions is recorded throughout history (Schultes & Hofman, 1992). Amongst native North American Indians for example datura (Angel's trumpet) is employed in initiation rites at puberty to induce mental images in individuals of their 'guardian spirit' – usually an animal. Medically, anticholinergic drugs employed in ophthalmology, cardiac disease or motion sickness, can in high doses or in susceptible individuals induce hallucinations (e.g. Fisher, 1991; also reviewed Perry & Perry, 1995). Reports often include visions of familiar animals or human figures rather similar to those reported by LBD patients. The young and elderly, with relatively low cholinergic activity in the temporal cortex, are particularly vulnerable to drug effects.

Many psychotropic agents acting on a variety of transmitter signalling systems lead to disturbances in consciousness. However, different kinds of chemicals are associated with different types of hallucinations (Table 30.1). Images are usually visual – perhaps because compared with the other senses, visual experience in most humans is the most active and varied. Monoaminergic enhancing agents such as mescaline are said to induce highly pleasurable visions of fantastic shapes, colours and content not generally familiar to the individual. Serotonergic agents such as LSD

Table 30.1. *Chemically-induced hallucinations*

Chemical	Subjective experiences	Transmitter based mechanisms
Indoleamines (e.g. LSD, DMT)	Synaesthesia; depersonalization; novel/mystical visions	5-HT_2 receptor
Phenylamines (e.g. mescaline)	Fantastic, usually pleasurable visions	Monoamine release
Tropane alkaloids (e.g. atropine)	Mainly visual images of familiar faces/animals	Muscarinic receptor
PCP/ketamine	Complex hallucinations; depersonalization; paranoid psychosis	NMDA receptor
Opiates	Dreamlike procession of thoughts and fantastic visions	Opiate receptor
Ethanol (withdrawal in alcoholics)	Mainly visual including small, threatening animals; paranoia	GABA receptor?

or DMT produce altered sensory perception including a degree of 'cross writing' or synaesthesia – hearing colours for example, and an often disturbing sense of depersonalization. Anticholinergic drugs tend, instead, to invoke images of familiar objects, animals or people. These distinctions are likely to be based on the relative distribution of the respective transmitter systems and their receptor subtypes in different regions of the brain – particularly cortex and striatum where muscarinic, 5HT_2 and monoaminergic receptors are concentrated.

Although it is not clear which of the five muscarinic receptor subtypes are involved in the psychomimetic action of antagonists such as atropine or scopolamine, there is some evidence that the M_4 subtype may be selectively involved. Clozapine, an atypical antipsychotic useful in schizophrenia, Parkinson's disease and an anecdotal case of LBD (Chacko et al., 1993), is a potent antagonist at cloned M_1, M_2, M_3 and M_5 subtypes (with K_i values of 2–20 nm) but a potent agonist (EC_{50} of 11 nm) at only the M_4 subtype (Zorn et al., 1994). Conversely then psychomimetic effects of atropine may relate to M_4 antagonism and this subtype is concentrated in primary visual cortex, lateral geniculate nucleus and striatum of marmoset brain (Ferrari-Dileo et al., 1994). If M_4 distribution in human brain is similar, the high density in primary visual cortex and thalamic relay nucleus concerned with vision would go some way to explaining antimuscarinic visual hallucinations. Why the images should tend to be of familiar faces or animals as opposed to other visual scenarios is a challenge to current concepts of neurotransmitter signalling. Presumably higher cortical association and information recall areas are also involved. In LBD the occipital cortex is not involved in Lewy body formation although loss of cholinergic activity occurs here as, though to a lesser extent than, in other neocortical areas.

Mechanistically, acetylcholine has been implicated in enhancing signal to noise ratios in the cortex (Sahakian, 1988). As a modulatory transmitter, acetylcholine enhances the effect of the excitatory amino acid glutamate and also promotes release of the inhibitory transmitter, GABA (Metherate et al., 1987; McCormick, 1989). The effect of acetylcholine may therefore be to promote or stabilize the 'on' or 'off' status of individual neurons, so increasing discrimination. In neural network terms, the interaction of the currently dominant set of neurons would be selectively enhanced. In terms of human consciousness, a role for acetylcholine in conscious awareness, enhancing awareness of the most immediately relevant material can be suggested. Loss of cortical acetylcholine could then lead to diminished awareness of currently relevant information and increased awareness of information which is normally suppressed, for example past memories, so giving rise to subjective experience which is not related to objective reality. The increased incidence of hallucinations in LBD patients on waking from sleep (Perry et al., in press) is consistent with this model although it also raises the question of the possible role of the reticular activating system (see below).

Other chemically induced psychotic states of particular interest in the context of LBD include 'delirium tremens', occurring in alcoholics on withdrawal. The actions of ethanol are complex – effects on GABA, glutamate, dopamine and acetylcholine have all been identified. Receptor interactions include the $GABA_A$ receptor and effects of benzodiazepines in LBD should be considered. Hallucinations and delirium, said to resemble anticholinergic induced states, also occur in a variety of toxic and metabolic disturbances. The concept of delirium as a 'syndrome of cerebral insufficiency' was proposed many years ago (Engel & Romano, 1959) and Blass et al. (1981) suggested that such impairments of oxidative metabolism in the brain reduce transmitter, especially acetylcholine, synthesis. Physostigmine successfully reverses delirium caused by a variety of drugs and situations (Lipowski, 1990). In summary, there is perhaps more evidence linking the psychosis of LBD to abnormalities of the cholinergic compared with other systems.

30.5 Is acetylcholine involved in schizophrenia?

Consideration of the neurochemical pathology of hallucinations and disturbances in consciousness in LBD would be incomplete without reference to schizophrenia. This is the most prevalent disorder of the human mind associated with hallucinations which, in contrast to LBD, are usually auditory (although visual experiences may occur later in the disease). The schizophrenic state also involves other disturbances in consciousness – thought disorder and thought insertion – which are not features of LBD, although in LBD delusional states also occur, probably as a secondary phenomenon in relation to hallucinatory experience.

Chemically tagged neuroimaging of the living brain or postmortem analysis in schizophrenia have not so far provided consistent evidence of any particular neurochemical (e.g. dopaminergic or glutamate receptor) disturbance. Current hypotheses in this disorder still depend primarily on psychopharmacology – neurochemical effects of drugs which induce or reduce psychotic features. In this respect it is interesting to note that phenocyclidine (PCP), considered by some to mimic schizophrenic psychosis most closely, is in addition to being a glutamate NMDA channel blocker also a muscarinic antagonist in vitro (Pechnick, 1993). Although the PCP binding affinity (K_i) at the muscarinic receptor (assessed using QNB which binds to all subtypes) is $10–100\times$ higher than that for the NMDA receptor, the fact that muscarinic receptors comprise more than five different molecular subtypes (Brann et al., 1993) allows for the possibility that PCP may be a more potent antagonist of one subtype – perhaps M_4. Clozapine, the atypical neuroleptic which successfully treats some schizophrenic patients, is in its plethora of pharmacological actions in vitro also an M_4 agonist (see above).

In a postmortem analysis conducted some years ago, significant reductions (up to 50%) in cortical muscarinic receptor binding (measured using QNB and therefore including all subtypes) were found in chronic schizophrenic cases (Perry & Perry, 1980). No attempt was made to relate this abnormality to specific symptomatology as it was originally considered likely to be a drug rather than disease effect. More recently muscarinic receptor binding has been investigated in LBD which, like schizophrenia, is commonly treated with neuroleptics. Receptor binding measured using N-methyl scopolamine which also binds to all subtypes was found to be increased in LBD (Perry et al., 1990c). The receptor loss in schizophrenia cannot therefore be attributed to drug treatment (the Achilles heel of all neurochemical analysis in this disease) and it would be

worth repeating the analysis, differentiating between muscarinic subtypes, especially in view of the speculation that M_4 (see above) or M_2
(Yeomans, 1995, see below) may be involved in psychosis. Although
presynaptic cholinergic activities are normal there may then be grounds
for considering an underactivity of cortical cholinoceptive neurons in
schizophrenia. Therapeutically tacrine and physostigmine have been
reported to reduce the severity of symptoms in schizophrenia (Gershon
& Olariv, 1960; Abood & Biel, 1962).

30.6 Possible role of noncortical areas

The involvement of the brainstem reticular activating system in REM
sleep and dreaming together with possible similarities between dreaming
and hallucinations in the awake state have stimulated hypotheses on the
role of particular brainstem neuronal systems in psychosis. The potential
role of tegmental cholinergic neurons has been highlighted by the finding
that in schizophrenic, or a proportion of schizophrenic cases there is a
higher than normal number of NADPH-dehydrogenase containing cholinergic neurons in the CH5 pedunculopontine tegmental nucleus (PPT)
related perhaps to abnormalities in programmed neuronal death during
development (Karson et al., 1991).

It has recently been suggested that the psychotic effects of antimuscarinic agents may be mediated by M_2 receptors in the PPT (Yeomans et
al., 1994). Since, Yeomans argues, anti-parkinsonian and anti-psychotic
antimuscarinics are M_1 and sometimes M_4 antagonists (but see effects of
clozapine above), psychotic effects could be due to M_2 or M_3 blockade.
Seventy per cent of muscarinic receptors in the brainstem are M_2 and
antipsychotic effects of muscarinic antagonists in man correlate with the
ability to induce hyperactivity in rats which is mediated mainly via PPT
muscarinic receptors (Yeomans et al., 1994). Blockade of M_2 autorecep-
tors in CH5 neurons would be associated with overactivity of these cholinergic neurons. This in turn, via thalamic activation would lead to poor
sensory filtering with concomitant hallucinations and psychosis and,
interestingly would also induce early onset REM sleep, which has been
noted in some schizophrenics, correlating with both positive and negative
symptoms (Tandon et al., 1992). Although interesting, this proposed M_2
action of antimuscarinic psychotics neglects the widespread distribution
of M_2 receptors throughout the brain – in archicortex, striatum and
thalamus as well as brainstem, where it tends to parallel the distribution
of presynaptic cholinergic activity. Moreover amongst cloned muscarinic

receptors, m_1, m_2 and m_4 have a higher affinity for atropine than m_2 (Buckley et al., 1989).

In focusing on a particular brain region which may be primarily involved in hallucinogenesis, the incidence of hallucinations associated with brain lesions is relevant. Temporal lobe epilepsy and peduncular infarction are examples of such lesions. Other areas such as the striatum may be indirectly involved. The striatum plays a major role in cortical integration as information from diverse cortical areas is relayed via striatum, globus pallidus and thalamus back to the frontal cortex. LBD patients with and without hallucinatory experiences have not so far been differentiated on the basis of striatal neurochemistry and the caudate nucleus in LBD and AD have similar cholinergic activity. Resolution of the argument as to which brain region, targeted by antimuscarinic agents is primarily involved in hallucinations may ultimately be resolved by in vivo scanning (e.g. glucose utilization in hallucinating individuals) although perhaps, like consciousness itself, such disturbances depend on disruption of integrative processing between diverse brain areas. In LBD, SPECT or PET imaging has indicated reductions in activity in temporal regions, as in Alzheimer's disease and also PD – even those without dementia (Brooks, in press). Preliminary findings of higher thalamic perfusion in LBD compared with AD (McKeith et al., in preparation) are interesting in relation to the possible role of the PPT cholinergic neurons. This population of cells is diminished in PD (Hirsch et al., 1987; Jellinger, 1988) but has not yet been investigated in LBD. Since other brainstem neurons, for example, locus coeruleus and substantia nigra are affected in LBD it would be surprising if the PPT neurons were spared. Neurochemical analysis of the thalamus in LBD, currently in progress, should be informative.

30.7 Neurotransmitter therapy may be particularly relevant in LBD

Relatively intact neuronal systems in the neocortex (few or absent neurofibrillary tangles compared with AD) provide a greater potential for transmitter oriented therapy than in AD (Perry et al., 1989). Reasons to suppose that cholinergic therapy may be of value can be summarized as follows:

1. Clinical symptoms are characteristically anticholinergic.
2. Neocortical cholinergic activities are extremely low.

3. Muscarinic receptors are upregulated in the cortex (Perry et al., 1990c).
4. Preliminary reports indicate some responders in tacrine trials of demented patients have Lewy bodies (Levy et al., 1994; Wilcock & Scott, 1994).
5. In tacrine trials of Alzheimer's disease the percentage of responders (generally 20–30%, Davis, 1995) is similar to the prevalence of patients with cerebral Lewy bodies.

The notion that acetylcholine is involved in psychotic features such as hallucinations, in addition to memory, may extend the future application of cholinergic therapy beyond cognitive disorders such as Alzheimer's disease to a variety of other psychiatric conditions. The involvement of the basal ganglia in LBD provides an important caveat to the potential value of cholinergic therapy. If cholinergic transmission in the striatum is enhanced therapeutically, this may, since dopamine levels are already below normal, exacerbate extrapyramidal symptoms – as do typical neuroleptics (Chapter 34). Recently reported deterioration of a suspected LBD patient on low levels of tacrine (Witjeratne et al., 1995) could relate to striatal effects. LBD provides the therapeutic paradox of requiring enhanced cortical and supressed striatal cholinergic function. Moreover, stimulation of brainstem cholinergic systems may increase psychosis (see above). Clearly anatomical targeting of cholinergic drugs is an important therapeutic goal.

Amongst alternative approaches to enhancing cholinergic transmission (cholinesterase inhibition or receptor stimulation for example), nicotinic receptor activation has its particular attractions. Nicotine increases attention and improves memory, presumably by enhancing cholinergic transmission in the cortex and also has beneficial effects on parkinsonism, enhancing dopamine release from the striatum (reviewed by Court & Perry, 1994). Nicotine or a related agonist may therefore provide dual benefit in LBD on symptoms arising from cortical cholinergic and nigrostriatal dopamine degeneration. Add to this the evidence, based on epidemiological data on tobacco use, of protective effects in both PD and AD (reviewed by Court & Perry, 1994) and the nicotinic receptor would appear to be a particularly rewarding focus for future therapeutic strategies in degenerative diseases affecting cognitive and motor processes. The nicotinic receptor, assessed using ^{3}H-nicotine, is diminished in both cortical areas and in the substantia nigra in LBD (Perry et al., 1995). In LBD the receptor loss in the nigra is as extensive as in PD, despite less extensive neuron loss suggesting that nicotinic down regulation may be a precursor of neuronal death. Nicotinic agonists which upregulate the receptor may then protect against neurodegeneration.

It is well established that nicotinic antagonists impair memory but whether, like muscarinic antagonists there are also psychotomimetic effects in man remains to be determined. Preliminary evidence (Perry & Perry, 1995) suggests hallucinating and nonhallucinating LBD cases are not distinguished on the basis of ^{3}H-nicotine binding to nicotine receptors in the neocortex. If antipsychotic muscarinic antagonists target the M_2 muscarinic subtype (Yeomans, 1995) then M_2 agonists could be useful in LBD. The peripheral, for example cardiovascular, side effects of such drugs are however notorious. The arguments in favour of the value of M_4 agonists are perhaps more convincing and novel ligands for this subtype will hopefully soon be available for clinical testing.

30.8 Unexplored areas

In addition to these therapeutic implications, brain imaging possibilities arise from the cortical cholinergic neuropathology of dementia as it is curently understood. These include distinguishing LBD from AD on the basis of more extensive presynaptic cholinergic deficits and elevated muscarinic receptor binding in the neocortex in patients with LBD.

Although much of the direct evidence from postmortem brain and indirect psychopharmacological evidence implicates acetylcholine in one of the principal clinical features of LBD, the role of other neuronal systems, e.g. GABA, neuropeptides such as somatostatin, and the monoamines noradrenaline, dopamine and 5-HT needs to be investigated further in relation to specific symptoms. This is particularly relevant in relation to therapy since atypical neuroleptics such as clozapine – which is not considered to be primarily cholinergic in action (although cholinergic actions are evident as discussed above) – may be most effective in controlling psychotic features such as hallucinations.

Another facet of the disorder that provides a singular challenge to neurobiologists is the fluctuating course of the symptoms. Following severe episodes of confusion, delirium, or hallucinations, the patient, at least in earlier stages of the disease, returns to normal or near normal. Given the ultimately progressive deterioration, it is reasonable to presume that these fluctuations are based on abnormalities in neurons which degenerate in the disease. Degenerative changes may initially trigger restorative activity which is ultimately overridden by extensive, irreversible neurodegeneration. It has been suggested that plasticity in relation to episodic symptomatology in schizophrenia may have its origins in the hippocampus involving adaptive mechanisms similar to those involved in long term potentiation (Port & Seybold, 1995). The presence of ubiquitinated (non-tau positive) 'Lewy neurites' (Chapter 18) in the CA2 region of the hippocampus – an area with a dense cholinergic input – may relate to some kind of plasticity associated with reactive regeneration. Mechanisms of receptor upregulation in response to deafferentation may also be involved in processes of neurophysiological rectification. Neither 'Lewy neurites' nor muscarinic supersensitivity (in terms of numbers of binding sites) are a feature of AD which does not generally follow the markedly fluctuating course of LBD. Interestingly delirium induced by anticholinergic agents is characterized by fluctuating consciousness (Lipowski, 1990). If transient restorative or compensatory mechanisms can be understood, perhaps they can also be stimulated therapeutically. An alternative explanation for periodic cortical dysfunction may be a disruption of the normal cyclical changes in brainstem cholinergic and monoaminergic activating systems which govern sleep/wake and REM/slow wave sleep cycles such that these fluctuations in neuronal activity somehow intrude into the waking state.

Whether any of these considerations of the neurochemical pathology of LBD in the context of hallucinogenesis contribute anything to understanding human consciousness is a matter of opinion. Degenerative diseases of the human brain associated with altered conscious awareness do at least provide the interested neuroscientist with potential material with which to explore the interface between consciousness and brain mechanisms. Intriguing aspects of other degenerative diseases, including the loss of volitional or intentional drive in PD and loss of conscious (explicit) but not subconscious (implicit) learning in AD, provide other opportunities for investigating the neurobiology of consciousness. In LBD, it is not so much the process of being consciously aware that is affected as the nature of information of which the patient is aware. Perhaps new insights into the fundamental process of conscious awareness itself will arise from examining the neurobiology of AD.

Acknowledgements

This review is partly based on collaborative research involving Ian McKeith, Elizabeth Marshall, Richard Harrison, Anthony Cheng,

Heather Melrose, Margaret Piggott, Mary Johnson and Peter Thompson. Many thanks also to Dawn Hinds for manuscript preparation.

References

Abood, L. G. & Biel, J. H. (1962). Anticholinergic psychotomimetic agents. *Int. Rev. Neurobiol.*, **4**, 217–73.

Blass, J. P., Gibson, G. E. & Duffy, T. E. (1981). Cholinergic dysfunction: a common denominator in metabolic encephalopathies. In *Cholinergic Mechanisms*, ed. G. Pepeu & H. Ladinsky, pp. 921–8. New York: Plenum Press.

Brann, M. R., Ellis, J., Jorgensen, H., Hill-Eubanks, D. & Jones, S. V. P. (1993). Muscarinic receptor subtypes: localization and structure/function. *Prog. Brain Res.*, **98**, 121–7.

Brooks, D. (in press). PET imaging in Parkinson's disease. *J. Neural Transm.*

Buckley, N. J., Bonner, T., Buckley, C. M. & Brann, M. R. (1989). Antagonist binding properties of five cloned muscarinic receptors expressed in CHO-K cells. *Mol. Pharmacol.*, **35**, 496–7.

Chacko, R. C., Hurley, R. A. & Jankovic, J. (1993). Clozapine use in Diffuse Lewy Body Disease. *J. Neuropsychiat. Clin. Neurosci.*, **5**, 206–8.

Cheng, A., Ferrier, I. N., Morris, C. M. et al. (1991). Cortical serotonergic S_2 receptor binding in Lewy body dementia, Alzheimer's and Parkinson's diseases. *J. Neurol. Sci.*, **106**, 50–5.

Court, J. A. & Perry, E. K. (1994). CNS receptors: therapeutic target in neurodegeneration. *CNS Drugs*, **2**, 216–33.

Davis, K. L. (1995). Tacrine. *Lancet*, **345**, 625–30.

Dickson, D. W., Davies, P., Mayeux, R. et al. (1987). Diffuse Lewy body disease. *Acta Neuropathol.*, **75**, 8–15.

Durkin, T., Galey, D., Micheau, J., Beslon, H. & Jaffard, R. (1986). The effects of intraseptal injection of haloperidol in vivo on hippocampal cholinergic function in the mouse. *Brain Res.*, **376**, 420–4.

Engel, G. L. & Romano, J. (1959). Delirium: a syndrome of cerebral insufficiency. *J. Chronic Dis.*, **9**, 260–77.

Ferrari-Dileo, G., Waelbroeck, M., Mash, D. C. & Flynn, D. D. (1994). Selective localization of the M_4 (m4) muscarinic subtype. *Mol. Pharmacol.*, **46**, 1028–35.

Fisher, C. M. (1991). Visual hallucinations on eyeclosure associated with atropine toxicity. *Can. J. Neurol. Sci.*, **18**, 18–27.

Gershon, S. & Olariv, J. (1960). J.B.329: A new psychotomimetic, its antagonism by tetrahydroaminocrin and its comparison with LSD, mescaline and sernyl. *J. Neuropsychiatry*, **1**, 283–92.

Haeske-Dewick, C. (1995). Hallucinations in Parkinson's disease: characteristics and associated clinical features. *Int. J. Geriatr. Psychiatry*, **10**, 487–95.

Hirsch, E. C., Graybiel, A. M., Duyckaerts, C. & Javoy-Agid, F. (1987). Neuronal loss in the pedunculopontine tegmental nucleus in Parkinson's disease and in progressive supranuclear palsy. *Proc. Natl. Acad. Sci. USA*, **84**, 5976–80.

Jellinger, K. (1988). The pedunculopontine nucleus in Parkinson's disease, progressive supranuclear palsy and Alzheimer's disease. *J. Neurol. Neurosurg. Psychiatry*, **5**, 540–3.

Karson, C. N., Garcia-Rill, E., Biedermann, J., Mrak, R. E., Husain, M. M. & Skinner, R. D. (1991). The brainstem reticular formation in schizophrenia. *Psychiatry Res.: Neuroimaging*, **40**, 31–48.

Langlais, P. J., Thal, L. & Hansen, L. (1993). Neurotransmitters in basal ganglia and cortex of Alzheimer's disease with and without Lewy bodies. *Neurology*, **43**, 1927–34.

Levin, E. D., McGurk, S. R., Roso, J. E. & Butcher, L. L. (1990). Cholinergic-dopaminergic interactions in cognitive performance. *Behav. Neural. Biol.*, **54**, 271–99.

Levy, R., Eagger, S., Griffiths, M. et al. (1994). Lewy bodies and response to tacrine in Alzheimer's disease. *Lancet*, **343**, 176.

Lipowski, Z. J. (1990). *Delirium: Acute Confusional States*. Oxford: Oxford University Press.

McCormick, D. A. (1989). Cholinergic and noradrenergic modulation of thalamocortical processing. *Trends Neurosci.*, **12**, 215–31.

McKeith, I. G., Perry, R. H., Fairbairn, A. F., Jabeen, S. & Perry, E. K. (1992). Operational criteria for senile dementia of Lewy body type (SDLT). *Psychol. Med.*, **22**, 911–22.

Metherate, R., Tremblay, N. & Dykes, R. W. (1987). Acetylcholine permits long term enhancement of neuronal responsiveness in cat primary somatosensory cortex. *Neuroscience*, **22**, 75–81.

Pechnick, R. N. (1993). Neurochemical substrates underlying the mechanism of action of phencyclidine (PCP). In *Biological Basis of Substance Abuse*, ed. S. G. Korenmah & J. D. Barchas, pp. 285–97. Oxford: Oxford University Press.

Perry, E. K. & Perry, R. H. (1980). The cholinergic system in Alzheimer's disease. In *Biochemistry of Dementia*, ed. P. Roberts, pp. 135–83. Chichester: John Wiley.

Perry, E. K. & Perry, R. H. (1995). Acetylcholine and hallucinations: disease-related compared to drug-induced alterations in human consciousness. *Brain and Cognition*, **28**, 240–58.

Perry, R. H., Irving, D., Blessed, G., Perry, E. K. & Fairbairn, A. F. (1989). Clinically and neuropathologically distinct form of dementia in the elderly. *Lancet*, **1**, 66.

Perry, R. H., Irving, D., Blessed, G., Fairbairn, A. F. & Perry, E. K. (1990a). Senile dementia of Lewy body type. A clinically and neuropathologically distinct form of Lewy body dementia in the elderly. *J. Neurol. Sci.*, **95**, 119–39.

Perry, E. K., Marshall, E., Kerwin, J. M. et al. (1990b). Evidence of a monoaminergic:cholinergic imbalance related to visual hallucinations in Lewy body dementia. *J. Neurochem.*, **55**(4), 1454–6.

Perry, E. K., Smith, C. J., Court, J. A. & Perry, R. H. (1990c). Cholinergic nicotinic and muscarinic receptors in dementia of Alzheimer, Parkinson and Lewy body types. *J. Neural. Transm.*, **2**, 149–58.

Perry, E. K., Irving, D., Kerwin, J. M. et al. (1993a). Cholinergic transmitter and neurotrophic activities in Lewy body dementia: similarity to Parkinson's and distinction from Alzheimer disease. *Alzheimer Dis. Assoc. Disord.*, **7**(2), 69–79.

Perry, E. K., Marshall, E., Thompson, P. et al. (1993b). Monoaminergic activities in Lewy body dementias: relation to hallucinosis and extrapyramidal features. *J. Neural. Transm.*, **6**, 167–77.

Perry, E. K., Haroutunian, V., Davis, K. L. et al. (1994). Neocortical cholinergic activities differentiate Lewy body dementia from classical Alzheimer's disease. *NeuroReport*, **5**, 747–9.

Perry, E. K., Morris, C. M., Court, J. A. et al. (1995). Alteration in nicotine binding sites in Parkinson's disease, Lewy body dementia and Alzheimer's disease; possible index of early neuropathology. *Neuroscience*, **64**, 385–93.

Perry, R. H., McKeith, I. G. & Perry, E. K. (in press). Lewy body dementia: clinical, pathological and neurochemical connections. *J. Neural. Transm.*

Port, R. L. & Seybold, K. S. (1995). Hippocampal synaptic plasticity as a biological substrate underlying episodic psychosis. *Biological Psychiatry*, **37**, 318–24.

Rodriguez-Puertas, R., Pazos, A. & Pascual, J. (1994). Cholinergic markers in degenerative Parkinsonism; autoradiographic demonstration of high affinity choline uptake carrier hyperactivity. *Brain Res.*, **636**, 329–32.

Sahakian, B. (1988). Cholinergic drugs and human cognitive performance. *Handbook of Psychopharmacology*, **20**, 393–424.

Schultes, R. E. & Hofman, A. (1992). *Plants of the gods*. Rochester: Healing Arts Press.

Sutherland, S. (1989). 'Consciousness'. In *Macmillan Dictionary of Psychology*. London: Macmillan.

Tandon, R., Shipley, J. E., Taylor, S. et al. (1992). Electroencephalographic sleep abnormalities in schizophrenia: relationship to positive/negative symptoms and prior neuroleptic treatment. *Arch. Gen. Psychiatry*, **49**, 185–94.

Wilcock, G. K. & Scott, M. I. (1994). Tacrine for senile dementia of Alzheimer's or Lewy body type. *Lancet*, **344**, 544.

Witjeratne, C., Bandyopadhay, D. & Howard, R. (1995). Failure of tacrine treatment in a case of cortical Lewy body dementia. *Int. J. Geriatr. Psychiatry*, **10**, 808.

Yanai, J., Roget-Fuchs, Y., Pick, C. G. et al. (1993). Septohippocampal cholinergic changes after destruction of the A10-septal dopamine pathways. *Neuropharmacology*, **32**, 113–17.

Yeomans, J. S. (1995). Role of tegmental cholinergic neurons in dopaminergic activation, antimuscarinic psychosis and schizophrenia. *Neuropsychopharmacology*, **12**, 1–16.

Yeomans, J. S., Mather, A., Shandarin, A. & Tampakeras, M. (1994). Locomotion and stereotyping induced by cholinergic agents via tegmental receptors. *Neuropsychopharmacology*, **10**, 1515.

Zorn, S. H., Jones, S. B., Ward, K. M. & Liston, D. R. (1994). Clozapine is a potent and selective muscarinic m4 receptor agonist. *Eur. J. Mol. Pharmacol.*, **264**, R1–2.

31

Cholinergic therapy and Lewy body dementia

P. LIBERINI, A. VALERIO, M. MEMO
and P. F. SPANO

Summary

The concept of heterogeneity of Alzheimer's disease is based on molecular, neuropathological, clinical and neuropsychological features. An additional expression of possible heterogeneity has been revealed by the observation that patients affected by Alzheimer's disease differ in their response to pharmacologic interventions. This finding is stimulating a new experimental approach aimed at correlating neurochemical-neuropathological dysfunctions with the capability of selective drugs to improve specific 'areas' of cognition. The pharmacologic approach may thus serve as a tool to define specific subgroups of patients differentially responsive to a given therapy and, at the same time, to define new nosographic entities. Recent investigations evaluating the therapeutic potential of cholinesterase inhibitors have disclosed the existence of at least two subsets of demented patients defined as responders and nonresponders to the 'cholinergic therapy'. The cluster of 'responders' to the cholinesterase inhibitors might include a significant number of subjects with a particularly severe dysfunction of the cholinergic system. The prominent vulnerability of the cholinergic system in the Lewy body dementia indirectly suggests that pharmacological treatments directly or indirectly enhancing cholinergic transmission might ameliorate some of the impaired cognitive functions.

31.1 The cholinergic deficit in degenerative dementia

Research on Alzheimer's disease (AD) over the past two decades has emphasized the dysfunctions of the basal forebrain cholinergic system.

414

Drachman and Leavitt (1974) reported that anticholinergic drugs produce an acute state of cognitive impairment similar to the memory deficit observed in patients with AD. Accordingly, a direct relationship between the cholinergic system and AD was originally hypothesized. Following studies (Davies & Maloney, 1976) demonstrating reduction of choline acetyltransferase (ChAT) activity, neuropathological investigations demonstrated a marked loss of the cholinergic neurons within the nbM and other regions of the basal forebrain complex in AD (Whitehouse et al., 1982). Thus, it has been suggested that the degeneration of basal forebrain neurons and the accompanying loss of cholinergic projections to the neocortex and hippocampus provide an important contribution to emerging cognitive deficits (Bartus et al., 1982). Although a large series of neuropathological data have clearly shown the disruption of the basal forebrain cholinergic neurons at the end-stage of AD, the genesis of such a phenomenon still remains a matter of discussion. The involvement of the forebrain cholinergic neurons in AD has been proposed as the consequence of the cortical degeneration resulting in a decrease of nerve growth factor (NGF) retrogradely transported to the nbM (Hefti & Weiner, 1986). This hypothesis is supported by experiments showing that cell degeneration and depletion of ChAT activity in the nucleus basalis of cortically injured laboratory animals is related to the primary cortical pathology and can be prevented by exogenous NGF (Cuello et al., 1989; Koliatsos et al., 1991; Tuszynski et al., 1991; Liberini et al., 1993b). Nevertheless, a direct transfer of these findings to the clinical setting is not immediate. Only indirect evidence, such as increased cortical NGF receptor mRNA levels (Mufson & Kordower, 1992), indicates changes of NGF expression in AD. The idea of NGF-dependence for nbM cholinergic neurons is balanced by the opposite hypothesis indicating the perturbation of these neurons as a primary event in AD (Coyle et al., 1982). This hypothesis was supported by neuropathological data showing a causal link between loss of cholinergic cortical innervation and plaque formation (Arendt et al., 1985). Nevertheless, the two hypotheses are not in conflict because the presence of atrophic cholinergic neurons in the basal forebrain is compatible with primary neurodegenerative processes or retrograde disruption secondary to cortical atrophy. A better understanding of the relative contribution of the two pathogenic processes in determining the cholinergic deficit may be relevant for the development of therapeutic strategies aimed at reducing the progression rate of the disease.

This body of research has indicated a pivotal role of cholinergic impairment in the pathology of cognitive dysfunction in AD. In analogy with the dopaminergic depletion in Parkinson's syndrome, a replacement or transmitter-mimetic therapeutic approach was thought to offer a significant step forward in the treatment of specific symptoms associated with AD. However, a number of criticisms questioning the relevance of the cholinergic deficit to AD have been recently raised (Fibiger, 1991). For example, the cholinergic deficit appears to be a minor neuropathological feature in comparison with other extensive degenerative phenomena affecting the hippocampus and the neocortex of AD patients (Selkoe, 1991). Amyloid plaques, neurofibrillary tangles and synaptic alterations are considered as the hallmarks of AD and the loss of synapses in midfrontal cortex appears to be the major correlate with the arising cognitive impairment (Terry et al., 1991). The contribution of degeneration of cholinergic system to the symptoms of AD has also been challenged (Fibiger, 1991) since the degree of correlation of either basal forebrain neuron loss or cortical ChAT activity with the presence and severity of dementia is still controversial (Perry et al., 1991; Liberini et al., 1993a).

Another element of discussion arises from experimental models of cholinergic disruption suggesting a role of the cholinergic system in the facilitation and modulation of cortical target structure activity rather than influencing learning and memory processes. Finally, based on the wide spectrum of neurotransmitter systems affected, AD has been assumed to be a multisystem disease. Glutamatergic, catecholaminergic, serotonergic and peptidergic neurons located in either cortical and subcortical regions are also affected in AD (Francis et al., 1993). From these data it appears likely that the cholinergic deficit can explain only a part of the entire clinical syndrome.

Incidentally, it should be noted that AD is a progressive neurodegenerative disorder which underlies evolving neuropathological and neurochemical changes. Almost all neuropathological studies were performed in postmortem tissue, possibly reflecting the end-point of the disease. Few, although pivotal, studies on biopsy material and ventricular cerebrospinal fluid in AD have provided information about neurotransmission in living patients during the early stage of the disease (Francis et al., 1993). One emerging indication of these studies is the circumscribed corticocortical glutamatergic deficit. Thus, molecules compensating the cortical glutamate deficit, either directly, such as glutamate receptor partial agonists, or indirectly, such as 5-HT$_A$ antagonists, may also succeed in AD.

31.2 Alzheimer's disease heterogeneity and responsiveness to cholinergic therapy

A number of clinical trials aimed at enhancing cholinergic neurotransmission in AD patients by administration of cholinergic agonists and cholinesterase inhibitors have been completed or are in progress. Up to now, the only palliative therapeutic agent approved by the FDA in AD is tetrahydroaminoacridine (tacrine).

Recent controlled clinical trials with the cholinesterase inhibitor tacrine have disclosed the existence of at least two subgroups of demented patients distinguishable as responders or nonresponders to the cholinesterase inhibitor treatment (Farlow et al., 1992; Forette et al., 1992; Davies et al., 1992; Knapp et al., 1994). Factors predicting cholinesterase inhibitors responsiveness have not yet been established: neither demographic data, such as age and sex, nor clinical characteristics such as the severity and the age of onset of the cognitive impairment, are clear predictors of drug efficacy (Forette et al., 1992). The variability of the response to cholinergic therapy may be related to individual differences in pharmacokinetics, such as rate of absorption, tissue distribution, permeability of blood brain barrier, and presence of cholinesterase isoforms less sensitive to tacrine. Alternatively, the differential response to tacrine may be related to the clinical heterogeneity of AD. Indeed, the latter still remains an open question since it is not even certain whether AD is a single pathological entity, a complex syndrome with a variety of clinical and neuropathological subtypes, or many different diseases with similar clusters of symptoms.

Recent investigations indicated that the Lewy body (LB) pathology represents the largest variant of AD (Byrne et al., 1989; Gibb et al., 1989; Perry et al., 1990; Förstl et al., 1993). This neuropathological condition, characterized by rounded eosinophilic inclusion bodies, Lewy bodies (LBs) (Lewy, 1912) in the neocortex, limbic areas and subcortical nuclei, is receiving increasing attention. Nevertheless, a correct identification of cortical LBs has not been possible until the recent introduction of ubiquitin-immunocytochemistry (Lennox et al., 1989). Much interest is growing about the possibility of considering LB dementia as an independent nosographic entity, although the clinical and neuropathological criteria for the identification of the LB dementia are not firmly established (Lippa et al., 1994). Based upon retrospective findings a cluster of clinical criteria have been proposed in order to differentiate LB dementia from AD (McKeith et al., 1994).

The postmortem examination of LB brain provides a set of neuropathologic features which more clearly, although not unequivocally, differentiate LB dementia from AD (Table 31.1). It is evident that some of the neuropathological findings reported in Table 31.1 highly correlate with the arising symptoms. For example, hallucinations have been associated with marked cortical cholinergic deficit (Perry et al., 1993) while extrapyramidal features and neuroleptic hypersensitivity are related to loss of dopaminergic neurons in substantia nigra. Interestingly, it has been recently reported that the neuronal damage in the nbM of LB patients is greater than that of AD cases (Förstl et al., 1993). In addition, recent neurochemical examination of autopsy material from LB cases showed an extensive cholinergic deficit in frontal, parietal and temporal cortices, with reductions in ChAT activity greater than those seen in AD (Perry et al., 1993; Langlais et al., 1993; Levy et al., 1994). The severity and topography of the neuropathological changes of the cholinergic neurons within the basal forebrain of LB patients follows a regional distribution which correlates with the regressive phenomena of the neocortex receiving the corresponding projections (Liberini et al., 1993c). Indeed, the anterior and intermediate nbM subregions provide the major cholinergic input to the frontal cortex (Mesulam & Geula, 1988). Therefore, the neuronal damage in the nbM of demented patients with LBs is likely to depend on the frontal accentuation of the cortical atrophy which in turn may cause a decrease of retrogradely transported trophic factors (Liberini et al., 1993c). In this context it would be important to determine whether the nbM damage consists of cholinergic cell loss, or cholinergic cell atrophy or both. In this regard we emphasize that when *neuronal size* was used in Nissl and haematoxylin/eosin preparations as the only criterion for detecting abnormality of the basal forebrain neurons, a great variability of cell loss was found in the nbM of LB cases in different studies. However, the cell atrophy occurring in the basal forebrain makes the size factor a less accurate criterion for the estimation of cell loss because shrunken but viable neurons may be missed (Liberini et al., 1994). In contrast, a more accurate assessment of the nbM status can be provided by quantitative analysis of neurons immunostained for cholinergic markers, such as ChAT or low affinity NGF receptors. In this case both large and atrophied cholinergic neurons of the basal forebrain are counted, thus nbM status is more precisely reflected (Liberini et al., 1994). This is of therapeutic relevance because atrophic but viable neurons may still be responsive to therapeutic interventions.

Table 31.1. *Neuropathological features differentiating Lewy body dementia (LBD) from Alzheimer's disease (AD)*

Feature	LBD	AD
Lewy bodies in neocortex, hippocampus and brainstem	Hallmark	Sparse or absent
Neurofibrillary tangles in neocortex and hippocampus (CA1 and subiculum)	Sparse or absent	Hallmark
Dystrophic neurites in CA2-3 hippocampal sectors	Common	Rare
Abnormally hyperphosphorylated tau proteins	Absent	Consistent
Loss of neurons in substantia nigra and locus coeruleus	Early and prominent, with presence of LBs	Relevant only in late stages
Atrophy/loss of cholinergic neurons in nucleus basalis of Meynert	Severe, with possible presence of LBs	Moderate to severe, with possible presence of NFTs
Decrease of neocortical choline acetyltransferase	Severe to dramatic	Moderate to severe
Spongiform vacuolization in the temporal lobe	Marked and frequent	Infrequent

After: Byrne et al., 1989; Gibb et al., 1989; Lennox et al., 1989; Perry et al., 1990; Förstl et al., 1993; Perry et al., 1993; Langlais et al., 1993; Lippa et al., 1994; Liberini et al., 1995.

31.3 Potential of cholinergic therapy in Lewy body disease

The prominent vulnerability of the cholinergic system in the LB dementia suggests that pharmacological treatments directly or indirectly enhancing cholinergic transmission might ameliorate some of the impaired cognitive functions (Liberini et al., 1995). Acetylcholine precursors, M_1 muscarinic receptor agonists and inhibitors of acetylcholinesterase are the most promising molecules (Table 31.2). In addition, successful demonstration of the NGF efficacy in primate models of neurodegeneration (Koliatsos et al., 1991; Tuszynsky et al., 1991; Liberini et al., 1993a) should encourage clinical investigators to consider the possibility of trophic therapy in cases of dementia (Liberini & Cuello, 1994). Behavioural and safety studies need to be completed in nonhuman primates, as indicated in the guidelines proposed by the *Ad Hoc Working Group on NGF and AD* (National Institute of Health, Bethesda, 1988) (Table 31.3).

Table 31.2. *Enhancing cholinergic activity (potentially valuable in the treatment of Lewy body disease)*

Acetylcholine precursors	Release and synthesis enhancers	Cholinergic agonists	Cholinesterase inhibitors	Neurotrophins
		Muscarinic		
Choline	Phosphatidyl-serine	Arecoline	Physostigmine	NGF
CDP-choline	4-Aminopyri-dine	Pilocarpine	Heptylphyso-stigmine	CEP 1347
Phosphatidyl-choline	Acetyl-1-carni-tine	Oxotremorine	Galanthamine	BDNF
Alfa-GFC	Linopirdine	Bethanecol RS-86	Metrifonate Tacrine	NJ-4/5
	Xanomeline	Velnacrine Suronacrine ENA 713 *Nicotinic* Nicotinic		

After: Traub & Freedman, 1992; Bowen et al., 1992; Alhainen & Riekkinen, 1993; Winblad et al., 1993; Levy et al., 1994; Liberini & Cuello, 1994; Winker, 1994

Table 31.3. *Methodological and basic research concerns to be solved before using recombinant human NGF (rhNGF) in the treatment of Alzheimer's disease patients (in accordance with the Ad Hoc Working Group on NGF and AD; N.I.A., Bethesda, 1988)*

- Identification of a reliable source of rhNGF in sufficient quantity for a comprehensive program of research
- Improvement of methods for chronic delivery of rhNGF
- Demonstration of the rhNGF efficacy on primate cholinergic neurons
- Animal dose-response evaluations to establish the minimal dose of rhNGF that has an effect on cholinergic functions
- Short- and long-term studies with rhNGF to identify toxicity and long term effectiveness in at least two animal species

It is tempting to speculate that the subgroups of AD patients who positively responded to the administration of cholinesterase inhibitors (Davis et al., 1992; Farlow et al., 1992; Forette et al., 1992; Knapp et al., 1994) included a significant number of LB patients. Studies evaluating the effects of cholinesterase inhibitors should try to consider possible correlations between response to the therapy and a standardized set of clinical criteria for the diagnosis of LB dementia. A demonstration of this hypothesis must await neuropathological confirmation. In this regard, the preliminary neuropathological study by Levy et al. (1994) showing LB neuropathology in three patients who met the diagnostic criteria for AD and specifically responding to tacrine is an interesting paradigm. Finally, it should be noted that LB patients with parkinsonian symptoms may be more exposed to side-effects of the cholinergic therapy (e.g. worsening of tremor and gait dysfunction) (Ott & Lannon, 1992). The appearance of these effects, although potentially dangerous and requiring additional pharmacological interventions, may be helpful in identifying clusters of LB patients.

31.4 Discussion

Correlations between selective drug responses and neuropathological and/or neurochemical substrates represent a new approach for the study of heterogeneity of degenerative dementia. Within this framework, several issues deserve clinical and experimental attention. Standardization of clinical and neuropathological criteria for the identification of LB pathology is a prerequisite for both epidemiological studies and development of therapeutic strategies. Neuropathological follow-up of those cases identified as LB patients on clinical and neuropsychological grounds is also essential. The variability of drug response demonstrated in demented patients argues in favour of the hypothesis that the disease is heterogeneous in many aspects including pathogenesis and biochemical profile. The group of responders might segregate a cluster of patients bearing LB pathology. Multivariate analysis may reveal whether the pharmacological efficacy of cholinergic therapy is related to minimal neurofibrillary degeneration or to severe cholinergic damage. The severe cholinergic deficit of the LB pathology needs to be further analysed; an *ad hoc* morphometrical analysis of the basal forebrain (including immunocytochemical studies with anti ChAT and anti $p75^{NGFR}$ antibodies) may provide information on functional relations between target areas and basal forebrain regions in LB pathology.

31.5 Conclusions

Pharmacologic approaches may be useful in defining specific subgroups of responsive patients and may help to define new nosographic entities.

The cluster of demented patients responding to the cholinesterase inhibitor tacrine may include a significant number of subjects with a particularly severe dysfunction of the cholinergic system, as in the case of LB pathology. A neuropathological demonstration of this correlation should provide new therapeutic perspectives.

Acknowledgements

The authors wish to thank Professor Ruggero Fariello and Stefano Cappa for critically revising the manuscript.

References

Alhainen, K. & Riekkinen, P. J. (1993). Discrimination of Alzheimer patients responding to cholinesterase inhibitor therapy. *Acta Neurol. Scand. Suppl.*, **149**, 16–21.

Arendt, T., Bigl, V., Tennsted, A. & Arendt, A. (1985). Neuronal loss in different parts of the nucleus basalis is related to neuritic plaque formation in cortical target areas in Alzheimer's disease. *Neuroscience*, **14**, 1–14.

Bartus, R. T., Dean, R. L., Beer, B. & Lippa, A. S. (1982). The cholinergic hypothesis of geriatric memory dysfunction. *Science*, **217**, 408–17.

Byrne, E. J., Lennox, G., Lowe, J. & Goldwin-Austen, R. B. (1989). Diffuse Lewy body disease: clinical features in 15 cases. *J. Neurol. Neurosurg. Psychiatry.*, **52**, 709–17.

Coyle, J. R., Price, D. L. & DeLong, M. R. (1982). Alzheimer's disease: a disorder of cortical cholinergic innervation. *Science*, **219**, 1184–90.

Cuello, A. C., Garofalo, L., Kenisberg, R. L. & Maysinger, D. (1989). Gangliosides potentiate in vivo and in vitro effects of nerve growth factor on central cholinergic neurons. *Proc. Natl. Acad. Sci. USA*, **86**, 2056–60.

Davies, P. & Maloney, A. J. F. (1976). Selective loss of central cholinergic neurons in Alzheimer's disease. *Lancet*, **2**(8000), 1403–4.

Davis, K. L., Thal, L. J. & Gamzu, E. R. for the Tacrine Collaborative Study Group (1992). A double-blind, placebo-controlled multicenter study of tacrine for Alzheimer's disease. *N. Engl. J. Med.*, **327**, 1253–9.

Drachman, D. A. & Leavitt, J. (1974). Human memory and the cholinergic system. A relationship to aging? *Arch. Neurol.*, **30**, 113–21.

Farlow, M., Gracon, S. L., Hershey, L. A. et al. & the Tacrine Study Group (1992). A controlled trial of tacrine in Alzheimer's disease. *JAMA*, **268**, 2523–9.

Fibiger, H. C. (1991). Cholinergic mechanisms in learning, memory and dementia: a review of recent evidence. *Trends Neurosci.*, **14**, 220–3.

Forette, F., Bert, P., Breuil, V. & Boller, F. (1992). Therapeutic drug trials and heterogeneity of Alzheimer's disease. In *Heterogeneity of Alzheimer's Disease*, ed. F. Boller, F. Forette, Z. S. Khachaturian, M. Poncet & Y. Christen, pp. 67–73. Berlin: Springer-Verlag.

Förstl, H., Burns, A., Luthert, P., Cairns, N. & Levy, R. (1993). The Lewy body variant of Alzheimer's disease. Clinical and pathological findings. *Br. J. Psychiatry*, **162**, 385–92.

Francis, P. T., Pangalos, M. N. & Stephens, P. H. (1993). Antemortem measurements of neurotransmission: possible implications for pharmacotherapy of Alzheimer's disease and depression. *J. Neurol. Neurosurg. Psychiatry*, **56**, 80–4.

Gibb, W. R. G., Luthert, P. J., Janota, I. & Lantos, P. L. (1989). Cortical Lewy body dementia: clinical features and classifications. *J. Neurol. Neurosurg. Psychiat.*, **52**, 185–92.

Hefti, F. & Weiner, W. J. (1986). Nerve growth factor and Alzheimer's disease. *Ann. Neurol.*, **20**, 275–81.

Knapp, M. J., Knopman, D. S., Solomon, P. R., Pendlebury, W. W., Davis, C. S. & Gracon, S. I., for the Tacrine Study Group. (1994). A 30-week randomized controlled trial of high-dose tacrine in patients with Alzheimer's disease. *JAMA*, **271**, 985–91.

Koliatsos, V. E., Clatterbuck, R. E. & Nauta, H. J. W. (1991). Human nerve growth factor prevents degeneration of basal forebrain cholinergic neurons in primates. *Ann. Neurol.*, **30**, 831–40.

Langlais, P. J., Thal, L. & Hansen, L. (1993). Neurotransmitter in basal ganglia and cortex of Alzheimer's disease with and without Lewy bodies. *Neurology*, **43**, 1927–34.

Lennox, G., Lowe, J., Morrell, K., Landon, M. & Mayer, R. J. (1989). Anti-ubiquitin immunocytochemistry is more sensitive than conventional techniques in the detection of diffuse Lewy body disease. *J. Neurol. Neurosurg. Psychiat.*, **52**, 67–71.

Levy, R., Eagger, S. & Griffiths, M. (1994). Lewy bodies and response to tacrine in Alzheimer's disease. *Lancet*, **343**, 176.

Lewy, F. H. (1912). Paralysis agitans. I: Pathologische anatomie. In *Handbuch der Neurologie*, 3rd edn, ed. M. Lewondowsky, pp. 920–33. Berlin: Springer.

Liberini, P. & Cuello, A. C. (1994). Effects of nerve growth factor in primate models of neurodegeneration: potential relevance in clinical neurology. *Rev. Neurosci.*, **5**, 1–16.

Liberini, P., Piccardo, P., Mena, R. & Cuello, A. C. (1993a). Aging and Alzheimer's. *Neurology*, **43**, 1624.

Liberini, P., Pioro, E., Maysinger, D., Ervin, F. R. & Cuello, A. C. (1993b). Long-term protective effect of human recombinant nerve growth factor and monosialoganglioside GM1 treatment on primate nucleus basalis cholinergic neurons after neocortical infarction. *Neuroscience*, **53**, 625–37.

Liberini, P., Spano, P. F. & Cuello, A. C. (1993c). Alzheimer's disease and Lewy body dementia. *Br. J. Psychiatry*, **163**, 693–4.

Liberini, P., Pioro, E., Maysinger, D. & Cuello, A. C. (1994). Neocortical infarction in subhuman primates leads to a restricted morphological damage of the cholinergic neurons in the nucleus basalis of Meynert. *Brain Research*, **648**, 1–8.

Liberini, P., Memo, M. & Spano, P. F. (1995). Cholinesterase inhibitors for Lewy body dementia? *JAMA*, **274**, 1199.

Lippa, C. F., Smith, T. W. & Swearer, J. M. (1994). Alzheimer's disease and Lewy body disease: a comparative clinicopathological study. *Ann. Neurol.*, **35**, 81–8.

McKeith, I. G., Fairbarn, A. F., Bothwell, R. A. et al. (1994). An evaluation of the predictive validity and inter-rate reliability of clinical diagnostic criteria for senile dementia of Lewy body type. *Neurology*, **872**, 872–7.

Mesulam, M. M. & Geula, C. (1988). Nucleus basalis (Ch4) and cortical cholinergic innervation in the human brain: observations based on the distribution of acetylcholinesterase and choline acetyltransferase. *J. Comp. Neurol.*, **275**, 216–40.

Mufson, E. J. & Kordower, J. H. (1992). Cortical neurons express nerve growth factor receptors in advanced age and Alzheimer disease. *Proc. Natl. Acad. Sci. USA*, **89**, 569–73.

Ott, B. R. & Lannon, M. C. (1992). Exacerbation of parkinsonism by tacrine. *Clin. Neuropharmacol.*, **15**, 322–5.

Perry, R. H., Irving, D., Blessed, G., Fairbairn, A. & Perry, E. K. (1990). Senile dementia of the Lewy body type: a clinically and neuropathologically distinct form of Lewy body dementia in the elderly. *J. Neurol. Sci.*, **95**, 119–39.

Perry, E. K., Irving, D. & Perry, R. H. (1991). Cholinergic controversies. *Trends Neurosci.*, **14**, 483–4.

Perry, E. K., Irving, D. & Kerwin, J. M. (1993). Cholinergic transmitter and neurotrophic activities in Lewy body dementia: similarity to Parkinson's and distinction from Alzheimer disease. *Alzheimer Dis. Assoc. Disord.*, **7**, 69–79.

Selkoe, D. J. (1991). The molecular pathology of Alzheimer's disease. *Neuron*, **6**, 487–98.

Terry, R. D., Masliah, E. & Salomon, D. P. (1991). Physical bases of cognitive alterations in Alzheimer's disease: synapse loss is the major correlate of cognitive impairment. *Ann. Neurol.*, **30**, 572–80.

Traub, M. & Freedman, S. B. (1992). The implication of current therapeutic approaches for the cholinergic hypothesis of dementia. *Dementia*, **3**, 189–92.

Tuszynski, M. H., Sang, U. H., Yoshida, K. & Gage, F. H. (1991). Recombinant human growth factor infusions prevent cholinergic neural degeneration in the adult primate brain. *Ann. Neurol.*, **30**, 625–36.

Whitehouse, P. J., Price, D. L., Struble, R. G., Clarke, A. W., Coyle, J. T. & DeLong, M. R. (1982). Alzheimer's disease and senile dementia loss of neurons in the basal forebrain. *Science*, **215**, 1237–9.

Winblad, B., Messamore, E., O'Neill, C. & Cowburn, R. (1993). Biochemical pathology and treatment strategies in Alzheimer's disease: emphasis on the cholinergic system. *Acta Neurol. Scand. Supp.*, **149**, 4–6.

Winker, M. A. (1994). Tacrine for Alzheimer's disease – Which patient, what dose? *JAMA*, **271**, 1023–4.

32

Clinical heterogeneity in dementia: responders to cholinergic therapy[*]

S. A. EAGGER and R. J. HARVEY

Summary

Clinical Alzheimer's disease (AD) is a heterogeneous disorder and it is possible to subgroup patients by a number of different criteria. One such subgrouping is those that have a positive response to cholinergic therapy and those who do not. This phenomenon has been clearly recognized in a number of therapeutic trials of cholinesterase inhibitors and is likely to be an issue in clinical practice. Tacrine, the first cholinesterase inhibitor to be licensed for the treatment of AD, has, at best, modest effects on 20–50% of patients and is associated with a high frequency of side effects which includes liver transaminitis. The potential of clinical tests or other investigations to identify those patients who are more likely to respond to cholinergic therapy would be a valuable aid in the clinical use of these therapies. In this paper we review the issue of heterogeneity in patient populations, in the design of trials and in the pharmacological compounds used in trials. We then summarize the findings of a number of small studies of potential response predictors which include the use of psychometric tests, orthostatic blood pressure, pupillary dilatation, the EEG, CSF neurochemistry and techniques involving functional imaging. Although some results are promising, generalizability is limited by the small numbers of patients studied, and the frequent open nature of the designs used. The main conclusion that can be drawn is that adequate doses are required to achieve therapeutic plasma levels before non-response is accepted.

[*] Reprinted with permission from *Alzheimer Disease and Associated Disorders*, 1995, **9**, Suppl 2: 37–42.

425

32.1 Introduction

The evidence for the role of the cholinergic system in Alzheimer's disease (AD) has developed from work begun in the late 1970s demonstrating reductions in the levels of cholinergic marker in the brains of patients with AD (Rossor et al., 1982; Bird et al., 1983; Davies & Maloney, 1988). These deficits correlate both with clinical severity and histological features of the disease (Perry et al., 1978; Wilcock et al., 1982). Neurochemically, the cholinergic deficit relates to damage in the ascending cholinergic projections from the nucleus basalis of Meynert to the cerebral cortex (Rossor et al., 1982; Bird et al., 1983). Many other transmitter systems are affected by the disease, but it is the cholinergic system that is most consistently affected and most studied, and now forms one of the targets for therapeutic intervention.

Several different strategies for the cholinergic therapy of AD have been explored. These include precursor loading (Cohen & Wurtman, 1976; Winblad et al., 1993) and direct agonism of muscarinic or nicotinic receptor sites, none of which have shown a consistently positive effect (Spiegel, 1991). The best developed approach to cholinergic therapy has been the use of cholinesterase inhibitors. The earliest studies with physostigmine were mixed but showed promise (Davis et al., 1978; Davis et al., 1983; Jotkowitz, 1983; Thal et al., 1983; Hallak & Giacobini, 1989), particularly when doses were optimized for individual patients (Jorm, 1986). Physostigmine has been limited by its very short duration of action, though longer acting controlled release forms are being developed.

Longer acting cholinesterase inhibitors such as tacrine (tetrahydroaminoacridine, THA, Cognex[®]), its metabolite velnacrine, and more recently a number of other new compounds have been studied in large multicentre trial. From the results of these trials, it has become clear that almost all have reported subgroups of patients who respond to therapy (Eagger et al., 1991; Davis et al., 1992; Farlow et al., 1992; Knapp et al., 1994), sometimes dramatically (Eagger et al., 1992). Similarly, they have shown other subgroups with no response to treatment even at high dose.

Tacrine has now become the first cholinesterase inhibitor to gain licensing approval and is available to the general population of AD patients in several countries world-wide. Trials with tacrine have shown that 20–50% of patients show a significant response, but up to half of all patients have to withdraw from treatment with significant adverse events, principally cholinergic side effects and elevation of liver transaminases (Harvey & Eagger, 1995). The liver transaminitis results in mandatory liver function test monitoring during treatment. The limited response combined with side effects and the requirement for monitoring makes tacrine a high-cost treatment. There is thus a considerable need to develop methods of selecting responders and thereby reducing the risks to nonresponders, and controlling treatment costs. In this chapter we will consider the issue of response to therapy in terms of the patient populations that have been involved in clinical trials, and will examine early work that has begun to address the issue of predicting response.

32.2 Heterogeneity

32.2.1 Clinical issues

Alzheimer's disease, by definition, is a diagnosis that can only be made with definite confidence at autopsy (McKhann et al., 1984). In clinical practice AD is a heterogeneous disorder and patient populations can be divided up into subgroups. Examples of subgroups include those with early versus late onset (Chang Chui et al., 1985), familial versus sporadic disease (Rossor, 1993, 1994), rapid versus slow progression (Nyth et al., 1991), and appearances on structural (Scheltens et al., 1992) and functional imaging (Haxby et al., 1988; Weinstein et al., 1991). Similarly, as the topic of this chapter, there are subgroups of responders and non-responders to cholinergic therapy. Within a clinical AD patient population being treated with cholinergic therapy, with even the most careful application of NINCDS–ADRDA criteria, 10–20% will have an alternate cause for their dementia (Dewan & Gupta, 1992). The treatment of patients with dementias other than AD may either improve or reduce the apparent effectiveness of the cholinergic drugs.

A particular case has been that of patients found to have Lewy bodies at autopsy. Lewy body dementia is now a well recognized clinico-pathological syndrome, although its diagnostic criteria and relationship to AD is still being defined. The neocortical cholinergic deficit seen in AD is much more extensive in the brains of patients where Lewy bodies are present (Perry et al., 1994). As patients who have participated in studies of cholinergic therapy have come to autopsy, early reports have suggested that those found to have Lewy bodies are more likely to have been responders (Levy et al., 1994). Considerable caution is necessary as these results are clinical observations rather than the results of a controlled study. Patients with Lewy bodies have a more rapid illness and earlier death (McKeith et al., 1994), and therefore might be expected to come to autopsy in advance of AD patients. Larger series of autopsies on trial patients, ideally as part of trial methodology, are needed to make this relationship clearer (Wilcock & Scott, 1994). However, this issue does highlight the importance of considering clinical heterogeneity in patient populations, and its possible effects on apparent treatment efficacy.

32.2.2 Clinical trial design issues

The data on effectiveness and response to cholinergic therapy has primarily come from double-blind, randomized, placebo-controlled trials. Unfortunately, until recently there has been little attempt to standardize methodology with the results of wide variations in design between studies. Firstly, in their choice of patients, studies have inevitably been restrictive in their inclusion and exclusion criteria, and have used varying diagnostic criteria. Patients in trials have tended to be Caucasian, in the middle stages of the disease and free of concomitant disease and behavioural symptoms. This results in a trial population that is unlikely to be representative of AD sufferers in general. Secondly, earlier trials used crossover designs which attracted methodological criticism, while more recent trials have used a more robust parallel group design (Farlow et al., 1992; Knapp et al., 1994). Thirdly, the length of treatment in studies has varied from as little as 1 week (Fitten et al., 1990) up to 30 weeks (Knapp et al., 1994).

Finally, the definition of response used in studies has also varied, different psychometric instruments have been applied and the magnitude of change required to define response has not been validated.

It is clear from the above that the methods used to test the efficacy of cholinesterase inhibitors in AD have also been heterogeneous. Most of the data cited as evidence for response versus non-response has been on the basis of post-hoc subgroup analysis of small numbers of patients and therefore the interpretation of these results need to be made with care.

32.2.3 Pharmacological issues

Finally under the topic of heterogeneity, it is important to consider the drug being used. Although a number of cholinergic therapies are now under development, published studies and other data available publicly mainly refer to physostigmine, tacrine and the metabolite of tacrine, velnacrine. Physostigmine is a fairly specific cholinesterase inhibitor, however, by contrast tacrine and velnacrine have a wide variety of pharmacological actions in addition to their ability to block acetylcholinesterase. In particular tacrine has a regulatory effect on muscarinic and nicotinic receptors, and on acetylcholine synthesis (Hakansson, 1993; Adem, 1993). It also inhibits GABA release, stimulates dopamine, histamine and 5-HT release (Freeman & Dawson, 1991), and inhibits MAO-A and MAO-B (Adem et al., 1989). In addition it has important abilities to block potassium, sodium and calcium channels (Adem, 1992), and in vitro can alter the secretion of beta-amyloid precursor protein in cultured cell lines (Lahiri et al., 1994). The neurotransmitter deficits in AD are not isolated to the cholinergic system, and it may well be that tacrine has its effect via actions on multiple transmitter systems.

An additional confounder when attempting to compare results from different trials is the dose of drug used. Earlier studies have tended to use lower doses (Davis et al., 1992; Farlow et al., 1992; Maltby et al., 1994), while later studies have recognized the need for higher doses to achieve maximal effect (Knapp et al., 1994). This improved response at higher dose is likely to be the result of achieving adequate serum levels with a drug that has varying bioavailability (Eagger & Levy, 1992). Further care is therefore needed when comparing results from one cholinergic therapy with another.

32.3 Predicting responders

32.3.1 Patient factors

The identification of clinical characteristics that could predict response to therapy would be valuable. Simple characteristics such as age, sex and duration and severity of illness have not been identified as predictors of response in those studies that have been of adequate statistical power to examine the effect (Davis et al., 1992; Farlow et al., 1992; Knapp et al., 1994).

Similarly for the stage of dementia, patients in a large, high dose study showed equivalent degrees of improvement regardless of the severity of their dementia (Knapp et al., 1994).

It is possible that the presence of behavioural symptoms such as hallucinations or delusions may predict response. A small double-blind, crossover study comparing haloperidol and physostigmine in AD patients with delusions showed that physostigmine was able to ameliorate the delusions (Cummings et al., 1993). However, as most general trial protocols have excluded such patients, it is impossible to assess how generalizable this effect is, and whether this group would also respond in terms of cognitive symptoms. Similarly, patients with Lewy bodies, who are known to have a more marked cholinergic deficit (Perry et al., 1994), have more psychotic phenomena and may be preferential responders. As discussed above they have been identified at autopsy follow-up of trial patients (Levy et al., 1994; Wilcock & Scott, 1994), and although caution is needed in interpreting the significance of these findings, the recent development of clinical criteria for Lewy body disease (McKeith et al., 1992; McKeith et al., 1994) may allow specific trials of cholinergic therapy in this group.

32.3.2 *Neuropsychological factors*

An attractive strategy for predicting response is to use the results of neuropsychological testing. Further analysis of data from patients who have participated in tacrine studies have suggested that it is attentional function rather than memory that improves during treatment (Sahakian et al., 1993). Two small studies have attempted to predict medium to long term treatment response for the neuropsychological effects seen with a single dose of tacrine. Both were open studies (Alhainen & Riekkinen, 1993; Alhainen et al., 1993), and therefore require caution in their evaluation, however, patients whose MMSE score and scores on tests of attention and working memory improved after the single dose were then subsequently more likely to respond to tacrine in a longer open study. If these results can be replicated in larger double-blind trials, then the use of short neuropsychological tests after a single dose of drug may be an effective clinical method of predicting response.

32.3.3 *Blood pressure*

Depressed nondemented elderly patients who show a drop in blood pressure of 10 mmHg or more on changing from lying to standing have been shown to be more likely to respond to antidepressant treatment (Schneider et al., 1986; Stack et al., 1988). The physiological basis of blood pressure regulation involves both parasympathetic and sympathetic autonomic activity via the central cholinergic system (Ewing et al., 1980). Patients with AD who have impaired cholinergic function may as a result also show a greater postural drop on standing, and that these may be the patients who will respond to cholinergic therapy.

The results of two small studies of this theory have been mixed. Pomara et al. (1991) measured orthostatic blood pressure in 23 AD patients entering a placebo controlled study of velnacrine. They found that conversely it was the non-responders in the study who had the greatest postural drop, although these findings were not repeated in a larger series of velnacrine treated patients (Murphy et al., 1991). Schneider et al. (1992) reported the preliminary findings from 40 patients entering a trial of tacrine, 22 of which were defined as responders at the end of the trial. They found that the responders showed a mean fall of 8.4 mmHg compared with only 2.1 mmHg in the nonresponder group. They also analysed the sample for age effects and found that both increasing age and fall in blood pressure contributed to predicting the response to tacrine. Their interpretation of this is that older patients with AD may have a more selective cholinergic deficit than younger onset patients.

The magnitude of these effects are small, and the findings currently contradictory, however, they do suggest that peripheral measures of central cholinergic function may be of use in predicting response to cholinergic therapy.

32.3.4 Pupillary dilatation

Recent reports have suggested that it may be possible to recognize AD by measuring the pupillary dilatation response to the anticholinergic agent tropicamide (Barinaga, 1994; Scinto et al., 1994). In this small study patients with clinical AD were found to have an exaggerated pupillary response. This may be the result of upregulation of cholinergic receptors, and might predict those most likely to respond to cholinergic therapy. The findings require replication in large numbers of patients, and in patients who subsequently enter treatment trials.

32.3.5 The EEG

Comparison of the EEG or quantitative-EEG (QEEG) before and after a single dose of tacrine is another method being evaluated as a predictor of subsequent response. Studies by Alhainen et al. (1991a, 1993) showed that a change from baseline of the alpha-theta ratio after a single dose of tacrine was the most sensitive method of predicting subsequent response to the drug.

The lack of EEG response in the non-responders may represent more advanced deafferation of the cortex from the basal forebrain afferants and brain stem inputs (Alhainen & Riekkinen, 1993).

The EEG has also been used to monitor response to tacrine treatment, during clinical trials (Perryman & Fitten, 1991; Minthon et al., 1993) and long-term treatment (Shigeta et al., 1993). In clinical trials variable effects have been shown which included an upward frequency shift in the dominant rhythm (Perryman & Fitten, 1991), a reduction in spectral power in the delta and theta bands in the parietal area (Perryman & Fitten, 1991), and a decrease in alpha power anteriorly and alpha and theta power posteriorly (Minthon et al., 1993). In a long term study of three individual cases (Shigeta et al., 1993), initial changes in the EEG of two patients returned to baseline levels on long-term treatment, while a third patient showed progressive improvement on long-term high dose treatment.

The EEG changes seen are likely to be due to effects on attention, arousal and cerebral blood flow. They offer some potential in predicting and monitoring treatment, but these small studies need replicating in larger numbers of patients before general conclusions or guidelines can be drawn.

32.3.6 CSF neurochemistry

Alhainen et al. (1993; 1991a) have also studied the CSF changes that occur before and during treatment with tacrine. Significant increases in CSF HVA and 5-HIAA were found in patients treated with tacrine, specially in the responder subgroup, indicating that the response may be mediated via dopaminergic and serotonergic systems in addition to cholinergic enhancement (Alhainen & Riekkinen, 1993). Changes in CSF somatostatin-like immunoreactivity (CSF SLI) also correlated with clinical response to tacrine, with a slight decrease in CSF SLI in the non-responder group, suggesting an additional response mediated via direct or indirect somatostatinergic mechanisms (Alhainen et al., 1991b; Alhainen & Riekkinen, 1993). The invasive nature of CSF sampling makes this method less likely to be used as a response prediction test. Tacrine treatment has also been shown to modify CSF neuropeptide levels in AD (Minthon et al., 1994).

32.3.7 Functional imaging

In addition to the EEG, functional imaging techniques such as positron emission tomography (PET) and single photon emission computerized tomography (SPECT) offer the possibility of directly measuring the cortical effects of dementia drug treatments. The PET (Rapoport, 1991; Kennedy et al., 1993) and SPECT (O'Brien et al., 1992) finding in AD are now well defined, and more recently the potential for visualizing treatment effects with these techniques has begun to be realized (Cohen et al., 1992; Nordberg et al., 1992; Nordberg, 1993). Treatment with tacrine in AD improves functional brain activity measured using PET scanning (Nordberg et al., 1992; Nordberg, 1993), with particular improvements in glucose metabolism and nicotine receptor binding mainly in patients with milder forms of the disease. These findings also correlated with neuropsychological and EEG measures, and were responsive to changes in dose (Nordberg, 1993).

Results using SPECT imaging have so far been mixed in studies of regional cerebral blood flow (rCBF) during treatment (Cohen et al., 1992; Minthon et al., 1993). The findings have generally been that treatment causes a general increase in rCBF, that may correlate with effects on cognition (Minthon et al., 1993).

32.4 Conclusions

With the first cholinesterase inhibitor now entering general use, the evidence is clear that this will not be a treatment that can be or should be used on every patient with AD. The effects are modest at best, and management is complicated by a high incidence of side effects, and a requirement for intensive monitoring during treatment.

Data from large scale clinical trials indicate that age and sex do not predict response, although there are clear cut groups of responders and nonresponders. This subgrouping by response seen in the highly selected trial population may be more marked in clinical practice. However, the exclusion of groups of patients with psychotic symptoms and other behavioural disturbance, which are common in AD (Burns et al., 1990), from trials may be excluding a group with a higher response rate. This group is likely to include those with Lewy bodies in whom a more pronounced cholinergic deficit is known to exist.

Individualized dosing, resulting in adequate plasma levels and thus cholinesterase inhibition is needed before nonresponse is concluded. A number of techniques have been studied for their ability to predict response, unfortunately, the small numbers of patients involved makes it difficult to generalize the results. Larger studies, and the incorporation of the more promising predictive tests into future clinical trial protocols will allow the sensitivity and specificity of these techniques to be better understood.

References

Adem, A. (1992). Putative mechanisms of action of tacrine in Alzheimer's disease. [Review]. *Acta Neurol. Scand. Suppl.*, **139**, 69–74.

Adem, A. (1993). The next generation of cholinesterase inhibitors. *Acta Neurol. Scand. Suppl.*, **149**, 10–12.

Adem, A., Jossan, S. S. & Oreland, L. (1989). Tetrahydroaminoacridine inhibits human and rat brain monoamino oxidase. *Neuroscience Letters*, **107**, 313–17.

Alhainen, K. & Riekkinen, P. J. (1993). Discrimination of Alzheimer patients responding to cholinesterase inhibitor therapy. *Acta Neurol. Scand. Suppl.*, **49**, 16–21.

Alhainen, K., Partanen, J., Reinikainen, K. et al. (1991a). Discrimination of tetrahydroaminoacridine responders by a single dose pharmaco-EEG in patients with Alzheimer's disease. *Neurosci. Lett.*, **127**, 113–16.

Alhainen, K., Sirvio, J., Helkala, E., Reinikainen, K. & Riekkinen, P. (1991b). Somatostatin and cognitive functions in Alzheimer's disease – the relationship of cerebrospinal fluid somatostatin increase with clinical response to tetrahydroaminoacridine. *Neurosci. Lett.*, **130**, 46–8.

Alhainen, K., Helkala, E. & Riekkinen, P. (1993). Psychometric discrimination of tetrahydroaminoacridine responders in Alzheimer patients. *Dementia*, **4**, 54–8.

Barinaga, M. (1994). Possible new test found for Alzheimer's disease. *Science*, **266**, 973.

Bird, T. D., Stranahan, S., Sumi, S. M. & Raskind, M. (1983). Alzheimer's disease: choline acetyltransferase activity in brain tissue from clinical and pathological subgroups. *Ann. Neurol.*, **14**, 284–93.

Burns, A., Jacoby, R. & Levy, R. (1990). Psychiatric Phenomena in Alzheimer's disease. I to IV Disorders of thought content. Disorders of Perception. Disorders of Mood. Disorders of Behaviour. *Br. J. Psychiatry*, **157**, 72–94.

Chang Chui, H., Lee Teng, E., Henderson, W. & Moy, A. C. (1985). Clinical subtypes of dementia of the Alzheimer type. *Neurology*, **35**, 1544–50.

Cohen, E. L. & Wurtman, R. J. (1976). Brain acetylcholine: increases after systemic choline administration. *Life Sciences*, **16**, 1095–102.

Cohen, M. B., Fitten, L. J., Lake, R. R., Perryman, K. M., Graham, L. S. & Sevrin, R. (1992). SPECT brain imaging in Alzheimer's disease during treatment with oral tetrahydroaminoacridine and lecithin. *Clin. Nucl. Med.*, **17**, 312–15.

Cummings, J. L., Gorman, D. G. & Shapira, J. (1993). Physostigmine ameliorates the delusions of Alzheimer's disease. *Biol. Psychiatry*, **33**, 536–41.

Davies, P. & Maloney, A. J. R. (1988). Selective loss of central cholinergic neurons in Alzheimer's disease. *Lancet*, **ii**, 1403.

Davis, K. I., Mohs, R. C., Davis, B. M. et al. (1983). Oral physostigmine in Alzheimer's disease. *Psychopharmacol. Bull.*, **19**, 451–3.

Davis, K. L., Mohs, R. C., Tinklenberg, J. R. et al. (1978). Physostigmine: improvement of long-term memory processes in normal humans. *Science*, **201**, 272–4.

Davis, K. L., Thal, L. J., Gamzu, E. R. et al. (1992). A double-blind, placebo-controlled multicenter study of tacrine for Alzheimer's disease. The Tacrine Collaborative Study Group. *New Engl. J. Med.*, **327**, 1253–9.

Dewan, M. J. & Gupta, S. (1992). Toward a definite diagnosis of Alzheimer's disease. [Review]. *Comp. Psychiatry*, **33**, 282–90.

Eagger, S. & Levy, R. (1992). Serum levels of tacrine in relation to clinical response in Alzheimer's disease. *Int. J. Geriatr. Psychiatry*, **7**, 115–19.

Eagger, S., Morant, N., Levy, R. & Sahakian, B. J. (1992). Tacrine in Alzheimer's disease. Time course of changes in cognitive function and practice effects. *Br. J. Psychiatry*, **60**, 36–40.

Eagger, S. A., Levy, R. & Sahakian, B. J. (1991). Tacrine in Alzheimer's disease. *Lancet*, **338**, 50–1.

Eagger, S. A., Levy, R. & Sahakian, B. J. (1992). Tacrine in Alzheimer's disease. *Acta Neurol. Scand. Suppl.*, **39**, 75–80.

Ewing, D. J., Hume, L., Campbell, I. W., Murray, A., Neilson, J. M. M. & Clarke, B. F. (1980). Autonomic mechanisms in the initial heart rate response to standing. *J. Appl. Physiol.*, **49**, 809–14.

Farlow, M., Gracon, S., Hershey, L. A., Lewi, K. W., Sadowsky, C. H. & Dolan-Ureno, J. (1992). A controlled trial of tacrine in Alzheimer's disease. The Tacrine Study Group. *JAMA*, **268**, 2523–9.

Fitten, L. J., Perryman, K. M., Gross, P. L., Fine, H. F., Cummins, J. & Marshall, C. (1990). Treatment of Alzheimer's disease with short- and long-term oral tetrahydroaminoacridine and lecithin: A double-blind study. *Am. J. Psychiatry*, **47**, 239–42.

Freeman, S. E. & Dawson, R. M. (1991). Tacrine: a pharmacological review. *Prog. Neurobiol.*, **36**, 257–77.

Hakansson, L. (1993). Mechanism of action of cholinesterase inhibitors in Alzheimer's disease. *Acta Neurol. Scand.*, **88**, 7–9.

Hallak, M. & Giacobini, E. (1989). Physostigmine, tacrine and metrifonate: the effect of multiple doses on acetylcholine metabolism in rat brain. *Neuropharmacology*, **28**, 199–206.

Harvey, R. J. & Eagger, S. A. (1995). The clinical efficacy of tacrine. *Rev. Contemp. Pharmacotherapy*, **6**, 335–48.

Haxby, J. V., Grady, C., Koss, E. et al. (1988). Heterogeneous anterio-posterior metabolic patterns in dementia of the Alzheimer type. *Neurology*, **38**, 1853–63.

Jorm, A. F. (1986). Effects of cholinergic enhancement therapies on memory function in Alzheimer's disease: a meta-analysis of the literature. *Aus. NZ J. Psychiatry*, **20**, 237–40.

Jotkowitz, S. (1983). Lack of clinical efficacy of chronic oral physostigmine in Alzheimer's disease. *Ann. Neurol.*, **14**, 690–1.

Kennedy, A. M., Newman, S. N., Warrington, E. K., Roques, P., Frackowiak, R. S. J. & Rossor, M. N. (1993). Familial alzheimer's disease versus sporadic alzheimer's-disease – a clinical, neuropsychological and pet study. *Neurology*, **43**, 192.

Knapp, M. J., Knopman, D. S., Solomon, P. R., Pendlebury, W. W., Davis, C. S. & Gracon, S. (1994). A 30-week randomized controlled trial of high-dose tacrine in patients with Alzheimer's disease. The Tacrine Study Group. *JAMA*, **271**, 985–91.

Lahiri, D. K., Lewis, S. & Farlow, M. R. (1994). Tacrine alters the secretion of the beta-amyloid precursor protein in cell lines. *J. Neurosci. Res.*, **37**, 777–87.

Levy, R., Eagger, S., Griffiths, M. et al. (1994). Lewy bodies and response to tacrine in Alzheimer's disease. *Lancet*, **343**, 176.

Maltby, N., Broe, G. A., Creasey, H., Jorm, A. F., Christensen, H. & Brooks, W. S. (1994). Efficacy of tacrine and lecithin in mild to moderate Alzheimer's disease: double blind trial. *BMJ*, **308**, 879–93.

McKeith, I. G., Perry, R. H., Fairbairn, A. F., Jabeen, S. & Perry, E. K. (1992). Operational criteria for senile dementia of Lewy body type (SDLT). *Psycholog. Med.*, **22**, 911–22.

McKeith, I. G., Fairbairn, A. F., Perry, R. H. & Thompson, P. (1994). The clinical diagnosis and misdiagnosis of senile dementia of Lewy body type (SDLT). *Br. J. Psychiatry*, **165**, 324–32.

McKhann, G., Drachman, D., Folstein, M., Katzman, R., Price, D. & Stadlan, E. M. (1984). Clinical diagnosis of Alzheimer's Disease: Report of the NINCDS–ADRDA work group under the auspices of Department of Health and Human Services Task Force on Alzheimer's Disease. *Neurology*, **34**, 939–44.

Minthon, I., Edvinsson, L. & Gustafson, L. (1994). Tacrine treatment modifies cerebrospinal-fluid neuropeptide levels in alzheimer's-disease. *Dementia*, **5**, 295–301.

Minthon, L., Gustafson, L., Dalfelt, G. et al. (1993). Oral tetrahydroaminoacridine treatment of Alzheimer's disease evaluated clinically and by regional cerebral blood flow and EEG. *Dementia*, **4**, 24–42.

Murphy, M. F., Hardiman, S. T., Nash, R. J. et al. (1991). Evaluation of HP 029 (velnacrine maleate) in Alzheimer's disease. *Ann. NY Acad. Sci.*, **640**, 253–62.

Nordberg, A. (1993). Effect of long-term treatment with tacrine (THA) in Alzheimer's disease as visualized by PET. *Acta Neurol. Scand., Suppl.*, **149**, 62–5.

Nordberg, A., Lilja, A., Lundqvist, H. et al. (1992). Tacrine restores cholinergic nicotinic receptors and glucose metabolism in Alzheimer patients as visualized by positron emission tomography. *Neurobiol. Aging*, **13**, 47–58.

Nyth, A. L., Gottfries, C., Blennow, K. et al. (1991). Heterogeneity of the course of Alzheimer's disease: A differentiation of subgroups. *Dementia*, **2**, 18–24.

O'Brien, J. T., Eagger, S. A., Syed, G. M. S., Sahakian, B. J. & Levy, R. (1992). A study of regional cerebral blood flow and cognitive performance in Alzheimer's disease. *J. Neurol. Neurosurg. Psychiatry*, **55**, 1182–7.

Perry, E. K., Tomlinson, B. E., Blessed, G., Bergmann, K., Gibson, P. H. & Perry, R. H. (1978). Correlation of cholinergic abnormalities with senile plaques and mental test scores in senile dementia. *BMJ*, **ii**, 1457–9.

Perry, E. K., Haroutunian, V., Davis, K. L. et al. (1994). Neocortical cholinergic activities differentiate Lewy body dementia from classical Alzheimer's disease. *Neuroreport*, **5**, 747–9.

Perryman, K. M. & Fitten, I. J. (1991). Quantitative EEG during a double-blind trial of THA and lecithin in patients with Alzheimer's disease. *J. Geriatr. Psychiatry & Neurology*, **4**, 127–33.

Pomara, N., Deptula, D. & Singh, R. (1991). Pretreatment postural blood pressure drop as a possible predictor of response to the cholinesterase inhibitor velnacrine (HP 029) in Alzheimer's disease. *Psychopharmacol. Bull.*, **27**, 301–7.

Rapoport, S. I. (1991). Positron emission tomography in Alzheimer's disease in relation to disease pathogenesis: a critical review. *Cerebrovascular & Brain Metab. Rev.*, **3**, 297–335.

Rossor, M. N. (1993). Molecular pathology of Alzheimer's disease. *J. Neurol. Neurosurg. Psychiatry*, **56**, 583–6.

Rossor, M. N. (1994). Clinical heterogeneity in familial alzheimer-disease. *Neurobiol. Aging*, **15**, 140.

Rossor, M. N., Garret, N. J., Johnson, A. L., Mountjoy, C. O., Roth, M. & Iversen, L. L. (1982). A post-mortem study of the cholinergic and GABA systems in senile dementia. *Brain*, **105**, 13–30.

Sahakian, B. J., Owen, A. M., Morant, N. J. et al. (1993). Further analysis of the cognitive effects of tetrahydroaminoacridine (THA) in Alzheimer's disease: assessment of attentional and mnemonic function using CANTAB. *Psychopharmacology*, **110**, 395–401.

Scheltens, P., Barkhof, F., Valk, J. et al. (1992). White matter lesions on magnetic resonance imaging in clinically diagnosed Alzheimer's disease. Evidence for heterogeneity. *Brain*, **115**, 735–48.

Schneider, L. S., Sloane, R. B., Staples, F. R. & Bender, M. (1986). Pretreatment orthostatic hypotension as a predictor of response to nortryptiline in geriatric depression. *J. Clin. Psychopharmacol.*, **6**, 172–6.

Scinto, L. F., Daffner, K. R., Dressler, D. et al. (1994). A potential noninvasive neurobiological test for Alzheimer's disease. *Science*, **266**, 1051–4.

Shigeta, M., Persson, A., Viitanen, M., Winblad, B. & Nordberg, A. (1993). EEG regional changes during long-term treatment with tetrahydroaminoacridine (THA) in Alzheimer's disease. *Acta Neurol. Scand. Suppl.*, **149**, 58–61.

Spiegel, R. (1991). Cholinergic drugs, affective disorders and dementia: problems of clinical research. *Acta Psychiatrica Scand. Suppl.* **366**, 47–51.

Stack, J. A., Reynolds, C. F., Perel, J. M., Houck, P. R., Hoch, C. C. & Kupfer, D. J. (1988). Pretreatment systolic orthostatic blood pressure (PSOP) and treatment response in elderly depressed inpatients. *J. Clin. Psychopharmacol.*, **8**, 116–20.

Thal, L. J., Fuld, P. A., Masur, D. M. & Sharpless, N. S. (1983). Oral physostigmine and lecithin improve memory in Alzheimer disease. *Ann. Neurol.*, **13**, 491–6.

Weinstein, H. C., Hijdra, A., & van Royen, E. A. (1991). SPECT in early- and late-onset Alzheimer's disease. *Ann. NY Acad. Sci.*, **640**, 72–3.

Wilcock, G. K. & Scott, M. I. (1994). Tacrine for senile dementia of Alzheimer's or Lewy body type [letter]. *Lancet*, **344**, 544.

Wilcock, G. K., Esiri, M. M., Bowen, D. M. & Smith, C. C. T. (1982). Alzheimer's disease. Correlations of cortical choline acetyltransferase activity with the severity of dementia and histological abnormalities. *J. Neurolog. Sci.*, **57**, 407–17.

Wilcock, G. K., Surmon, D. J., Scott, M. et al. (1993). An evaluation of the efficacy and safety of tetrahydroaminoacridine (THA) without lecithin in the treatment of Alzheimer's disease. *Age & Ageing*, **22**, 316–24.

Winblad, B., Messamore, E., O'Neill, C. & Cowburn, R. (1993). Biochemical pathology and treatment strategies in Alzheimer's disease: Emphasis on the cholinergic system. *Acta Neurol. Scand.*, **88**, 4–6.

33

Tacrine and symptomatic treatment in Lewy body dementia

F . LEBERT , L . SOULIEZ and F . PASQUIER

Summary

Two characteristics of senile dementia of the Lewy body type (SDLT) compared with Alzheimer's disease (AD) are relevant to treatment management: relative hypocholinergic activities and behavioural disturbances such as psychotic manifestations with neuroleptic hypersensitivity. A better tacrine responsiveness of SDLT patients has been proposed. An open trial with tacrine (120 mg/day) prescribed in 22 probable AD patients (meeting NINCDS–ADRDA criteria) resulted in no memory improvement in the four patients meeting SDLT criteria. The potential of GABAergic agents, particularly carbamazepine, in the management of delirium and psychotic symptoms in SDLT is discussed.

33.1 Introduction

In recent years there has been an increasing interest in behavioural disorders in dementia since psychiatric disturbance is considered to be one of the most troublesome aspects of the disease by many relatives of demented patients. They are an important risk factor for institutionalization. On the other hand, behavioural abnormalities are not usually considered in the diagnosis of degenerative dementia although psychotic symptoms and mood disorders may be the earliest signs of frontal lobe dementia or Lewy body disease. Episodic confusion, depressive and psychotic symptoms are frequently observed in senile dementia of Lewy body type (SDLT). Hallucinations are more often reported in SLDT than in dementia of Alzheimer type (AD) (Ballard et al., 1995). Dopamine hyperactivity is a putative neurochemical basis for psychosis and cholinergic/dopaminergic imbalance with relative dopamine excess linked to hallucinations in different neurological diseases such as Parkinson's disease. Moreover, physostigmine reduced delusions in two AD patients (Cummings et al., 1993). In SLDT, in which hallucinations are frequent, cholinergic hypometabolism (e.g. choline acetyltransferase decrease) has been reported (Perry et al., 1993). Tetrahydroaminoacridine (THA) is used in the treatment of AD, although results are variable. The discrepancy between studies may be due to the heterogeneity of AD defined by NINCDS–ADRDA criteria. McKeith et al. (1994) have reported that, in their experience, 15% of SDLT patients meet NINCDS–ADRDA criteria for 'probable' AD, with up to 50% fulfilling criteria for 'possible' AD. There is a need to develop criteria for response to THA treatment and to assess its efficacy in SDLT meeting criteria for AD.

Therapeutic management of noncognitive symptoms is difficult in SDLT because of the neuroleptic sensitivity (McKeith et al., 1992). Further data on atypical neuroleptic medications in the management of behavioural disturbances would be particularly valuable in SLDT.

33.2 Tacrine in SLDT

A great variability in response has been found in trials of cholinesterase inhibitors in AD. The lower activity of the choline acetyltransferase in brains of patients with SLDT, compared with those of AD patients suggests that SLDT patients could be responders to THA (Perry et al., 1994). In addition, muscarinic receptor 'supersensitivity' in SDLT may reflect the relative preservation of intrinsic cortical systems (Perry et al., 1994). Moreover, at necropsy, three 'responder' cases in the THA trial from the London Institute of Psychiatry series had Lewy bodies in addition to Alzheimer changes (Levy et al., 1994).

Since October 1994, THA has been prescribed in French hospitals for probable mild or moderate AD. The aim of the following study was to determine whether a subtype would discriminate responders and non-responders to THA treatment at a daily dose of 120 mg.

Twenty-two patients with mild or moderate probable AD (NINCDS–ADRDA criteria) assessed with the CERAD protocol, were treated with THA (Table 33.1). Patients with suspected frontal lobe dementia were excluded on the basis of Lund and Manchester criteria (1994). Patients were divided into three groups according to clinical presentation and the SPECT pattern; AD-P typical Alzheimer's disease syndrome with parietotemporal hypoperfusion ($n = 13$); AD-F, patients with frontal behavioural features ($n = 4$); and SDLT patients fulfilling McKeith et

Table 33.1. *Characteristics of the patients*

Sex (M/F)	10/12
Mean age (SD)	72.7 (7.4)
Mean MMSE (SD)	18.6 (4.1)

al. (1992) criteria ($n = 5$). The characteristics of these three groups are shown in Table 33.2. None received psychotropic medication except serotonin reuptake inhibitors prescribed for at least one month pretrial in six patients. Psychotic symptoms were assessed by semi-structured interview with the carer.

The trial was an open study. Patients started with the same dose of THA, 40 mg/day. The THA dosage was increased every 6 weeks, if treatment was well tolerated, up to 120 mg/day.

Before treatment, a battery of neuropsychological tests was performed including the Mattis Dementia Rating Scale (DRS), the digit span subtest of the Wechsler Memory scale, and the Grober and Buschke Selective Reminding test (Grober & Buschke, 1987). The same assessment with parallel forms was performed post-treatment. A patient was regarded as a responder if there was an increase of at least one memory task score compared with the baseline.

Four patients were regarded as responders to THA, 4/9 AD-P, 0/4 AD-F, 0/5 SDLT. Improvement in memory tasks scores was observed in the memory subtest of the DRS, and on learning subscores of the Grober and Buschke test. An increase in the Concept subscore was also observed. The increase in the various subscores was consistent in these patients. The responder and the nonresponder groups did not differ with respect to age, duration of the disease, MMSE and DRS scores at baseline (Table 33.3). There was no relation between hallucinations, serotonergic treatment and THA responsiveness.

Of the 22 probable AD patients, four (18%) fulfilled criteria of probable SDLT. All were male, in agreement with the literature data which report male predominance (McKeith et al., 1994). Efficacy of THA in improving long-term memory has already been reported (Alhainen & Riekkinen, 1993). No cognitive improvement post-THA treatment in AD-F patients is in agreement with the cerebral blood flow study in Lund (Minthon et al., 1993) which showed that patients with frontal hypometabolism had less improvement with THA than those with a

Table 33.2. *Characteristics of three groups of patients treated with 120 mg of THA*

	DTA-P (n = 13)	DTA-F (n = 4)	SDLT (n = 5)
Age mean (SD)	73.3 (6.9)	71.7 (11.8)	71.8 (5.8)
M/F	4/9	1/3	5/0
MMSE mean (SD)	19.3 (4.1)	16.0 (4.5)	19.0 (3.8)
Mattis score mean (SD)	109.0 (4.0)	91.7 (21.8)	98.0 (15.8)

There were no significant differences between groups in any of the above

Table 33.3. *Characteristics of the THA responders and nonresponders*

	THA responders	THA nonresponders	Stat
Age mean (SD)	71.2 (2.5)	73.0 (2.1)	NS
Duration of the disease mean (SD)	3.0 (0.8)	3.5 (1.1)	NS
M/F	3/1	7/11	NS
MMSE score mean (SD)	20 (0.8)	18.3 (4.5)	NS
Mattis score mean (SD)	112.5 (11.4)	101.5 (16.6)	NS

typical parietotemporal pattern. In the present study, the four responders did not fulfil SDLT criteria. The hypothesis of a specific relation between the presence of Lewy bodies and the efficacy of THA was not confirmed in all autopsy proven cases reported by Wilcock and Scott (1994). A relation between hallucinations and hypocholinergic activities has been reported in SDLT (Perry et al., 1993). In our preliminary study, no relation was found between hallucinations and THA responsiveness. Two points are worth noting: first, the SDLT patients were originally diagnosed as probable AD and did not meet 'diffuse Lewy body disease' criteria, and second, patients were regarded as responders only on memory performance, whereas THA could improve attention (Alhainen & Riekkinen, 1993). Perry et al. (1993) also reported a serotonergic-cholinergic imbalance in SLDT. No relation was found in the present study between serotonergic reuptake inhibitors and THA responsiveness. However, the small number of patients limits the value of these results, which need to be confirmed with a larger population.

33.3 Symptomatic treatment in SLDT

33.3.1 Neuroleptics

SLDT patients have frequent, severe and sometimes fatal, neuroleptic sensitivity (McKeith et al., 1992). In SDLT, two patterns of neuroleptic sensitivity have been described: exaggerated extrapyramidal symptoms and features suggesting neuroleptic malignant syndrome (McKeith et al., 1992). However, all SLDT patients do not develop neuroleptic sensitivity. No variable such as daily dose, route or duration appears to predict the subsequent development of neuroleptic sensitivity: atypical neuroleptics defined by their low extrapyramidal side-effects are likely to be a useful alternative therapeutic strategy. Lee et al. (1994) have demonstrated a positive effect of risperidone, a neuroleptic with potent serotonin 5-HT2 and dopamine D2 antagonist activity, titrated up to 1 mg b.i.d., on psychotic symptoms (visual hallucinations, paranoid delusions) in one SLDT patient.

Clozapine has a greater affinity for D1 and D4 receptors relative to its affinity for D2 receptors and is more selective for mesolimbic and mesocortical pathways, which accounts for its relative lack of extrapyramidal side-effects. Clozapine is used in Parkinson's disease but rarely in demented elderly. Oberholzer et al. (1992) have shown, in an open study, the efficacy of clozapine on antisocial behaviour in demented patients. Recently, Pitner et al. (1995), reported beneficial effect of clozapine in three elderly psychotic demented patients. The criteria of diagnosis used in these two studies do not exclude SDLT in demented patients with psychotic symptoms. Adverse effects of clozapine, frequent and severe, occurred in four cases in the study of Pitner et al. (1995): falls, bradycardia and delirium, were reported immediately after the first dose. Clozapine must therefore be used with caution. Moreover, the efficacy of clozapine is decreased in Parkinson's disease with psychosis and cognitive decline (Factor et al., 1994). The use of clozapine in SDLT is of interest because of its lack of extrapyramidal side-effects, although its anticholinergic action, including muscarinic M1 antagonist activity, could promote delirium and memory disorders. On the other hand, clozapine is a potent and selective muscarinic M_4 receptor agonist (Zorn et al., 1994). This action might contribute to its specific antipsychotic effect by altering the cholinergic–dopaminergic balance.

33.3.2 GABAergic agents

SLDT differs from AD in several respects: frequent episodic confusion, early EEG abnormalities and different location of neuropathological lesions in limbic structures. These characteristics prompted us to try carbamazepine in SDLT. Carbamazepine is an anticonvulsant agent with antikindling effects on the limbic system of value in cyclothymic disorders. It had been prescribed in demented patients with beneficial effects on agitation (Gleason & Schneider, 1990). The responses of two patients with probable SDLT were so striking that we include the following descriptions:

Case 1

A 71-year-old man with a 12-month history of mild cognitive impairment presented with long-standing fluctuations of his cognitive state and severe episodes of hallucinations (he had Capgras delusions). He was admitted to a behaviour acute care unit for agitation. His MMSE score was 4/30. Daily life dependency was 95%. Physical and biological assessments were normal. No cause for delirium was found. Moderate asthma was treated with theophyline. Psychiatric manifestations were not affected by haloperidol (1 mg t.i.d., p.o. for one week, trazodone 50 mg t.i.d. p.o. for 2 weeks, and lorazepam 1 mg t.i.d. for 2 weeks). One month before, the patient was able to use his credit card and his MMSE score was 17/30. EEG measurements indicated posterior bradykinesia. Internal temporal atrophy and mild periventricular hyperintensities were the only abnormalities observed on MRI. The patient did not fulfil NINDS–AIREN criteria for vascular dementia.

The clinical features were in agreement with SDLT (McKeith et al., 1992). Carbamazepine (100 mg qid. p.o.) was prescribed. At baseline Brief Psychiatric Rating Scale (BPRS) score was 43/72. One week later, behavioural abnormalities were decreased. BPRS score was 19/72. He ate alone again. He had no more urinary incontinence. MMSE score was only 9/30. Two weeks later, serum concentration of carbamazepine was 5 μ/ml. He had no side-effects and at 7-month follow-up did not manifest confusion.

Case 2

A 75-year-old woman with a 2-year history of cognitive impairment presented with frequent episodic confusions and severe hallucinations (visual hallucinations of children and dogs). She was admitted to a behaviour acute care unit on account of insomnia. Her MMSE score was 6/30. Daily life dependency was 60%. She was treated by her general practitioner with haloperidol (doses unknown) for the previous month without positive effects on hallucinations but with side-effects, including moderate extrapyramidal features. The caregiver reported three unexplained falls. Six weeks before, the MMSE score obtained in a screening for THA treatment initiation was 17/30. Physical and biological assessments were normal. The CT scan showed only bilateral temporal atrophy. There was no past psychiatric history. The patient fulfilled SDLT criteria of McKeith et al. (1992). Haloperidol was discontinued and extrapyramidal signs decreased, but psychotic symptoms continued unabated. Her BPRS score was 31/72. Carbamazepine was initiated at a dose of 100 mg/day. Four months later, the patient did not report any hallucinations or episodic confusion. Her MMSE score was 10/30 and her BPRS score was 13/72.

33.4 Discussion

These cases of probable SDLT indicate the efficacy of carbamazepine on behavioural abnormalities (Lebert et al., 1995). Carbamazepine appears superior to neuroleptics, benzodiazepines, and trazodone, the latter being particularly efficient in DAT (Lebert et al., 1994). Carbamazepine decreases anxiety, tension, hostility, hallucinations, agitation and confusion. These are the same symptoms as those reported in studies on the efficacy of carbamazepine in AD patients (Gleason & Schneider, 1990).

Moreover, carbamazepine may be useful in relation to episodic confusion in SDLT as well as on cyclothymic mood disorders.

Carbamazepine has complex actions including: anti-kindling effect on limbic system; action on amino acid transmitter systems (NMDA receptors and reduction of GABA turnover); and modulation of somatostatin levels. GABA and somatostatin are neurotransmitters implicated in delirium (Ross, 1991). In SDLT somatostatin levels and metabolism of some amino acid transmitters are affected, for example kynurenine (Langlais et al., 1993) which has an action on NMDA receptors. Thus, several biological mechanisms could explain the effects of carbamazepine in SDLT. Beneficial effects of another GABAergic agent, chlormethiazole, have been reported in SDLT (McKeith et al., 1992). GABA interneurons receive terminals from cholinergic basal forebrain nuclei. In SDLT, wherein cholinergic metabolism is decreased, GABAergic agents could regulate behavioural abnormalities.

33.5 Conclusion

Whereas at present psychopharmacological investigations do not provide support for the efficacy of cholinesterase inhibition in SDLT, they indicate other approaches that may be worth investigating. These include carbamazepine which, amongst its complex pharmacology may affect GABA neurotransmission. The need to examine patients primarily diagnosed as SDLT (as opposed to those fulfilling AD clinical criteria) is highlighted as is the need for placebo-controlled trials in view of the natural fluctuations associated with the disorders.

Acknowledgements

We wish to thank Professor Henri Petit, and Laurence Grymonprez. This work was supported by ER 153 from the direction de la recherche et des études doctorales du Ministère de l'Enseignement Supérieur et de la Recherche, by the Conseil Général and the Mairie de Lille and by Grant 93 06 from the commission mixte CHRU-Faculté de Médecine de Lille.

References

Alhainen, K. & Riekkinen, P. J. (1993). Discrimination of Alzheimer patients responding to cholinesterase inhibitor therapy. *Acta Neurol. Scand. Suppl.*, **149**, 16–21.

Ballard, C. G., Saad, K., Patel, A. et al. (1995). The prevalence and phenomenology of psychotic symptoms in dementia sufferers. *Int. J. Geriatr. Psychiatry*, **10**, 477–86.

Cummings, J. L., Gorman, D. G. & Shapira, J. (1993). Physostigmine ameliorates the delusions of Alzheimer's disease. *Biol. Psychiatry*, **33**, 536–41.

Factor, S. A., Brown, D., Molho, E. S. et al. (1994). Clozapine: a 2-year open trial in Parkinson's disease patients with psychosis. *Neurology*, **44**, 544–6.

Gleason, R. P. & Schneider, L. S. (1990). Carbamazepine treatment of agitation in Alzheimer's outpatients refractory to neuroleptics. *J. Clin. Psychiatry*, **51**, 115–18.

Grober, E. & Buschke, H. (1987). Genuine memory deficits in dementia. *Dev. Neuropsychol.*, **3**, 13–36.

Langlais, P. J., Thal, L., Hansen, L. et al. (1993). Neurotransmitters in basal ganglia and cortex of Alzheimer's disease with and without Lewy bodies. *Neurology*, **43**, 1927–34.

Lee, H., Cooney, J. M. & Lawlor, B. A. (1994). The use of risperidone, an atypical neuroleptic, in Lewy body disease. *Int. J. Geriatr. Psychiatry*, **9**, 415–17.

Lebert, F., Pasquier, F. & Petit, H. (1994). Behavioral effects of trazodone in Alzheimer's disease. *J. Clin. Psychiatry*, **55**, 536–8.

Lebert, F., Pasquier, F. & Petit, H. (1995). The use of carbamazepine in senile dementia of Lewy body: a case study. *Alzheimer's Res.*, **1** (Suppl 1), 51.

Levy, R., Eagger, S., Griffiths, M. et al. (1994). Lewy bodies and response to tacrine in Alzheimer's disease. *Lancet*, **343**, 176.

Lund & Manchester Groups (the) (1994). Clinical and neuropathological criteria for frontotemporal dementia. *J. Neurol. Neurosurg. Psychiatry*, **57**, 416–18.

McKeith, I. G., Perry, R. H., Fairbairn, A. F. et al. (1992). Operational criteria for senile dementia of Lewy body type. *Psychol. Med.*, **22**, 911–22.

McKeith, I. G., Fairbairn, A. F., Bothwell, R. A. et al. (1994). An evaluation of the predictive validity and inter-rater reliability of clinical diagnostic criteria for senile dementia of Lewy body type. *Neurology*, **44**, 872–7.

Minthon, L., Gustafson, L., Dalfelt, G. et al. (1993). Oral tetrahydroaminoacridine treatment of Alzheimer's disease evaluated clinically and by regional cerebral blood flow and EEG. *Dementia*, **4**, 432–42.

Oberholzer, A. F., Hendriksen, A. U., Monsch, B. H. et al. (1992). Safety and effectiveness of low-dose clozapine in psychogeriatric patients: a preliminary study. *Int. Psychogeriatrics*, **4**, 187–95.

Perry, E. K., Marshall, E., Thompson, P. et al. (1993). Monoaminergic activities in Lewy body dementia: relation to hallucinosis and extrapyramidal features. *J. Neural. Transm.*, **6**, 167–77.

Perry, E. K., Haroutunian, V., Davis, K. L. et al. (1994). Neocortical cholinergic activities differentiate Lewy body dementia from classical Alzheimer's disease. *NeuroReport*, **5**, 747–9.

Pitner, J. K., Mintzer, J. E., Pennypacker, L. C. et al. (1995). Efficacy and adverse effects of clozapine in four elderly psychotic patients. *J. Clin. Psychiatry*, **56**, 180–5.

Ross, C. A., Peyser, C. E., Shapiro, I. et al. (1991). Delirium: phenomenologic and etiologic subtypes. *Int. J. Psychogeriatr.*, **3**, 135–47.

Wilcock, G. K. & Scott, M. I. (1994). Tacrine for senile dementia of Alzheimer's or Lewy body type. *Lancet*, **344**, 544.

Zorn, S. H., Jones, S. B., Ward, K. M. et al. (1994). Clozapine is a potent and selective muscarinic M4 receptor agonist. *Eur. J. Pharmacol.*, **269**, R1–2.

34

Neurochemical correlates of pathological and iatrogenic extrapyramidal symptoms

M. A. PIGGOTT and E. F. MARSHALL

Summary

Several aspects of movement control by neuronal pathways in the basal ganglia are summarized. Evidence from neurochemical analyses in various neurodegenerative disorders is presented to demonstrate that a severe loss of dopamine in the putamen does not of itself represent a necessary condition for the appearance of extrapyramidal symptoms, and that the appearance of extrapyramidal symptoms or sensitivity to antipsychotics eliciting extrapyramidal symptoms is not solely dependent on a lack of striatal dopamine. The strategies of reduction of cholinergic activity and of reduction of the firing rate of the serotonergic neurons are alternatives to the traditional dopamine replacement therapy in the management of extrapyramidal symptoms. Inhibition of dopaminergic activity by dopamine D2 receptor blockers, as a means of controlling psychotic symptoms is considered inappropriate in disorders such as Lewy body dementia with a potential for increased sensitivity to such medication.

34.1 Introduction

The major extrapyramidal features of resting tremor, cogwheel rigidity, akinesia and disturbance of posture are most commonly regarded as clinical symptoms of Parkinson's disease (PD), and neurochemically are associated with lesions of the dopaminergic projections to the corpus striatum from the zona compacta of the substantia nigra. However, these abnormal motor movements also occur in Lewy body dementia (LBD) and in other categories of patients, examples of which are listed in Table 34.1.

Table 34.1 *Classification of disorders*

	Disorders	Clinical	Pathological/neurochemistry
Group 1	Parkinson's disease (PD) Postencephalitic Parkinson's disease (PEPD) Progressive supranuclear palsy (PSP)	Extrapyramidal symptoms	Loss in nigral cell numbers >60%
Group II	Lewy body dementia (LBD)	Mild extrapyramidal symptoms Dementia Fluctuating cognitive impairment Sensitivity to anti-psychotic medication	Loss in nigral cell numbers <60%
Group III	Tardive dyskinesia in schizophrenia Neuroleptic sensitivity in Lewy body dementia	• Persistent when discontinued • May lead to increased mortality even following withdrawal	Loss in nigral cell numbers <60%
Group IV	Corticobasal degeneration Olivopontocerebellar atrophy Meige syndrome	No extrapyramidal symptoms No extrapyramidal symptoms No extrapyramidal symptoms	Loss in nigral cell numbers >60% No loss in nigral cell numbers No loss in nigral cell numbers

In considering these disorders, the questions under discussion are whether extrapyramidal features are always a result of loss of dopaminergic neurotransmission and, if not, what neurochemical environment is responsible for the absence or presence of parkinsonian symptoms in patients with variable losses of nigrostriatal dopaminergic function.

To assist in understanding the balance of neurotransmitter activities which predispose to the appearance of extrapyramidal symptoms, a simplified version of the circuitry of the basal ganglia is presented in Fig. 34.1 as a framework in which the details of these disorders may be envisaged. Figure 34.1 focuses on the direct and indirect pathways (Flaherty & Graybiel, 1994) from the various regions of the cerebral cortex to the striatum, through the thalamus to the frontal cortex. The direct pathway appears to be mediated by excitatory D1 receptors in the striatum acting on one or two inhibitory γ-aminobutyric acid (GABA)-pathways through the internal segment of the pallidum or the pars reticulata of the substantia nigra to the thalamic nuclei. The indirect pathway consists of a GABA-containing projection from the striatum to the external segment of the globus pallidus, followed by a series of inhibitory and excitatory pathways involving GABA or glutamate, respectively, in the external segment of the pallidus, the subthalamic nucleus, the internal segment of the pallidum and thence to the thalamus. The sum effect of the indirect pathway is an inhibition of movement, which can, in turn be inhibited by stimulation of D2 receptors in the striatum. Thus dopamine acts optimally to promote movement when stimulating both D1 and D2 receptors. Dopamine release stimulated by acetylcholine may be mediated by the nicotinic receptor but cholinergic interneurons are possibly also targets of the dopaminergic and glutamatergic inputs to the striatum (Starr, 1995). Dopamine controls acetylcholinergic activity both indirectly through D1 receptors acting on the corticostriatal glutamatergic pathway which stimulates release of acetylcholine, and by acting directly through D2 receptors to suppress the release of acetylcholine. The precise interconnections of the serotonergic projection from the dorsal raphe in the striatum have not been fully resolved, but serotonin (5HT) appears to exert a tonic inhibition of dopaminergic activity. It could be anticipated that a loss in 5HT would balance deficits in the dopaminergic pathways, but the proportion of D1/D2 receptors may play a critical role in the effects of serotonin.

Thus, functional activity of the basal ganglia can be envisaged as an interaction between several different neuronal tracts, deficits in any one of which may be responsible for behavioural dysfunction. The classification

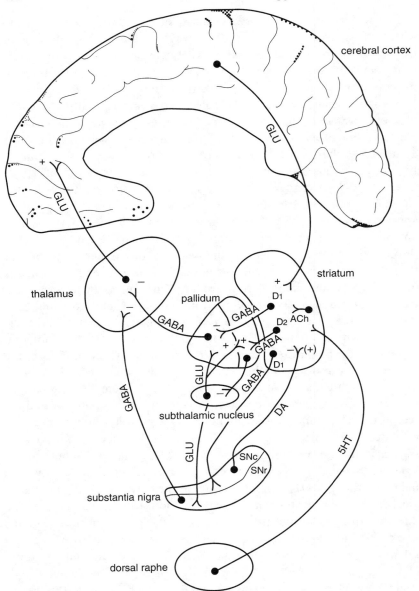

Fig. 34.1 Simplified basal ganglia circuitry.

of the disorders considered in this study (Table 34.1) is made according to their clinical and neuropathological attributes. Of the two probable dopaminergic projection areas from the substantia nigra, we have focused our discussion on neurochemical evidence primarily from the putamen as this appears to be the area most affected in Parkinson's disease (Bernheimer et al., 1973).

Group I. Diseases associated with greater than 60% loss of nigral neurons

Cell losses in the substantia nigra of the first group of conditions are well established (Jellinger, 1987; Pascual et al., 1992), and greater than 60% loss, compared with age-matched controls, is regarded as a prerequisite for the appearance of extrapyramidal symptoms. Neurochemically such cell loss is indicated in PD by decreases in activities of the synthetic enzymes tyrosine hydroxylase and dihydroxyphenylalanine decarboxylase in substantia nigra and striatum (Rinne et al., 1979) with associated losses of dopamine (DA) and its metabolites, homovanillic acid (HVA) and dihydroxyphenylacetic acid (DOPAC) (Perry et al., 1992). It is clear that there are particular patterns of change in the putamen from PD and postencephalitic PD (PEPD) with regard to neurotransmitters and metabolites (Figs 34.2 and 34.3), and to numbers of dopamine uptake sites and dopamine D1 and D2 receptors (Fig. 34.4). In the putamen of PD, dopaminergic denervation is indicated by a 65% reduction in neuron density in the substantia nigra (Fig. 34.5), by decreases of dopamine and DOPAC greater than 80%, 50% losses of HVA, and dopamine uptake sites with corresponding increases in the turnover index HVA/DA and upregulation of D2 receptors. The increase in the ratio of HVA/DA, which also represents functional release, suggests that there is an enhanced firing of the remaining dopamine neurons and a down regulation of D2 receptors should be expected. It must be assumed that the observed increase in D2 receptors in the putamen from Parkinson's disease, reminiscent of the development of D2 receptor supersensitivity in rats having nigrostriatal lesions (Creese & Snyder, 1979), indicates that the dopamine deficits are partially compensated by the upregulation of dopaminergic activity.

In agreement with previous studies (Bernheimer et al., 1973), dopamine deficiency in a recently investigated case of PEPD is more severe than in idiopathic parkinsonism, with extreme losses in DA, HVA and DOPAC (Fig. 34.2). Although not detailed here the decreases in the caudate were similar to those in the putamen and the cell loss in substantia nigra was greater than in PD. The high HVA/DA ratio indicates a very fast firing rate for the few remaining dopamine-containing neurons,

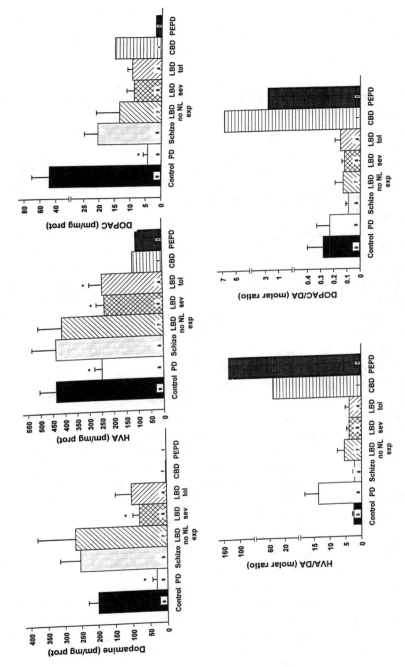

Fig. 34.2 Concentrations of DA, HVA, DOPAC and the molar ratios of HVA/DA and DOPAC/DA in putamen of neuropsychiatric disorders. The numbers in the columns are sample sizes (*$p < 0.05$ vs. control).

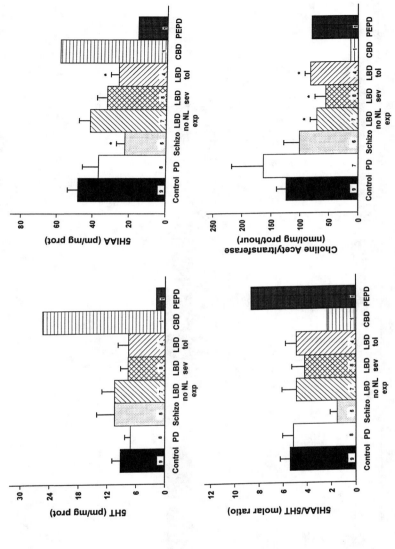

Fig. 34.3 Concentrations of 5HT, 5HIAA, the molar ratio of 5HIAA/5HT and choline transferase activity in putamen of neuro-psychiatric disorders. The numbers in the columns are sample sizes (*$p < 0.05$ vs. control).

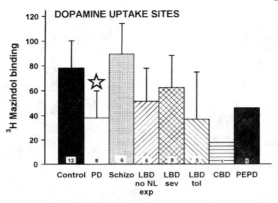

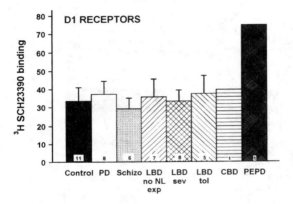

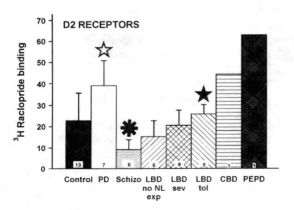

Fig. 34.4 3H-Mazindol binding (dopamine uptake sites, fmol/mg), 3H SCH23390 binding (D1 receptor, fmol/mg) and 3H-raclopride binding (D2 receptor, fmol/mg) in putamen of neuropsychiatric disorders. White star and black asterisk $= p < 0.05$ vs. controls, and the black star $= p < 0.05$ vs. the other LBD groups.

Substantia nigra neuron density

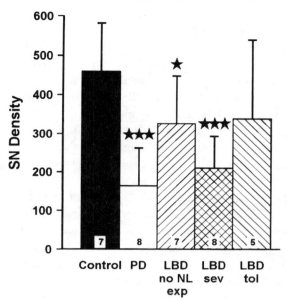

Fig. 34.5 Neuronal cell densities in controls, PD and LBD; *** $p<0.001$ vs. controls, *p<0.05 vs. controls (one-tailed t-tests).

but the severe loss of DOPAC and the comparatively well preserved number of dopamine uptake sites, with decreases of less than 50% compared with normal, suggest that the nerve ending structure survives, to some extent, but retains no capacity for dopamine storage within it. In contrast to the findings from PD, the increase in D2 receptors is paralleled by an increase in D1 receptors, a change which was also noted in symptomatic and recovered cats after being made parkinsonian with 1-methyl-4-phenyl-1,2,3,6-tetrahydropyridine (MPTP) (Frohna et al., 1995) and believed to be caused by the extensive DA losses in an environment of a successfully compensating striatum. D1 receptor upregulation in striatum was also reported in subjects suffering from narcolepsy, a disorder with some similarities to encephalitis lethargica and possibly a similar aetiology, having been almost unknown before the 1920s. In this case of PEPD, age 70 at death, excessive sleepiness in youth was a feature, with lethargy and slowness developing later. A diagnosis of PEPD was not made in life and the patient did not receive levodopa until his last decade when it improved the parkinsonian symptoms but induced hyperactivity, aggressiveness and disinhibition. Facial dyskinesia and protrusion of the tongue also occurred. It may be that these characteristics are mediated by D1 receptor activation.

In progressive supranuclear palsy (PSP) the ratio of HVA/DA is significantly lower in the putamen compared with PD and only slightly higher than the normal range for both areas of the striatum (Kish et al., 1985). D2 receptor numbers are reduced in caudate nucleus and putamen both postmortem and in vivo in patients with PSP, clearly representing a loss of dopaminoceptive cells and perhaps providing a part explanation for the fact that PSP patients do not respond to levodopa treatment. D1 receptors remain intact in the striatum although in accord with the loss of nigral cells, there is a considerable loss of nigral D1 receptors (Pascual et al., 1992).

Although cholinergic neurons, present as large aspiny interneurons in the striatum, represent a small percentage of the total neuronal population of the striatum, they appear to have an important role in motor control. Pharmacologically, the extrapyramidal symptoms of Parkinson's disease may be controlled by the administration of anti-cholinergic drugs. However, there is no evidence that there is any change in choline acetyltransferase (ChAT) activity, a cholinergic marker, in either the striatum (Fig. 34.3) or the substantia nigra (Dubois et al., 1983) in Parkinson's disease. A hypothesized hyperactivity of cholinergic inervation caused by the release from inhibitory control by the dopaminergic input has not been confirmed, which may be explained by the increase in D2 receptor numbers inhibiting release of acetylcholine. Changes in cortical cholinergic activity in PD is generally considered to be associated with the intellectual impairment seen in some of these patients. ChAT activity in the case with PEPD is within the normal range (Fig. 34.3), as would be expected if increases in both D1 and D2 receptor numbers balance out the effects of residual dopamine on cholinergic activity.

Decreases of 40–60% in ChAT activity found in the caudate, putamen and nucleus accumbens of patients with PSP (Ruberg et al., 1985) were not in agreement with the modest reductions found by Kish et al. (1985). Neither result is consistent with the decrease in D2 receptor numbers found by Pascual et al. (1992) which should allow for an increase in cholinergic activity by activation of D1 receptors. It is possible that the very few remaining dopamine-containing neurons do not make available sufficient dopamine to activate the D1 receptors of the glutamatergic corticostriatal pathway.

The decreases of 5HT and its metabolite, 5-hydroxyindoleacetic acid (5HIAA) in the putamen of the subjects with PD are rarely greater than

50% (Fig. 34.2) and not significantly different from normal. The densities of the 5HT1 and 5HT2 receptors have not been shown to be abnormal in the striatum or the cortex from subjects with PD (Perry et al., 1984; Rinne et al., 1980). As mentioned above a loss of serotonergic input would be expected to counteract the subnormal dopamine transmission. However, there is probably no direct interaction between 5HT and acetylcholine-containing neurons, as the loss of 5HT and 5HIAA in the subject with PEPD is profound while ChAT activity in the putamen in that patient is normal. The nonsignificant increase in serotonin turnover in the putamen of PEPD is probably not great enough to counteract the severe loss in serotonin, which may contribute to the dyskinesia previously noted in this patient. In PSP, 5-HT and 5HIAA has been reported to be normal in basal ganglia, hypothalamus and temporal cortex (Kish et al., 1985).

Group II. Diseases associated with less than 60% loss of nigral neurones

These subjects with LBD have recently been described neuropathologically (Perry et al., 1990) and clinically (McKeith et al., 1992). It is a condition which presents with dementia, fluctuating cognitive impairment, and mild parkinsonian symptoms with a high proportion of patients experiencing visual hallucinations. Previously, we noted that the neurochemical deficit in the caudate from a group of patients with Lewy body dementia, unclassified in terms of their neuroleptic sensitivity, lay, most probably, with the storage of dopamine as reflected in concentrations of DOPAC and the ratio DOPAC/DA (Marshall et al., 1994). The cases studied here are classified according to their neuroleptic medication and sensitivity. In those patients who did not receive neuroleptic medication, there was a trend for the DOPAC concentration and the ratio DOPAC/DA in the putamen to be lower than normal, although DA and HVA concentrations are normal (Fig. 34.2). There is no up-regulation in dopamine activity, and despite a tendency for D2 receptors to be lower than in controls, there is no significant change in the numbers of either D1 or D2 receptors. Thus, although there is evidence of a decrease in nigral cell density (Fig. 34.5), the extent of dopaminergic denervation is limited. There is a tendency for the serotonergic markers to be lower than normal. Significantly lower ChAT activity (Fig. 34.3) in the putamen from the cases with LBD compared with controls may reflect changes in glutamatergic activity, and may contribute to the mild extrapyramidal symptoms exhibited.

Group III. Conditions showing sensitivity to antipsychotic medication

In Group III, LBD may again be considered on the basis of an increased sensitivity to neuroleptics resulting in increased mortality in about 80% of this population. LBD subjects had significantly lower ChAT activity in the putamen compared with normals. When comparing the LBD subjects according to their treatment with and reaction to antipsychotics, there are no measures of neurotransmitters or metabolites which differentiate one group from another, although DA and HVA concentrations in the putamen are lowest in those patients most sensitive to antipsychotics and are significantly lower than in controls. In the same age group of patients the nigral neuronal density is quite severely diminished (Fig. 34.5). In those patients who tolerated antipsychotics, despite there being no significant loss of dopamine or decrease in turnover in putamen compared with either control or the neuroleptic sensitive LBD subjects, D2 receptor numbers are significantly higher than in the neuroleptic sensitive and neuroleptic naive groups (Fig. 34.4 and Piggott et al., 1994). The lack of upregulation of D2 receptors in those subjects who were intolerant of antipsychotics cannot be attributed to either the concentration or turnover of dopamine in the striatum, but it may contribute to the increased sensitivity to antipsychotics by causing the dopaminergic block to be more complete. The significant decrease of 5HT in the putamen of neuroleptic-tolerant patients may be relevant in terms of removing an inhibition of dopaminergic activity.

The level of dopamine denervation identified in this group of patients is not as severe as that found in a group of Lewy body dementia cases believed to have no neuroleptic sensitivity (Langlais et al., 1993). However, the concentration of dopamine in the putamen of the controls, as measured by Langlais et al. (1993), is much lower than that found by Hornykiewicz or our group (Hornykiewicz, 1993; Marshall et al., 1994) although the molar loss of dopamine in the neuroleptic tolerant LBD is of the same order. It may be that methodological differences are accountable for these discordances in values which lead to disagreements in interpretation. Another factor may be the duration of mild extrapyramidal symptoms reported to be present in the patients with LBD from the study by Langlais et al. (1993). They may have suffered extrapyramidal disorder for a long period of time as the symptoms are reported as appearing early in their illness which had a mean duration of six years.

In schizophrenic patients with tardive dyskinesia following many years of antipsychotic treatment which continued until death, measures of dopaminergic activity in the putamen (Fig. 34.2) are not abnormal. The 5HIAA concentration in the putamen is lower than controls and the index of 5HT turnover, 5HIAA/5HT is significantly lower than normal values (Fig. 34.3). Furthermore, despite there being no change in the turnover of dopamine, there are significant decreases in D2 receptor numbers in putamen from schizophrenics (Fig. 34.4). These data are not in agreement with those obtained in a study by Toru et al. (1988) in which a hyperdopaminergic state was identified in both the caudate and the putamen, in terms of D2 receptor binding and tyrosine hydroxylase activity. However, they did not report if their patients were suffering from tardive dyskinesia.

Despite the fact that all the patients in this group of disorders have received neuroleptics until or nearly until death, the profile of their neurotransmitter and metabolite concentrations, and their receptor numbers are quite different. Schizophrenics with a neuroleptic sensitivity leading to tardive dyskinesia, have, apart from decreased numbers of D2 receptors, near normal measures of dopaminergic activity and a decreased index of 5HT turnover. On the other hand, the LBD patients with neuroleptic sensitivity have normal D2 receptor numbers, increased turnover index, and lower concentrations of neurotransmitter and metabolite. Given that the effects of chronic administration of neuroleptic to rats leads to increases in dopamine turnover and increases in D2 numbers, but no change in 5HT turnover, it is evident that the effects of chronic administration of neuroleptics in humans is dependent on their illness and to a smaller extent the nature of their sensitivity.

Group IV. Diseases with no parkinsonism having nigrostriatal dopaminergic deficits

This group of disorders, in which there is evidence of low striatal dopaminergic activity with no accompanying extrapyramidal symptoms, is included by way of contrast with the previous groups in which extrapyramidal symptoms of varying severity were exhibited. They offer another dimension in considering the neurochemistry of movement control.

In one recently reported case of corticobasal degeneration (CBD) (Marshall et al., 1995), presenting primarily with a dementing syndrome having no extrapyramidal symptoms, lower concentrations of dopamine in the putamen compared with PD are accompanied by a higher turnover index, HVA/DA and an extremely high DOPAC/DA ratio (Fig. 34.2). Together with the reduced numbers of dopamine uptake sites and raised

D2 receptor numbers (Fig. 34.4), the data point to a severe dopaminergic denervation consistent with the neuropathological picture of reduced cell numbers in the substantia nigra. In contrast with the normal values obtained for ChAT in the one other reported case in which these data have been previously reported (Riley et al., 1990), there is a marked loss of cholinergic activity in the putamen of this case (Fig. 34.3) of CBD which may be partially responsible for the absence of classical extrapyramidal symptoms. In addition, we have no support for the contention (Hornykiewicz, 1993) that the upregulation of dopamine activity in cases of striatal dopamine loss is under cholinergic control. Another possible explanation for the absence of extrapyramidal symptoms is that the increase in D2 receptors in the putamen, which must be on noncholinergic cells, represents a compensatory mechanism increasing the activity of the GABAergic projections (Fig. 34.1) through the indirect pathway. The fourfold increase in 5-HT in the putamen with a concomitant decrease in the turnover index, 5HIAA/5HT, is in line with a decreased inhibition of dopaminergic activity but possibly reveals a control by a 5HT pathway which is critical for preservation of motor control, as these changes in serotonergic activity are not found in PD.

Dominantly inherited olivopontocerebellar atrophy (OPCA) is a progressive autosomal dominant neurodegenerative disorder presenting clinically with ataxia and characterized histologically with loss of neurones in the inferior olives, pons and cerebellum. Although there are significantly reduced levels of dopamine, HVA and DOPAC in both caudate and putamen (Kish et al., 1992) there is, except in two of 14 patients, no evidence of nigral cell loss and none of upregulation of dopaminergic activity. None of the patients had been diagnosed as having PD and none had received antiparkinsonian treatment, although, retrospectively it was noted that the two patients with nigral cell loss had exhibited parkinsonian signs. No measure of cholinergic function was made so the possibility remains that in hereditary OPCA, at least, as a consequence of the reduction in dopaminergic activity, there is a reduction in cholinergic function, which may account, in part, for the absence of parkinsonian symptoms.

A similar phenomenon may be responsible for the absence of extrapyramidal symptoms in a condition known as Meige syndrome (Mark et al., 1994) in which HVA concentration was found to be low despite normal dopamine concentrations in both caudate and putamen. In this case, although 5HT was reported as normal there was no measure of turnover and no measure of cholinergic activity is made.

34.2 Discussion

In describing the neurochemical characteristics of several disorders exhibiting more or less extrapyramidal symptoms, it is clear that there is not an absolute correlation between lack of dopamine or even dopaminergic activity and the appearance of extrapyramidal features of behaviour.

The data from each of the disorders examined in the study can be considered in terms of the balance represented in Fig. 34.6. For PD and PEPD, the reduction of dopamine leading to the increased activity in the indirect pathway and decreased activity in the direct pathway leads to a shift in the direction of akinesia. The increase in HVA/DA ratio and the number of D2 receptors represents a compensatory increase in dopaminergic activity and permits a greater inhibition of the indirect pathway in an environment of reduced dopamine. Thus the effect of the medication received by these patients should lessen these changes and promote inhibition of the indirect pathway; however, replacement therapy is clearly not sufficient as extrapyramidal features remain a feature. The data should be interpreted as representing a continuing compensation against the loss of dopamine. The increase in D1 receptors in PEPD points to a potential increase in the direct pathway, possibly augmented by the increased turnover of 5HT, leading to an easy precipitation of dyskinesia. The situation with PSP is somewhat different in that there is no upregulation of dopaminergic activity and the loss of D2 receptors would lead to an increase in activity of the direct pathway explaining the predominance of dyskinesia in PSP.

The tardive dyskinesia associated with schizophrenia in the patients of this study could be a consequence of an increased activity in the direct pathway, following a decrease in D2 receptor numbers. It would be enhanced by the lowered turnover of 5HT allowing greater release of dopamine. For all patients with LBD, the decrease in cholinergic activity would reduce the indirect pathway activity and partly compensate for the loss of dopamine to result in less severe extrapyramidal symptoms. In those receiving neuroleptic treatment, the anticipated increase in D2 receptor numbers would allow the indirect pathway to be more easily inhibited. Clearly, the sensitivity of those LBD patients in whom the D2 receptors fail to upregulate, stems from a resultant incapacity to inhibit the activity of the indirect pathway.

In the event of such sensitivity being identifiable premortem, effective pharamacological treatment of these patients would be more usefully focused on the other transmitters involved in the balance. In cases such

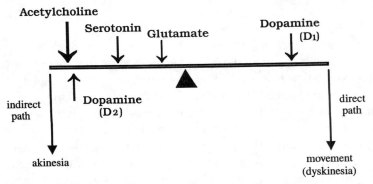

Fig. 34.6 A schematic balance of the interaction of neurotransmitters in the striatum.

as CBD, for whom EPS is not a problem, the profound loss of striatal dopamine is counteracted by some mechanism which could be interpreted as self-medicating. The most obvious features are the very large increase in the HVA/DA and DOPAC/DA ratios accompanied by decreases in D1/D2 ratio, choline acetyltransferase and 5HT turnover primarily caused by a lack of 5HT release, changes which together promote activity in the direct pathway away from akinesia.

Reported increases in serotonergic turnover in OPCA may appear at first to be inconsistent with an inhibitory action on the dopamine pathways. However, when it is realized that there is no upregulation of dopaminergic activity in the striatum of OPCA patients, then the pattern of increased serotonin turnover might be expected. Thus, the maintenance of the status quo in terms of dopamine activity despite loss of neurotransmitter, may extend to a balanced action on the direct and indirect pathways of Fig. 34.1 resulting in neither extrapyramidal symptoms nor dyskinesia.

Activities of other neurotransmitters, such as glutamate and GABA could be altered in these conditions to prevent the occurrence of EPS. The evidence from one case of CBD that glutamate is decreased by 50% in striatum is in accord with an enhanced stimulation of the direct pathway and away from the appearance of EPS. Our own evidence is limited to a finding of reduced numbers of NMDA receptors in the putamen of the schizophrenic patients. Such a reduction could contribute to the appearance of dyskinesia. Thus it is clear that further study on the role played by GABA and glutamate is required to determine the specific role played by these transmitters in the control of movement as opposed to the general role of information processing.

34.3 Conclusion

The data presented in this study confirm that a severe loss of dopamine in the putamen does not necessarily lead to the appearance of extrapyramidal symptoms and conversely that extrapyramidal symptoms or sensitivity to EPS-producing antipsychotics are not solely dependent on a profound lack of striatal dopamine. In the face of basal ganglia pathology, with decreased but compensating striatal activity, the measures in the putamen which come out most consistently in favour of reducing extrapyramidal symptoms, are a reduced choline acetyltransferase activity indicating lowered cholinergic activity and a low 5HIAA/5HT ratio representing reduced firing rate of serotonergic neurones. By comparing disorders exhibiting sensitivity to neuroleptic treatment, such as LBD and schizophrenia with tardive dyskinesia, the neurochemical effects of the neuroleptic are seen to be dependent on the disorder and the behavioural outcome represents an inability to control the balance of the direct and indirect pathways in the basal ganglia. Thus, in the absence of a means to identify the neuroleptic-sensitive from the neuroleptic-tolerant form of LBD, it would appear inappropriate to treat psychotic behaviour in LBD, having a tendency to exhibit parkinsonian symptoms and a potential for neuroleptic sensitivity, with pharmacological agents which exacerbate the inability to upregulate dopaminergic activity. In the management of extrapyramidal symptoms, other approaches such as focusing on muscarinic receptors in the striatum with a specific cholinergic receptor antagonist, or on reducing the firing rate of the serotonergic pathway may prove more effective.

Acknowledgements

The authors would like to acknowledge their colleagues Elaine K. Perry, Robert H. Perry, Ian G. McKeith, Evelyn Jaros, Mary Johnson, Heather L. Melrose, Jennifer A. Court, Stephen Lloyd, Mel Leitch, Andrew Fairbairn, Andrew Brown, Peter Thompson who contributed greatly to the data collections detailed in this survey.

References

Bernheimer, H., Birkmayer, W., Hornykiewicz, O., Jellinger, K. & Seitelberger, F. (1973). Brain dopamine and the syndromes of Parkinson and Huntington – Clinical morphological and neurochemical correlations. *J. Neurol. Sci.*, **20**, 415–55.

Creese, I. & Snyder, S. H. (1979). Nigrostriatal lesions enhance striatal 3H-apomorphine and 3H-spiroperidol binding. *Eur. J. Pharmacol.*, **15**, 277–81.

Dubois, B., Ruberg, M., Javoy-Agid, F., Plaska, A. & Agid, Y. (1983). A subcortico-cortical cholinergic system is affected in Parkinson's disease. *Brain Res.*, **288**, 213–18.

Flaherty, A. & Graybiel, A. (1994). Anatomy of the basal ganglia. In *Movement Disorders 3*, ed. C. Marsden & S. Fahn, pp. 3–27. Oxford: Butterworth-Heinemann Ltd.

Frohna, P., Rothblat, D., Joyce, J. & Schneider, J. (1995). Alterations in dopamine uptake sites and D1 and D2 receptors in cats symptomatic for and recovered from experimental Parkinsonism. *Synapse*, **19**, 46–55.

Hornykiewicz, O. (1993). Parkinson's disease and the adaptive capacity of the nigrostriatal dopamine system: Possible neurochemical mechanisms. *Adv. Neurol.*, **60**, 140–7.

Jellinger, K. (1987). The pathology of parkinsonism. In *Movement Disorders 2*, ed. C. Marsden & S. Fahn, pp. 124–65. London: Butterworth.

Kish, S., Chang, L., Mirchandani, L., Shannak, K. & Hornykiewicz, O. (1985). Progressive supranuclear palsy: relationship between extrapyramidal disturbances, dementia and brain neurotransmitter markers. *Ann. Neurol.*, **18**, 530–6.

Kish, S., Robitaille, Y., El-Awar, M. et al. (1992). Striatal monoamine neurotransmitters and metabolites in dominantly inherited olivopontocerebellar atrophy. *Neurology*, **42**, 1573–7.

Langlais, P. J., Thal, L., Hansen, L., Galasko, D., Alford, M. & Masliah, E. (1993). Neurotransmitters in basal ganglia and cortex with and without Lewy bodies. *Neurology*, **43**, 1927–34.

Mark, M., Sage, J., Dickson, D. et al. (1994). Meige syndrome in the spectrum of Lewy body disease. *Neurology*, **44**, 1432–6.

Marshall, E. F., Perry, E. K., Perry, R. H., McKeith, I. G., Fairbairn, A. F. & Thompson, P. (1994). Dopamine metabolism in post-mortem caudate nucleus in neurodegenerative disorders. *Neurosci. Res. Commun.*, **14**, 17–25.

Marshall, E. F., Thompson, P., Perry, E. et al. (1995). Preservation of motor function despite extensive striatonigral degeneration in a case of corticobasal degeneration. *J. Psychopharmacol.*, **9**, A25.

McKeith, I. G., Perry, R. H., Fairbairn, A. F., Jabeen, S. & Perry, E. K. (1992). Operational criteria for senile dementia of Lewy body type (SDLT). *Psychol. Med.*, **22**, 911–22.

Pascual, J., Berciano, J., Grijalba, B. et al. (1992). Dopamine D1 and D2 receptors in progressive supranuclear palsy: An autoradiographic study. *Ann. Neurology*, **32**, 703–7.

Perry, E. K., Perry, R. H., Candy, J. M. et al. (1984). Cortical serotonin-S2 receptor binding abnormalities in patients with Alzheimer's disease: comparison with Parkinson's disease. *Neurosci. Lett.*, **51**, 353–7.

Perry, R. H., Irving, D., Blessed, G., Fairbairn, A. F. & Perry, E. K. (1990). Senile dementia of Lewy body type: a clinically and pathologically distinct form of Lewy body dementia of the elderly. *J. Neurol. Sci.*, **95**, 119–39.

Perry, E. K., Marshall, E. F., Cheng, A., Edwardson, J. & Perry, R. H. (1992). Neurodegenerative changes in aging and dementia: A comparison of Alzheimer and Lewy body type pathology. *Neurodevel., Aging and Cognition*, 199–214.

Piggott, M. A., Perry, E. K., McKeith, I. G., Marshall, E. & Perry, R. H. (1994). Dopamine D2 receptors in demented patients with severe neuroleptic sensitivity. *Lancet*, **343**, 1044–5.

Riley, D., Lang, A., Lewis, A., Resch, L., et al. (1990). Cortico-basal ganglionic degeneration. *Neurology*, **40**, 1203–12.

Rinne, U. K., Sonninen, V. & Laaksonen, H. (1979). Responses of brain neurochemistry to levodopa treatment in Parkinson's disease. *Adv. Neurol.*, **24**, 259–74.

Rinne, U. K., Koskinen, V. & Lonneberg, P. (1980). Neurotransmitter receptors in the Parkinsonian brain. In *Parkinson's disease: current Progress, Problems and Management*, ed. U. K. Rinne, M. Klinger & G. Stamm, pp. 93–107. Amsterdam: Elsevier North Holland Press.

Ruberg, M., Javoy-Agid, F., Hirsch, E., Scatton, B. et al. (1985). Dopaminergic and cholinergic lesions in progressive supranuclear palsy. *Ann. Neurol.*, **18**, 523–9.

Starr, M. (1995). Glutamate/dopamine D1/D2 balance in the basal ganglia and its relevance to Parkinson's disease. *Synapse*, **19**, 264–93.

Toru, M., Watanabe, S., Shibuya, H. et al. (1988). Neurotransmitters, receptors, and neuropeptides in post-mortem brains of chronic schizophrenic patients. *Acta Psychiatr. Scand.*, **78**, 121–37.

35
Neurotrophins and the cholinergic system in dementia

G. K. WILCOCK

Summary

There is considerable evidence to support a role for neurotrophins as a strategy for treating chronic neurodegenerative conditions causing dementia, especially Alzheimer's disease and probably others including senile dementia of Lewy body type. In particular, a wealth of animal and tissue culture research points to the potential of nerve growth factor (NGF) as a means of supporting subcortical cholinergic cells, thereby retarding the disease process. Very early pilot work in human subjects has already been undertaken and attempts are under way to try and improve the drug delivery systems needed to allow such peptides to enter the brain and reach their predominantly subcortical targets. If successful, this approach would have a wider application to a number of neurodegenerative disorders, not necessarily confined to cholinergic cell systems.

35.1 Introduction

The concept of neurotrophic support for developing neurons was first suggested in the 1950s when Levi-Montalcini described the effect of transplanted mouse sarcoma tissue on the developing sensory and sympathetic nervous system of chick embryos. (This is reviewed by Levi-Montalcini, 1987.) Work in this field has moved on rapidly, especially in the last five years, and now much is known about a whole family of neurotrophic molecules and also their receptor systems in both normal development and disease. It is clear that members of this family can act in a neuroprotective role in the central as well as the peripheral nervous system. NGF and its receptors are the neurotrophin system most explored, espe-

468

cially in relation to Alzheimer's disease (AD), as far as dementia is concerned. It appears to be released by cells in the 'target area' of the efferent projections from the deeper lying cholinergic subcortical structures such as the basal nucleus of Meynert. The NGF is then internalized via specific receptors and transported back to the neuronal nucleus, exerting a growth or survival effect.

In general, the neurotrophin family relevant to the cholinergic system in dementia appears to have a common low-affinity receptor of approximately 75 kD, and in addition each neurotrophin has a high-affinity receptor of approximately twice this molecular weight with which it specifically binds. The high-affinity receptors, the trk family, are a proto-oncogene product whose catalytic domains are very similar to that of known members of the tyrosine kinase receptor family which, when activated, are autophosphorylated on tyrosine residues leading to a cascade of different cellular responses. The specific receptor for NGF is trkA, while trkB is specific for brain derived neurotrophic factor (BDNF) and trkC for neurotrophin-3 (NT-3), these latter two neurotrophins being described in more detail below.

There is now an extensive knowledge base supporting the evaluation of neurotrophins in a number of neurological conditions affecting both the peripheral and the central nervous system. As mentioned above, most of our knowledge in relation to dementia has centred on the investigation of the role of NGF and the cholinergic system in Alzheimer's disease. This account will draw heavily upon our knowledge in this field, referring to other members of the neurotrophin family in relation to different dementias as and when appropriate.

35.2 Neuroprotection and neurotrophins

Most, if not all readers, will be aware of the evidence linking NGF in animal and tissue culture models, to the protection of cholinergic cells, especially those in the basal forebrain. Such approaches have included the cellular production of acetylcholine with and without NGF and the benefits of NGF in a number of different lesioning studies. More recently work in this field has included the ability to link improvements in memory with extracellular acetylcholine level in the parietal cortex and hippocampus of aged rats (Scali et al., 1994). Although ageing rodents may not in themselves provide a good model for Alzheimer's disease, this nevertheless links improvement in memory with an NGF related up-regulation of acetylcholine release apparently directly affecting behavioural performance, and has many features in common with the basis of the cholinergic hypothesis for developing treatments for Alzheimer's disease.

Brain derived neurotrophic factor is another neurotrophic factor, which in common with the other members of this family, has a molecular structure that is highly conserved in all members, although each contains distinct variable domains that probably define their different receptor specificity. Unlike NGF which is more widely distributed, BDNF appears to be predominantly located within the CNS, especially within neurons, and is present in particularly high levels within the hippocampus, a primary site of degeneration in AD. BDNF mRNA is known to be reduced in the hippocampus in Alzheimer's disease and may therefore have a part to play in the disease process. In general however, although BDNF occurs in the target area for the cholinergic projections from the basal nucleus, the available evidence demonstrates that its effect upon these neurons is less pronounced than that of NGF (Dekker et al., 1994). It may have a more important role on the survival of dopaminergic neurons.

Neurotrophin-3 was the third member of the family to be identified but has little or no effect on cholinergic neurons (Koliatsos et al., 1994). It is important for other groups of cells, including those in the locus ceruleus. It may, therefore, have a part to play in the symptoms and disease progression of a number of dementia disorders but not specifically via the cholinergic system, at least not directly so.

Neurotrophin-4/5 is known to protect neurons from calcium-mediated injury, and neurotrophin-6 has a less effective but NGF-like action on sympathetic and sensory neurons (Cheng et al., 1994; Gotz et al., 1994). Whether or not these new additions to the family have a part to play in human neurodegenerative disorders of the brain, including the dementias, has yet to be determined.

35.2.1 *Pathophysiology of NGF in relation to Alzheimer's disease*

It has been appreciated for many years that the number of cholinergic cells at subcortical sites is reduced in some dementias, including Alzheimer's disease. It is however clear from a number of studies (Pearson et al., 1983; Allen et al., 1990) that the number of remaining neurons is probably larger than previously estimated. It is also clear that most of the remaining neurons express the low affinity NGF receptor, implying that the more specific trkA receptor is also present, providing a substrate upon which exogenous neurotrophin could exert a neuroprotective effect. This is further supported by the presence of similar levels of low affinity NGF receptor mRNA in both the normal and AD basal forebrain (Goedert et al., 1989).

A therapeutic hypothesis based upon the provision of exogenous NGF could be taken to imply that there is a lack of endogenous NGF in the Alzheimer brain. In general this is not true although it is not known whether specific regions, for example, the cholinergic cells in the basal forebrain, receive sufficient target-derived neurotrophin. There are several studies in which NGF levels have been found to be normal, both within the brain, for example, hippocampus, parietal, frontal and temporal cortex, and in terms of serum and CSF levels as well (Allen et al., 1991; Murase et al., 1993; Jette et al., 1994). Why then might the administration of exogenous neurotrophins prove helpful? Whilst production of neurotrophin at the target site appears to be normal, there is as yet no evidence that this is satisfactorily transported retrogradely to the neuronal cell body. The neurofibrillary tangles of Alzheimer's disease, for instance, represent a significant disruption of the cytoskeleton with all that this implies for intraneuronal transport. In one study (Mufson et al., 1995) evidence was found to indicate that there may indeed be defective retrograde transport of NGF to the basal nucleus. Using NGF immunohistochemistry combined with quantitative optical densitometry, Mufson and colleagues reported that in normal aged humans the majority of the cholinergic basal forebrain neurons stained for NGF. In contrast, cases of Alzheimer's disease displayed fewer neurons, each with diminished or undetectable NGF immunoreactivity. There are a number of interpretations of this when linked to the apparently normal production of target derived neurotrophin, including disruption of trkA production or function, as well as the actual process of intraneuronal retrograde transport.

There is therefore a considerable body of evidence upon which to base a therapeutic strategy using exogenous NGF as a possible treatment for Alzheimer's disease, probably more in hope of preventing further deterioration and degeneration in people in whom the diagnosis has been made early, rather than in trying to rectify the clinical picture that arises later in the course of the disease, reflecting a significant level of neuronal death. The similarity of the general molecular structure of different members of the neurotrophin family, the specificity inherent within the variable domains, and the parallels that can be drawn in the pathophysiology of different causes of dementia make it likely that this approach may well be applicable to a number of different conditions that cause dementia, if it is shown to be successful in Alzheimer's disease. The significant cholinergic impairment in Lewy body dementia, and also the response of the symptoms to anticholinesterase treatments such as tacrine, imply that senile dementia of Lewy body type is as important a potential target for such strategies as is Alzheimer's disease. The supporting role of other neurotrophins to different neurotransmitter systems may also be important both in relation to preserving other vulnerable groups of neurons in conditions like AD, but also as a potential therapeutic manoeuvre in some of the other conditions in which there are neurotransmitter deficits in addition to or without a cholinergic loss.

35.2.2 Neurotrophins in relation to dementias other than Alzheimer's disease

Much less is known about the neurotrophic background in relation to other conditions that cause dementia. Senile dementia of Lewy body type (SDLT), as already mentioned, is the area most explored in this context. Whether the principles emerging from this growing field are also relevant to diffuse Lewy body disease is uncertain, and more information is required about the interrelationships of these two conditions, and also the substrate of the dementia in Parkinson's disease.

Much of the pioneering work in this field has been undertaken by Perry and colleagues, and it is now quite clear that as well as sharing nicotinic receptor deficits with a number of dementias associated with cortical cholinergic loss, SDLT also exhibits changes in the low affinity muscarinic receptors, at least at a cortical level, as well as being associated with a significant and extensive cholinergic deficit, especially in those subjects with visual hallucinations (Perry et al., 1990a,b; Perry et al., 1991). There are of course abnormalities in a number of transmitter systems in Lewy body dementia, including the dopaminergic system in the basal ganglia. Less is known about the neurotrophin system in Lewy body dementia but it would appear from the immunocytochemical studies of the low affinity (P75) receptor that this is decreased to at least some extent in SDLT (Perry et al., 1993).

Whether or not there are problems with neurotrophic factor transport in Lewy body-associated dementias, or whether there are abnormalities of different aspects of the neurotrophic support system is unclear. In Alzheimer's disease it is easy to envisage, probably over-simplistically so, a defect of retrograde transport of target derived NGF because of the obvious disruption to the endoskeleton that accompanies the production of neurofibrillary tangles. The dementias associated with Lewy bou formation are however usually much less affected by neurofibrillary tangle formation, and although the Lewy body itself may be composed of altered endoskeletal constituents, the pathophysiology of the cholinergic malfunction may be very different to that of AD.

Neurotrophic treatment strategies may well be relevant to a number of neurodegenerative conditions, including Huntington's disease. Intravenous injection of NGF conjugated to an antibody directed against the transferrin receptor in an animal model of Huntington's disease, that is intrastriatal injection of quinolinic acid, prevented the loss of striatal choline acetyltransferase-immunoreactive neurons which normally occurs in this rodent model (Kordower et al., 1994). This is preliminary data and requires confirmation, but it does indicate a very significant potential for neurotrophin related cholinergic strategies as part of the treatment approach to yet another dementia, and hence possibly also to a wider variety of conditions.

35.2.3 Treatment options

The only therapeutic strategy so far evaluated in human neurodegenerative disease associated with dementia has been the use of intracerebroventricular NGF in a small number of subjects with Alzheimer's disease, one of which is published (Olson et al., 1992), and in which there was some minor improvement in some of the parameters assessed. This approach is fraught with difficulty, is clearly not of long-term clinical relevance, and a significant side-effect profile has been reported.

Related approaches that have been investigated in animal models have included the use of polymer-encapsulated human NGF-secreting fibroblasts, and conjugates of NGF with monoclonal antibodies directed against the transferrin receptor, since these appear to carry the NGF across the blood brain barrier. There is experimental evidence to indicate that each of these approaches has potential benefit.

The intravenous injection of NGF has also been considered but one has to take into account the effect of this upon the peripheral endocrine and immune systems, as well as the peripheral nervous system. It seems unlikely that this will be potentially useful in treating pathology that affects the CNS lying on the other side of the blood brain barrier, although it may well prove to have application for the treatment of certain conditions such as some peripheral neuropathies.

Attempts are in hand to produce a 'pan-neurotrophin'. This is a synthetic neurotrophic factor engineered by combining the active domains of NGF, BDNF and NT-3 into a single molecule (Ilag et al., 1995). In tissue culture and animal models this compound has been shown to have potent and multi-specific neurotrophic properties and may be of value in the treatment of peripheral neuropathies and nerve damage. Whether or not its actions will extend to the central nervous system remains to be seen.

Other and less specific approaches to neurotrophic support have involved the use of drugs that have been found in animal experiments to stimulate the production of NGF. These have included idebenone and propentofylline which improve cognitive function in ageing rats. These are presently under evaluation in clinical trial and the results are awaited. It will be interesting to see whether or not such a non-specific approach is of therapeutic value.

35.2.4 Potential adverse effects of NGF

The attempt to develop NGF, and similar neurotrophic support strategies for treating conditions like Alzheimer's disease and some of the other dementias has not been without its critics. NGF in particular increases the mRNA level of the prion protein, albeit of the normal non-infectious form and has also been shown to increase the production of mRNA for the beta amyloid protein precursor (APP). Although neither of these is necessarily potentially harmful such findings do of course emphasize the need for caution in taking this strategy forward. Clinical use has been associated with weight loss, pain and other possible adverse reactions but, since experience is extremely limited, as of yet it is difficult to know how relevant these findings will be once we have advanced our knowledge about the relevant pharmacological issues, for example, dose strategy, etc.

35.3 Conclusion

There is clearly considerable evidence upon which to base at least early pilot therapeutic studies of neurotrophic support in Alzheimer's disease using NGF, with Lewy body dementia following on close behind it. It is likely that within the next 12 to 24 months a significant number of pilot studies of NGF will be undertaken, initially employing an intracerebroventricular route such as that originally used by Olson et al. (1992). In parallel with this are studies to develop better drug delivery systems that would allow more extensive clinical evaluation if the early pilot studies yield promising results. If successful this will probably be but the first stage in a development of a wide programme of neurotrophic support for many neurodegenerative conditions.

References

Allen, S. J., Dawbarn, D., MacGowan, S. H., Wilcock, G. K., Treanor, J. J. S. & Moss, T. H. (1990). A quantitative morphometric analysis of basal forebrain neurons expressing B-NGF receptors in normal and Alzheimer's disease brains. *Dementia*, **1**, 125–37.

Allen, S. J., MacGowan, S. H., Treanor, J. J., Feeney, R., Wilcock, G. K. & Dawbarn, D. (1991). Normal beta-NGF content in Alzheimer's disease cerebral cortex and hippocampus. *Neurosci. Lett.*, **131**, 135–9.

Cheng, B., Goodman, Y., Begley, J. G. & Mattson, M. P. (1994). Neurotrophin-4/5 protects hippocampal and cortical neurons against energy deprivation- and excitatory amino acid-induced injury. *Brain Res.*, **650**, 331–5.

Dekker, A. J., Fagan, A. M., Gage, F. H. & Thal, L. J. (1994). Effects of brain-derived neurotrophic factor and nerve growth factor on remaining neurons in the lesioned nucleus basalis magnocellularis. *Brain Res.*, **639**, 149–55.

Goedert, M., Fine, A., Dawbarn, D., Wilcock, G. K. & Chao, M. V. (1989). Nerve growth factor receptor mRNA distribution in human brain: normal levels in basal forebrain in Alzheimer's disease. *Mol. Brain Res.*, **5**, 1–7.

Gotz, R., Koster, R., Winkler, C. et al. (1994). Neurotrophin-6 is a new member of the nerve growth factor family. *Nature*, **372**, 266–9.

Ilag, L. L., Curtis, R., Glass, D. et al. (1995). Pan-neurotrophin 1: a genetically engineered neurotrophic factor displaying multiple specificities in peripheral neurons in vitro and in vivo. *Proc. Natl. Acad. Sci. USA*, **92**, 607–11.

Jette, N., Cole, M. S. & Fahnestock, M. (1994). NGF mRNA is not decreased in frontal cortex from Alzheimer's disease patients. *Brain Res. Mol. Brain Res.*, **25**, 242–50.

Koliatsos, V. E., Price, D. L., Gouras, G. K., Cayouette, M. H., Burton, L. E. & Winslow, J. W. (1994). Highly selective effects of nerve growth factor, brain-derived neurotrophic factor, and neurotrophin-3 on intact and injured basal forebrain magnocellular neurons. *J. Comp. Neurol.*, **343**, 247–62.

Kordower, J. H., Charles, V., Bayer, R. et al. (1994). Intravenous administration of a transferrin receptor antibody-nerve growth factor conjugate prevents the degeneration of cholinergic striatal neurons in a model of Huntington disease. *Proc. Natl. Acad. Sci. USA*, **91**, 9077–80.

Levi-Montalcini, R. (1987). The nerve growth factor 35 years later. *Science*, **237**, 1154–62.

Mufson, E. J., Conner, J. M. & Kordower, J. H. (1995). Nerve growth factor in Alzheimer's disease: defective retrograde transport to nucleus basalis. *Neuroreport*, **6**, 1063–6.

Murase, K., Nabeshima, T., Robitaille, Y., Quirion, R., Ogawa, M. & Hayashi, K. (1993). NGF levels is not decreased in the serum, brain-spinal fluid, hippocampus, or parietal cortex of individuals with Alzheimer's disease. *Biochem. Biophys. Res Commun.*, **193**, 198–203.

Olson, L., Nordberg, A., von Holst, H. et al. (1992). Nerve growth factor affects 11C-nicotine binding, blood flow, EEG, and verbal episodic memory in an Alzheimer patient (case report). *J. Neural. Transm. Park. Dis. Dem. Sect.*, **4**, 79–95.

Pearson, R. C. A., Sofroniew, M. V., Cuello, A. C. et al. (1983). Persistence of cholinergic neurones in the basal nucleus in a brain with senile dementia of Alzheimer's type demonstrated by immunohistochemical staining for choline acetyl transferase. *Brain Res.*, **289**, 375–9.

Perry, E. K., Smith, C. J., Court, J. A. & Perry, R. H. (1990a). Cholinergic nicotinic and muscarinic receptors in dementia of Alzheimer, Parkinson and Lewy body types. *J. Neural. Transm. Park. Dis. Dement. Sect.*, **2**, 149–58.

Perry, E. K. et al. (1990b). Cerebral cholinergic activity is related to the incidence of visual hallucinations in senile dementia of Lewy body type. *Dementia*, **1**, 2–4.

Perry, E. K., McKeith, I., Thompson, P. et al. (1991). Topography, extent, and clinical relevance of neurochemical deficits in dementia of Lewy body type, Parkinson's disease, and Alzheimer's disease. *Ann. NY Acad. Sci.*, **640**, 197–202.

Perry, E. K., Irving, D., Kerwin, J. M. et al. (1993). Cholinergic transmitter and neurotrophic activities in Lewy body dementia: similarity to Parkinson's and distinction from Alzheimer disease. *Alzheimer Dis. Assoc. Disord.*, **7**, 69–79.

Scali, C., Casamenti, F., Pazzagli, M., Bartolini, L. & Pepeu, G. (1994). Nerve growth factor increases extracellular acetylcholine levels in the parietal cortex and hippocampus of aged rats and restores object recognition. *Neurosci. Lett.*, **170**, 117–20.

36

Relevance of Lewy bodies to alterations in oxidative stress in Lewy body dementia and Parkinson's disease

A. D. OWEN, A. H. V. SCHAPIRA,
P. JENNER and C. D. MARSDEN

Summary

Degeneration of the substantia nigra with Lewy bodies in remaining neurones is a key pathological marker of Parkinson's disease (PD). A number of observations suggest that processes of oxidative stress are taking place within substantia nigra in PD. Oxidative stress, and the associated finding of reduced activity of complex I of the mitochondrial respiratory chain, might be a primary cause of the pathology of PD. We have tested this hypothesis by examining indices of oxidative stress and mitochondrial enzyme activity in another brain region in which Lewy bodies are known to occur in PD, namely the substantia innominata. We have also examined similar indices in cingulate cortex of brains from patients with senile dementia of the Lewy body type. Tissues from Alzheimer's disease (SDAT) have also been included for comparison. These studies have shown that oxidative stress and altered mitochondrial activity do not necessarily occur in the other regions containing Lewy bodies, although there is evidence for oxidative stress in the same brain regions in SDAT. Oxidative stress and reduced mitochondrial complex I activity appear to be confined to the substantia nigra in PD, and may reflect the peculiar vulnerability of the substantia to such processes.

36.1 Introduction

The primary pathology of Parkinson's disease (PD) is the degeneration of the dopamine containing, pigmented neurones of the substantia nigra pars compacta, with Lewy bodies in remaining neurones. Neuronal loss with Lewy bodies is however more widespread involving a range of pigmented catecholamine-containing brain stem nuclei, such as the locus coerulus, as well as non-pigmented, non-catecholamine containing nuclei, such as the substantia innominata. Lewy bodies are also evident in the cerebral cortex in PD, and to much greater extent in cortical regions in the related condition known as senile dementia of the Lewy body type (SDLT). This form of dementia is believed to be second only to senile dementia of the Alzheimer's type (SDAT) as a cause of dementia.

Lewy body pathology in substantia nigra in PD is associated with biochemical evidence for oxidative stress and reduced activity of complex I of the mitochondrial respiratory chain. Here we have examined whether such changes occurs in the substantia innominata in PD or whether a similar sequence of events occurs in the cortex in SDLT. In this paper, biochemical indices of oxidative stress and mitochondrial activity are examined in affected brain regions in PD, SDAT and SDLT.

36.2 Evidence for oxidative stress in substantia nigra in Parkinson's disease

The occurrence of oxidative stress in substantia nigra in PD is shown by increases in total iron levels, a decrease or lack of change in ferritin, and loss of reduced glutathione (GSH) content. Inhibition of complex I of the mitochondrial respiratory chain and inhibition of the key TCA cycle enzyme, α-ketoglutarate dehydrogenase (α-KGDH) have also been found. Direct evidence of oxidative damage stems from reports of increased lipid peroxidation and DNA damage. Key factors appear to be the increase in iron levels, decrease in GSH content and inhibition of complex I, so consequently these parameters form the basis of the present discussion.

36.2.1 Iron

In PD elevated level of iron occur within the substantia nigra, that do not occur in other brain regions (Dexter et al., 1989; Youdim et al., 1989). Levels of the iron binding protein, ferritin, are unchanged or decreased in substantia nigra (Dexter et al., 1990). This suggests that the increase in iron is in a free, reactive form (Fig. 36.1a and b) able to increase free radical production. Alterations in iron levels are not specific to PD. Increased iron levels are found in substantia nigra in multiple system atrophy and progressive supranuclear palsy. Iron also accumulates in brain in multiple sclerosis, Huntington's chorea, tardive dyskinesia, spastic paralysis and Hallervorden–Spatz syndrome. Indeed, iron

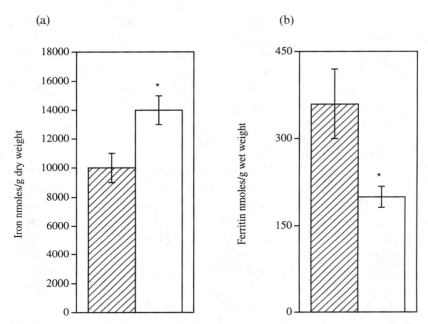

Fig. 36.1 Levels of (a) iron and (b) ferritin in substantia nigra in PD (□) and age-matched controls (▧). Values are expressed as mean ± standard error of the mean (SEM). *$p < 0.05$ compared with control subjects; Students t test. Adapted from Jenner, 1991.

accumulation appears to be generally associated with occurrence of pathological changes in brain. So changes in iron levels are unlikely to specifically initiate nigra cell death in PD but may form an important component of a cascade leading to the acceleration of nigral cell loss.

36.2.2 Glutathione

Loss of reduced glutathione in the substantia nigra of PD was first reported in 1982 by Perry and coworkers, who suggested that the depletion was due to the accumulation of an unidentified toxin. However, the reported ratio between the reduced and oxidized forms of glutathione was not compatible with the oxidative state of the brain and there was a complete absence of GSH in the PD brains. This led to criticism that methodological problems or postmortem artifacts was responsible for the results. However, subsequently a reduction in total glutathione in the substantia nigra in PD was reported which increased with disease severity (Riederer et al., 1989). More recently using an accepted method a specific loss in GSH in substantia nigra in PD was confirmed (Sian et al., 1994; Figs. 36.2a and b). The loss of glutathione only occurs in the substantia nigra of PD and not in multiple system atrophy or progressive supranuclear palsy patients (Sian et al., 1994). So this change in GSH is disease and brain region specific alteration in PD, which may be of importance to the underlying pathological process.

36.2.3 *Mitochondrial function*

In the substantia nigra in PD the activity of NADH CoQ$_1$ reductase (complex I) is decreased. There are no confirmed observations of decreases in complex II/III or IV or in the nonrespiratory enzyme citrate synthesase. The decrease in complex I is specific to substantia nigra, it does not occur in other areas of the brain in PD and no alterations occur in substantia nigra in multiple system atrophy (Schapira, 1994; Fig. 36.3). The lack of changes in multiple system atrophy also suggest the decrease is not due to levodopa treatment since both patient groups are treated with the drug. An immunohistochemical study shows the key TCA cycle

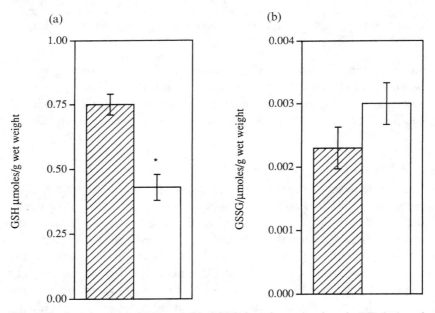

Fig. 36.2   Levels of (a) GSH and (b) GSSG in substantia nigra in PD (□) and age-matched controls (▨). Values are expressed as mean ± SEM. *$p < 0.01$ compared with control subjects; Students t test. Adapted from Sian et al., 1994.

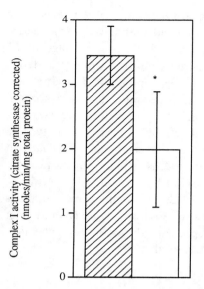

Fig. 36.3 Complex I activity in substantia nigra in PD (□) and age-matched controls (▨). Values are expressed as mean ± standard deviation, *$p < 0.005$ compared with control subjects; Mann-Whitney U test. Adapted from Schapira, 1994.

enzyme α-KGDH to be inhibited (Mizuno et al., 1994). α-KGDH indirectly provides reducing equivalent to both complex I and complex II and so may compound mitochondrial inhibition in PD. Interestingly, both complex I and α-KGDH are also inhibited by the nigral toxin MPP^+.

There would appear not to be any defect in mitochondrial DNA encoding complex I (Schapira, 1994). Mitochondrial defects are inherited maternally and this does not occur in PD. An alternative explanation is that complex I is inhibited by a toxin similar in its action to MPP^+. Candidate toxins include endogenously formed isoquinolines and β-carbonyl derivatives.

36.2.4 Oxidative stress: A primary cause of neuronal death or a secondary result?

From the postmortem studies in PD, there is no evidence as to whether oxidative stress is a primary cause of the neuronal loss in substantia nigra or a secondary result of cell death. Indeed, it is not possible to define whether these changes occur early or late in the course of the illness. For this reason, we have examined cases of incidental Lewy body disease (ILBD). In about 10–15% of normal individuals over the age of 65 years Lewy bodies and nigral cell loss are found at autopsy and this can be considered to be indicative of presymptomatic PD. In brain from ILBD iron and ferritin levels in the substantia nigra are normal, supporting the concept that changes in iron metabolism are late and secondary to the primary disease process. Complex I activity was reduced, but not significantly. However, the extent of cell death in ILBD is much less marked than in late PD, so it may not be possible to measure changes against a background of healthy cells. There is however a marked fall in GSH levels in ILBD and to the same degree as found in advanced PD. So, alterations in GSH are an early marker of pathological change and currently represents the earliest biochemical marker of oxidative stress in PD (Dexter et al., 1994).

36.3 Relevance of the Lewy body to oxidative stress in Parkinson's disease

Oxidative stress clearly occurs in the substantia nigra in PD but its relationship to the presence of Lewy bodies remains unknown. Consequently, we have examined alterations in the levels of iron, GSH and complex I levels in substantia innominata, as a nondopaminergic area pathologically affected in PD where Lewy bodies also appear.

In contrast to substantia nigra, levels of iron in the substantia innominata of PD patients are not different to those of age-matched controls. Similarly, GSH levels in the substantia innominata are unchanged compared to control values and there are no alterations in the activity of complex I. These results initially suggest that oxidative stress does not occur in substantia innominata in PD. It also suggests that there is no obvious connection between the formation of Lewy bodies and the occurrence of oxidative stress and vice versa. However, the extent of pathology in substantia innominata is not as marked as in substantia nigra in PD, so it is possible that small changes in indices of oxidative stress cannot be detected. However, the extent of pathology occurring in ILBD is also much less than PD yet a significant decrease in GSH levels are detected. This observation raises the possibility that either oxidative stress in PD is a phenomenon restricted to the substantia nigra or that dopamine itself may be an integral part of the mechanism responsible for initiating oxidative processes.

36.4 Oxidative stress in the substantia innominata in Alzheimer's disease

In contrast to PD, substantia innominata shows marked pathological changes in SDAT associated with the presence of neurofibrillary plaques and tangles. Loss of cholinergic cells in substantia innominata is believed to be the primary cause of dementia in SDAT. Similarly, damage to this region may also explain the dementia often observed in PD. Since the substantia innominata is affected in both SDAT and PD, but by different pathologies, it forms a useful comparison on the role of oxidative stress. Data for iron and GSH levels, but not complex I, are currently available. In the substantia innominata in SDAT, there is no significant difference in iron level compared to control tissues. However, GSH levels are significantly reduced in SDAT tissues. So, in contrast to the substantia innominata from PD cases a key index of oxidative stress is altered in SDAT tissues. There are several ways in which oxidative stress may be involved in SDAT. Iron is increased in neurons which contain neurofibrillary tangles, microglia cells are activated and increased in number and represent a major source of free-radicals. Increased aluminium levels are thought to have a stimulatory effect on iron-induced lipid peroxidation and it is suggested that amyloid-β fragments spontaneously form free-radical peptides. Perhaps GSH levels are the most sensitive index of oxidative stress currently measured, although it is surprising that iron accumulation does not occur considering the extent of substantia innominata pathology. Some but not all GSH is contained in neurons and so the degree of cell loss may potentially correlate to the GSH depletion observed. Clearly, it is now important to determine mitochondrial function in these tissues.

36.5 Relationship between the cortical Lewy body and oxidative stress in Lewy body dementia

SDLT is characterized by the presence of Lewy bodies in the cortex rather than the senile plaques and neurofibrillary tangles observed in SDAT. The presence of Lewy bodies again provides an opportunity to assess the relationship between oxidative stress and the Lewy body. So, we have compared cingulate cortical tissues from PD, SDAT and SDLT patients for alterations in indices of oxidative stress.

36.5.1 Parkinson's disease

Examination of the cingulate cortex of PD patients showed no differences in levels of iron, GSH or complex I. This indicates that oxidative stress is unlikely to have occurred in this region as expected since there is little or no pathology in the cingulate cortex in PD.

36.5.2 Alzheimer's disease

In cingulate cortex from SDAT, iron levels were significantly increased while the levels of GSH were significantly decreased. This indicates that oxidative stress is occurring within the region, although complex I was unaltered. There is already a great deal of supporting evidence that oxidative stress occurs in the cortex in SDAT. It has been shown that there is a selective increase in lipid peroxidation in the inferior temporal cortex (Palmer & Burns, 1994) and that increased oxidative damage to mitochondrial DNA takes place in the parietal cortex (Mecocci et al., 1994). Both of these are indexes of oxidative damage taking place within the cortex. In addition there is also data which shows that the mitochondrial enzymes may be compromised with reductions in the activities of α-KGDH (Mastrogiacomo et al., 1993) and cytochrome c oxidase (Parker & Parks, 1995). The activity of the antioxidant enzymes catalase and superoxide dismutase may also be altered, with a reduction in the activity of catalase (Gsell et al., 1995) and a possible upregulation in the expression of copper/zinc superoxide dismutase (Ceballos et al., 1991), although this last change has not been consistently found in SDAT tissues (see Gsell et al., 1995). These reports all support the conclusion that oxidative stress takes place in the cortex in SDAT. The source of this oxidative stress remains unknown, but current thinking suggests it may be related to the production of β-amyloid within the degenerating tissues (Friedlich & Butcher, 1994).

36.5.3 Lewy body dementia

In SDLT iron levels in the cingulate cortex were increased, but GSH levels and complex I activity were not altered. The rise in iron levels cannot be easily explained in the absence of changes in the level of GSH and the activity of complex I, but may be a consequence of the presence of Lewy bodies although why this should be the case in these tissues and not in the substantia innominata in PD, where there is a slight fall in iron levels, is unknown. It is possible that it may be indicative of the pathology, as seen in other neurodegenerative diseases such as multiple system atrophy and progressive supranuclear palsy, and is not related to processes inducing oxidative stress. Overall, the results suggest that oxidative stress has not occurred in this region of the brain and that again the presence of Lewy bodies is not linked to oxidative stress.

36.6 Conclusion

We have hypothesized that presence of oxidative stress and Lewy bodies are two factors which may be intimately linked in PD. This has been tested by the assay of iron, GSH and complex I, which are known indexes of oxidative stress. From our results it does not appear to be the case that these two phenomena must occur together, as illustrated by the result that oxidative stress does not occur in substantia innominata in PD or in cingulate cortex in SDLT, both of which contain Lewy bodies. Oxidative stress does however occur in these regions in SDAT. A possible explanation for the lack of evidence for oxidative stress is that the degree of pathology is not great enough for it to be measured against a background of healthy cells. This is possibly the case, although it would not explain why decreases in GSH levels are seen in ILBD, where pathology is not extensive. From the evidence which is currently available it is our conclusion that oxidative stress and the Lewy body are caused by processes which although possibly linked are not intimately connected.

Acknowledgements

The support of the Medical Research Council, the Parkinson's Disease Society and the National Parkinson Foundation are gratefully acknowledged. We would also like to acknowledge the help of the Neuropathology Department at Newcastle General Hospital, also the MRC Neurochemical Pathology Unit, for supplying SDLT brain materials for this study.

References

Ceballos, I., Javoy-Agid, F., Delacourte, A. et al. (1991). Neuronal localization of copper-zinc superoxide dismutase protein and mRNA within the human hippocampus from control and Alzheimer's disease brains. *Free Rad. Res. Commun.*, **12–13**, 571–80.

Dexter, D. T., Wells, F. P., Lees, A. J. et al. (1989). Increased nigral iron content and alterations in other metal ions occurring in brain in Parkinson's disease. *J. Neurochem.*, **52**, 1830–6.

Dexter, D. T., Carayon, A., Vidailhet, M. et al. (1990). Decreased ferritin levels in brain in Parkinson's disease. *J. Neurochem*, **55**, 16–20.

Dexter, D. T., Sian, J., Rose, S. et al. (1994). Indices of oxidative stress and mitochondrial function in individuals with incidental Lewy body disease. *Ann. Neurol.*, **35**, 38–44.

Friedlich, A. L. & Butcher, L. L. (1994). Involvement of free oxygen radicals in b-amyloidosis: An hypothesis. *Neurobiol. Aging*, **15**, 443–55.

Gsell, W., Conrad, R., Hickethier, M. et al. (1995). Decreased catalase activity but unchanged superoxide dismutase activity in brains of patients with dementia of Alzheimer's type. *J. Neurochem.*, **64**, 1216–23.

Jenner, P. (1991). Oxidative stress as a cause of Parkinson's disease. *Acta Neurol. Scand. Suppl.*, **136**, 6–15.

Mastrogiacomo, F., Bergeron, C. & Kish, S. J. (1993). Brain α-ketoglutarate dehydrogenase complex activity in Alzheimer's disease. *J. Neurochem.*, **61**, 2007–14.

Mecocci, P., MacGarvey, U. & Flint-Beal, M. (1994). Oxidative damage to mitochondrial DNA is increased in Alzheimer's disease. *Ann. Neurol.*, **36**, 747–51.

Mizuno, Y., Matuda, S., Yoshina, H., Mori, H. & Hattori, N. (1994). An immunohistochemical study of α-ketoglutarate dehydrogenase complex in Parkinson's disease. *Ann. Neurol.*, **305**, 204–10.

Palmer, A. M. & Burns, M. A. (1994). Selective increase in lipid peroxidation in the inferior temporal cortex in Alzheimer's disease. *Brain Res.*, **645**, 338–42.

Parker, W. D. & Parks, J. K. (1995). Cytochrome c oxidase in alzheimer's disease brain: Purification and characterization. *Neurology*, **45**, 482–6.

Perry, T. L., Godin, D. M. & Hansen, S. (1982). Parkinson's disease: A disorder due to nigral glutathione deficiency. *Neurosci. Lett.*, **33**, 305–10.

Riederer, P., Sofic, E., Rausch, W.-D. et al. (1989). Transition metals, ferritin, glutathione and ascorbic acid in Parkinson's disease. *J. Neurochem.*, **52**, 381–9.

Schapira, A. H. V. (1994). Evidence for mitochondrial dysfunction in Parkinson's disease – A critical appraisal. *Mov. Disord.*, **9**, 125–38.

Sian, J., Dexter, D. T., Lees, A. J. et al. (1994). Alterations in glutathione levels in Parkinson's disease and other neurodegenerative disorders affecting the basal ganglia. *Ann. Neurol.*, **36**, 348–55.

Youdim, M. B. H., Ben Schachar, D. & Riederer, P. (1989). Is Parkinson's disease a progressive siderosis of substantia nigra resulting in increased iron and melanin induced neurodegeneration. *Acta Neurol. Scand.*, **126**, 47–54.

Résumé of treatment workshop sessions

H. J. SAGAR, E. N. H. JANSEN and
E. K. PERRY

Contributors to the chapters on treatment issues met together with other interested participants in the Workshop (Owen Collins, Alan Cross, Murat Emre, Ernst Jansen, Amos Korczyn, John O'Brien, Arjun Sahgal, and Peter Thompson) for a morning discussion of key areas relating to therapy. The group explored the biological basis for four symptom clusters in dementia with Lewy bodies (DLB): psychosis, cognitive deficits, affective and motor disorders. An important issue relating to therapy was considered to be the nature and extent of interactions between these different symptoms and the way in which they vary with time. Therapeutic strategies were discussed from several viewpoints: in terms of clinical experience with currently available pharmaceuticals in treating these symptoms in other disorders; anecdotal experience with DLB patients; and theoretically based hypothesis-driven designs for future treatment. The group concentrated on neurotransmitter-orientated intervention since this was considered the most immediately relevant in relation to symptoms (neuroleptics or cholinergics for psychosis or dementia). It was appreciated that in the longer term, with increased understanding of aetiology and development of new preventative or neuroprotective approaches, therapeutic objectives would expand beyond the symptomatic range. Examples of such strategies include the potential of neurotrophins (Chapter 35) or antioxidants (Chapter 36).

The hypothesis that psychotic features such as hallucinations in DLB are associated with depleted neocortical cholinergic activities (Chapters 30 and 31) was considered in the light of present preliminary and conflicting evidence on the effects of anticholinesterases. Most of this evidence is based on trials of tacrine in clinically diagnosed cases of Alzheimer's disease (AD) which inevitably include some cases of DLB. Whilst some responders in the separate trials of Sarah Eagger and

Gordon Wilcock and co-workers (see Chapter 32) were confirmed DLB
cases at autopsy, other responders were AD and in nonautopsy confirmed cases Florence Lebert noted no response in four cases meeting
DLB criteria (see Chapter 33). These trials included DLB patients initially diagnosed as AD who are likely to be atypical and clinical outcome
was assessed using ratings of dementia devised for AD rather than
assessments more appropriate to DLB which need to include psychosis.
It was agreed that, before discarding the original hypothesis, patients
primarily meeting newly devised DLB diagnostic criteria need to be
tested with particular emphasis on the course of psychotic features
and taking proper account of the fluctuating nature of symptoms in
DLB. Cholinergic strategies should include other cholinesterase inhibitors, with more selective actions on the cerebral cortex and with less
severe toxicity restrictions on effective upper dose limits, and also, since
acetylcholinesterase is likely to be depleted (as in AD), direct receptor
stimulation via muscarinic or nicotinic agonists. It was considered curious that tacrine treatment is not associated with the induction of extrapyramidal symptoms in those patients treated and subsequently
confirmed as having cortical Lewy bodies. This would be expected on
the basis of compromised dopamine function in the striatum in DLB
and anti-parkinsonism effects of anticholinergics such as muscarinic
antagonists in PD. Extrapyramidal effects are seen with physostigmine
in AD. Tacrine is therefore either a less effective anticholinesterase in
general or specifically less active on the enzyme as it occurs in the
striatum.

The hypothesis that psychotic features originate from hyperactive
monoaminergic (e.g. dopaminergic and/or 5-HT function) receives
more experimental support psychopharmacologically. Clinicians in the
group agreed that both typical and atypical neuroleptics are generally
effective in controlling psychosis in DLB patients (including cases confirmed at autopsy). The particular sensitivity of DLB patients to dopamine D2 receptor antagonism, frequently resulting in a reaction closely
resembling the neuroleptic malignant syndrome, is however a major
problem (Chapters 31 and 34). The atypical neuroleptic risperidone
shares with typical neuroleptics, via dopamine D2 receptor blockade,
the risk of inducing parkinsonism. Despite restrictions in its use, the
atypical neuroleptic clozapine (with lower D2 affinity) was considered
by many to be the most appropriate of currently available neuroleptics,
especially if dose levels are increased gradually to circumvent the problem
of somnolence. With respect to such side-effects, olanzapine was consid-

ered by Ernst Jansen to be superior and just as efficacious. Clinical experience with 5-HT antagonists were more limited and it was considered worthwhile to test ondansetron which, despite its lack of efficacy in AD, might be of value in DLB through its 5-HT$_3$ receptor control of acetylcholine release. In principle dopaminergic D4 receptor antagonism, targetting cortical (limbic) as opposed to motor dopamine systems would also be expected to be a valuable approach to controlling psychosis in DLB.

The question of whether psychotic features and cognitive deficits share a common biological basis which could be targetted in the same medication was addressed. Cholinergic therapy directed towards the cerebral cortex should in theory act synergistically, as antipsychotic and cognition enhancing. There is some theoretical basis derived from inhibitory effects of dopamine on the septal cholinergic system (see Chapter 30) for expecting that appropriate dopamine antagonists might have cognition enhancing as well as antipsychotic activity. During trials simultaneously monitoring outcome measures of both clinical features not only in DLB but also in AD should generate practical and theoretically useful information.

The basis and treatment of affective disorder were not discussed in any detail by the group who did not consider this to be a major component of DLB – less than 30 per cent of patients, as in AD, suffering from depression. Anecdotal reports of clozapine bringing a smile to the face of previously tearful patients (including a case of diffuse Lewy body disease, Chacko et al., 1993) are worth considering in relation to possible combined antidepressive and antipsychotic effects of the same medication. Antidepressant therapy based on enhancing synaptic 5-HT (e.g. via reuptake inhibition) might however be expected to exacerbate psychosis.

The question of how to restore motor function in DLB patients with extrapyramidal features without altering mental function was considered. In view of the psychotomimetic hazards of levodopa or dopamine receptor stimulation in Parkinson's disease and tendency of deprenyl (monoamine oxidase inhibition) to induce confusion, various other approaches were suggested. These included nicotinic agonists which have antiparkinsonism and cognitive enhancing (particularly increasing arousal) effects. Such agents as nicotine could be administered alone or combined with muscarinic (e.g. M1) agonists which should enhance cognition. A recent report suggests nicotine may relieve both motor and some of the mental symptoms in elderly cases of Parkinson's disease (Fagerström et al., 1994).

In attempting to design an ideal drug trial in DLB based on compounds such as those identified above, several important issues specific to this disorder were identified. These were: (a) the need to include appropriate assessment tools – some distinct from those used in AD trials; (b) the problem of fluctuation which could readily generate both false positive and false negative impressions; and (c) the likely need to intervene with additional medication (e.g. antipsychotic) for periodic behavioural disturbances in some patients. In addition to conventional measures of cognition employed in AD, a psychosis rating scale would be a necessary clinical assessment. A trial period of at least three months was considered essential as would the standard use of placebo control with crossover to allow for natural fluctuations in the disease. Over the trial period some patients would need maintenance, for example conventional antipsychotic therapy as required, and provided this was documented, patients should continue to be included. It was also suggested that a day to day carer's diary would be a great asset over the trial period.

The close relationship between DLB and patients presenting with Parkinson's disease who develop psychosis and/or dementia provides the treatment of DLB with valuable precedents. As Harvey Sagar (Chapter 28) pointed out from his knowledge of dementia and psychosis in Parkinson's disease the pathology contributing to any one symptom cluster in DLB is likely to be multiple and interactive. Nevertheless neurochemical deficits are at least amenable to standard and exploratory pharmacological therapy. It was the consensus of the group that with newly refined clinical criteria for DLB concerted efforts should now be made to initiate controlled pharamaceutical trials as a first step towards establishing effective and nontoxic therapy. The need for such progress in DLB is in some respects even greater than in other forms of dementia such as AD, on account of the increased burden placed on carers by the high incidence of noncognitive/behavioural abnormalities.

References

Chacko, R. C., Hurley, R. A. & Jankovic, J. (1993). Clozapine use in diffuse Lewy body disease. *J. Neuropsychiatry Clin. Neurosci.*, **5**, 206–8

Fagerström, K. O., Pomerleau, O., Giordani, B. & Stelson, F. (1994). Nicotine may relieve symptoms of Parkinson's disease. *Psychopharmacology*, **116**, 117–19.

Appendix 1

Consensus criteria for the clinical diagnosis of dementia with Lewy bodies (DLB)*

These criteria are proposed as being able to predict with high likelihood that dementia is associated with cortical Lewy bodies. They represent a refinement of earlier criteria proposed for Lewy body dementia. They are potentially applicable to patients with idiopathic Parkinson's disease who subsequently develop dementia. These criteria do not exclude the presence of concomitant Alzheimer pathology and many patients may simultaneously meet guidelines for the clinical diagnosis of Alzheimer's disease.

1. The central feature required for a diagnosis of DLB is progressive cognitive decline of sufficient magnitude to interfere with normal social or occupational function. Prominent or persistent memory impairment may not necessarily occur in the early stages, but is usually evident with progression. Deficits on tests of attention and of frontal-subcortical skills and visuospatial ability may be especially prominent.

2. **Two** of the following core features are **essential** for a diagnosis of *probable* DLB, **one** is **essential** for *possible* DLB.

   (a) Fluctuating cognition with pronounced variations in attention and alertness.
   (b) Recurrent visual hallucinations which are typically well formed and detailed.
   (c) Spontaneous motor features of parkinsonism.

3. Features **supportive** of the diagnosis

   (a) Repeated falls
   (b) Syncope
   (c) Transient loss of consciousness
   (d) Neuroleptic sensitivity
   (e) Systematised delusions
   (f) Hallucinations in other modalities

*Consensus guidelines for the clinical and pathological diagnosis of dementia with Lewy bodies (DLB): Report of the Consortium on DLB International Workshop. McKeith, I. G., Galasko, D., Kosaka, K., Perry, E. K. et al. (in press) *Neurology*, with permission.

4. A diagnosis of DLB is **less likely** in the presence of

  (a) Stroke disease evident as focal neurological signs or on brain imaging.
  (b) Evidence on physical examination and investigation of any physical illness, or other brain disorder, sufficient to account for the clinical picture.

Appendix 2

Guidelines for the selection of cortical areas for the evaluation of Lewy body distribution and proposed diagnostic rating protocol[*]

Guidelines for brain sampling

Brain sampling

(i)   Centres should continue current practice regarding which side of the cerebral hemisphere is sampled for histology (e.g. routinely from the right or left hemisphere, or alternatively right then left).

(ii) For cerebral hemisphere dissection the recommended coronal plane should be perpendicular to a line joining the inferior frontal and inferior occipital poles.

Neocortical regions

Coronal levels (CL) are indicated – see Fig. 1.

(i)   Frontal BA8/9   The middle frontal gyrus in the superior frontal sulcus at the plane just rostral to the temporal tip **CL8/9**

(ii) Temporal BA21   The superior sulcal margin (superior temporal sulcus) of the middle temporal gyrus at the plane of the amygdaloid and mammillary body. **CL14/15**

(iii) Parietal BA40   The superior sulcal margin (intraparietal sulcus) of the parietal lobule at the plane 1 cm caudal to the posterior pole of the splenium. **CL24/25**

Limbic or paralimbic regions

(i)   Anterior cingulate BA24   At a plane rostral to the anterior commissure approximately 1.5 cm caudal to the anterior pole of the genu. **CL10/11**

(ii) Transentorhinal BA29   The sulcal margin (collateral sulcus) of the parahippocampal gyrus at the plane of the red nucleus. **CL17/18**.

[*]Consensus guidelines for the clinical and pathological diagnosis of dementia with Lewy bodies (DLB): Report of the Consortium on DLB International Workshop. McKeith, I. G., Galasko, D., Kosaka, K., Perry, E. K. et al. (in press) *Neurology*, with permission.

493

Brain stem regions

The CERAD Neuropathological Assessment sampling protocols are
recommended for the substantia nigra, locus coeruleus, and dorsal nucleus of
vagus.

Guidelines for evaluation of Lewy body distribution and frequency

Cortical Lewy body frequency

Assessment is on a semiquantitative scale. In each region the total number of
Lewy bodies (LB) in the designated area are counted in either H&E or
ubiquitin-stained sections (cases with concomitant Alzheimer's disease may
need additional stains to discriminate Lewy bodies and globose neurofibrillary
tangles). The numerical score is converted as follows:

Score	Count (LB/area)
0	0
1	up to 5
2	> 5

Cortical areas for LB assessment are defined as follows:

(i)   Neocortex   The sulcal margin of the selected gyrus from the base
                         of the sulcus to the crest (external lip) of the sulcus.
(ii) Cingulate   The whole gyrus
(iii) Transentorhinal   The cortical ribbon from the depth to the surface of the
                         collateral sulcus.

Tissue blocks should be selected such that the cortex is not sectioned
tangentially.

Guidelines for diagnostic rating protocol

Lewy body scores and regionally defined categories

The Lewy body scores for individual areas are summated to give a final score and anatomical distribution as follows:

Category	Lewy body score						Total
	Transentorhinal	Cingulate	Temporal	Frontal	Parietal		
Brainstem predominant	0–1	0–1	0	0	0		0–2
Limbic (transitional)	1–2	1–2	1	0–1	0		3–6
Neocortical*	2	2	1–2	1–2	1–2		7–10

*Scores higher than 1 in any neocotical area generally indicate neocortical category.

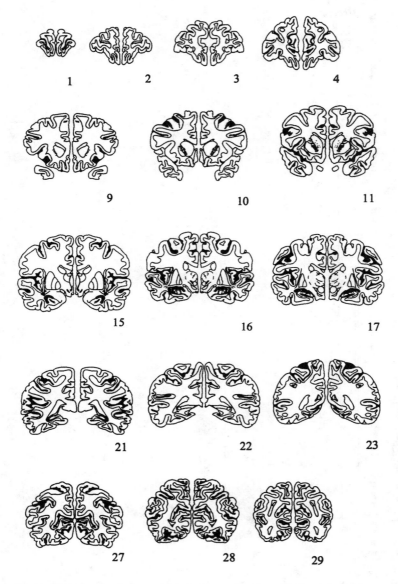

Fig. 1a Standardized coronal levels (intercommissural plane) in the human cortex related to internal brain landmarks and cortical Brodmann regions.

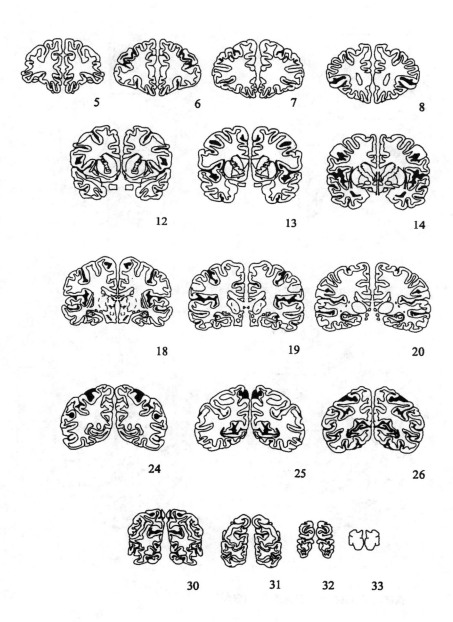

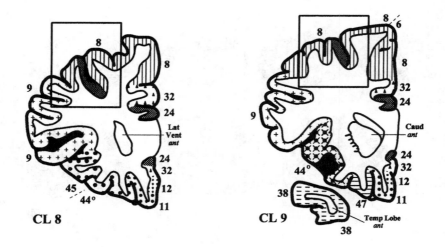

FRONTAL (middle frontal gyrus BA 8/9)

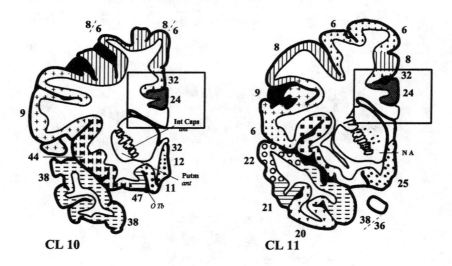

ANTERIOR CINGULATE (BA 24)

Fig. 1b. Rectangular blocks demarcate areas to be sampled for Lewy bodies in frontal, cingulate, temporal, parietal and transentorhinal cortex (one block should be taken from each area, two levels are shown to allow host matching).

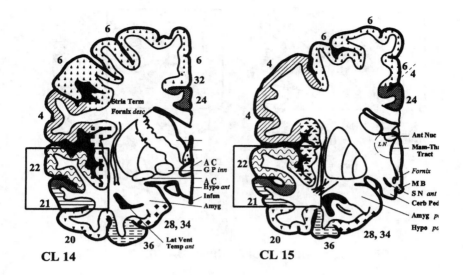

TEMPORAL (middle temporal gyrus BA 21)

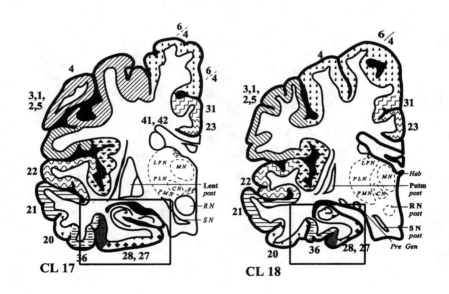

TRANSENTORHINAL (parahippocampal gyrus BA 28)

Fig. 1b (*Continued*)

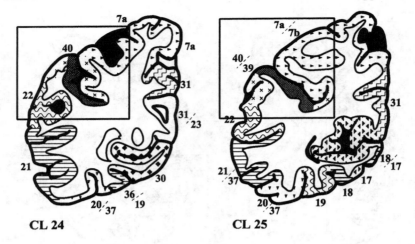

CL 24

CL 25

PARIETAL (inferior parietal lobule BA 40)

Fig. 1b (*Continued*)

Index